Developmental Anatomy and Physiology of Children

For Elsevier

Senior Commissioning Editor: Sarena Wolfaard/Ninette Premdas
Project Development Manager: Dinah Thom
Project Manager: Derek Robertson/Emma Riley
Designer: Judith Wright
Illustration Manager: Bruce Hogarth

Developmental Anatomy and Physiology of Children

A Practical Approach

Carol A. Chamley BA MA CertEdFE DipNursing DipGroupManagementSkills
ENBN51 RGN RSCN ONC RCNT RNT

Senior Lecturer, School of Health and Social Sciences, Coventry University, Coventry, UK

Pauline Carson BSc(Hons) MSc(ChildHealth) PGCE(HE) RGN RSCN

Senior Lecturer, University of Wolverhampton, Wolverhampton, UK

Duncan Randall BSc(Hons) CHN PGCE RGN RSCN RHV RNT

Lecturer, University of Birmingham, Birmingham, UK

Mary Sandwell BSc(Hons) DipNursing DNCert JBNS405 RSCN RGN RCNT

Senior Lecturer, School of Health and Social Sciences, Coventry University, Coventry, UK

Foreword by
Helen Langton BA(Hons) MSc RGN RSCN RCNT RNT

Associate Dean, Director of Research, School of Health and Social Sciences, Coventry University, Coventry, UK

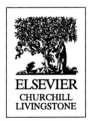

ELSEVIER
CHURCHILL
LIVINGSTONE

EDINBURGH   LONDON   NEW YORK   OXFORD   PHILADELPHIA   ST LOUIS   SYDNEY   TORONTO   2005

ELSEVIER
CHURCHILL
LIVINGSTONE

An imprint of Elsevier Limited

First published 2005
Reprinted 2007

ISBN 13: 978 0 443 07341 0
ISBN 10: 0 443 07341 4

British Library Cataloguing in Publication Data
A catalogue record for this book is available from the British Library

Library of Congress Cataloging in Publication Data
A catalog record for this book is available from the Library of Congress

Notice
Medical knowledge is constantly changing. Standard safety precautions must be
followed, but as new research and clinical experience broaden our knowledge, changes
in treatment and drug therapy may become necessary or appropriate. Readers are
advised to check the most current product information provided by the manufacturer of
each drug to be administered to verify the recommended dose, the method and duration
of administration, and contraindications. It is the responsibility of the practitioner, relying
on experience and knowledge of the patient, to determine dosages and the best treatment
for each individual patient. Neither the Publisher nor the authors assume any liability
for any injury and/or damage to persons or property arising from this publication.

The Publisher

 your source for books,
journals and multimedia
in the health sciences
www.elsevierhealth.com

The
Publisher's
policy is to use
**paper manufactured
from sustainable forests**

Transferred to Digital Printing in 2010

Contents

Foreword

I am delighted to have been asked to write the foreword to this excellent textbook. The gap in the market for a textbook for children's nurses—especially student nurses—on developmental anatomy and physiology related totally and specifically to children has been crying out to be filled. I am pleased that Carol Chamley and her colleagues have risen to the challenge.

The text is comprehensive and systematic in its approach. Each physiological system is described separately from the other systems but also as a part of the larger whole, thus giving an integrated and harmonious overview to the body as a complete entity. A strength of the book is that each chapter commences with a detailed exploration of the embryological development of the system under review. This clear focus on embryology demonstrates the importance for children's nurses of understanding the origins of human development if sense is to be made of both development after birth and the causes when things go wrong.

The other clear focus of the text is on normal anatomy and development. There are many good texts that apply the anatomy and physiology of children with great success. However, the strength of this text is its focus purely on enabling children's nurses to develop their knowledge base of the normal development of children, thus providing clear underpinning knowledge for practice. This approach thus lends itself to being used by lecturers for children's nursing courses when in-depth teaching of the knowledge base surrounding developmental anatomy and physiology is required.

An unusual and welcome feature of the book is the chapter on dentition. This chapter recognizes that changes in society have raised the profile of health and dentition, identifying dentition not simply as an extension of the body but as significant in its own right. The inclusion of a chapter focused on dentition is a natural sequel to this. The chapter identifies the significance of embryological development to good dentition as well as describing the normal development expected from birth to adulthood. Furthermore, the discussion of dentition is linked to other chapters, for example the digestive and integumentary systems, thus providing a good example of the way in which each chapter in this book not only stands alone but integrates well with others to promote a whole-systems approach.

The authors have been courageous in covering the range of development, from embryo to adult. Quite often, texts aimed at children's nurses focus on either pre-adolescents or adolescents, and seem to shy away from discussing the emerging adult. However, as children's nurses know, in practice the age range of patients in their care is from the newborn (including those born very prematurely) right through to young adults who may have been utilizing health care from an early age. Both healthcare professionals and patients in this older age group may be unsure about making the transition from child to adult services, so it is useful to find a text that embraces the whole range, as this reflects the reality of paediatric nursing practice.

The book uses an assortment of features to guide the reader through the text in a logical and learning fashion. Each chapter commences with learning outcomes and an overview of the content. For students who are used to learning with clear outcomes, this emulates their experience on their courses and will help them to use this text to meet wider learning outcomes set in other arenas. Another feature is the use of clinical link notes. Although the focus of the text is predominantly pure knowledge, this direction of the reader to areas where the knowledge may be applied in practice is to be commended, and may be particularly valuable for readers who struggle with the application of theory to practice. Each chapter concludes with opportunities for self-assessment against the learning outcomes, and includes details for further reading if required.

In conclusion, the authors are to be congratulated on providing a comprehensive text that is likely to be standard reading for pre-registration child nursing courses in the future and also of value for qualified staff who need to update their knowledge in this area as they enhance skills in particular arenas. As all systems are covered, the majority of children's nurses in all areas of practice should find it of use. In a wider context there are other healthcare professionals who may benefit from this textbook, and I would commend it as a comprehensive underpinning text for all those for whom knowledge of the developmental anatomy and physiology of children is a prerequisite to practice. Furthermore, it is exciting that this book has been developed through a whole-team approach within the child nursing team at Coventry University, providing a clear example of how innovation and working together can enhance the resources for pre-registration nursing courses while offering personal development for all team members and encouraging team working in the process. I commend this text to you and look forward to watching its value in children's nursing being recognized.

Helen Langton
Coventry 2005

Preface

Child development has captivated scholars, academics, researchers and practitioners for many centuries. With increasing advances in technology, research, science and medicine we can now enter the aquatic world that the embryo and fetus inhabit for 280 days, and witness biological events as they unfold.

The prenatal period remains one of the most fascinating yet curious periods of human development, the end of which is marked by a beginning, that is the birth of a unique human being. But many societies award this stage an age of zero, as if nothing of any relevance or interest has occurred before this time.

Human development begins with the fertilization of an oocyte (ovum) no bigger than a full stop on this page. Through highly complex and dramatic processes, a specialized totipotent cell is transformed into an extraordinary, unique multicellular human being that is eventually capable of sustaining independent life outside the womb. *Developmental Anatomy and Physiology of Children* attests to the remarkable anatomical and physiological processes that shape our growth and development from our earliest primordial beginnings, through childhood and maturity into adulthood.

THE ORGANIZATION AND CONTENT OF THIS BOOK

The study of human embryology provides the link between human anatomy and physiology, and within the context of this book the developing human is described using a systems approach that combines the sciences of anatomy, physiology, embryology, growth development and maturation of systems. However it is important to stress that whilst each system is reviewed separately, they are integrated and function in harmony together.

THE FORMAT OF THE CHAPTERS

Each chapter follows the same systematic approach and contains the following headings:

- Chapter outcomes
  - The chapter outcomes outline and emphasize the major elements that can be learned and reinforced from reading the chapter.
- Chapter overview
  - The chapter overview outlines the normal embryonic and fetal development of the system, explaining its normal structure and functioning, and drawing the reader's attention to key perspectives in relation to its development and maturation.
- Clinical notes
  - Each chapter contains several boxes headed 'Clinical notes' that are relevant to the system being studied. Clinical notes address issues of clinical relevance and potential interest to the reader, and exemplify the transition from theory to practice.
- Illustrations
  - Studying developmental anatomy and physiology of children is both a visual and descriptive exercise. Within the context of each chapter, illustrations, tables, figures and flow charts bring to life the written text in an effort to help students visualize the development of embryological and anatomical structures and relate these to normal physiological functioning.
- Self-assessment exercises
  - At the end of each chapter there is a self-assessment exercise to test and reinforce learning from the chapter. These exercises take a variety of different forms and help the reader to reflect upon the chapter, assess individual learning and harness the relationship between theory and practice.
- References
  - Each chapter gives full citations of the literature used to support the chapter, together with a short bibliography that gives the reader further opportunity to explore the literature in more detail.

Carol A. Chamley
Coventry 2005

Acknowledgements

This book is testament to all children who have been the inspiration and driving force behind this first edition of *Developmental Anatomy and Physiology of Children: A Practical Approach*. In particular, we are indebted to Helen Langton for contributing the foreword, Dr Roger Watson and Susan Law for their diligence and technical expertise in reading and commenting upon the draft manuscript, and for their sustained enthusiasm for the concept of this book.

I would like to thank my co-writers for their commitment to this project and for their continuing encouragement and staying power, which enabled us to successfully complete this project. Furthermore, gratitude is extended to the Editorial and Production teams at Elsevier for their advice, support and investment in this first edition.

This first edition is dedicated to our families and their support as we laboured over the finer details of each chapter. Without them, the deadlines may never have been realized. A very special dedication to our own wonderful children, for permitting us to use their photographs, and for asking those questions that only children can ask.

Carol A. Chamley 2005

Glossary

Abnormality: Away from the norm; a condition that differs from the usual cultural or scientifically accepted norms.

Acini: Masses of cells in the pancreas that secrete digestive enzymes.

Acne: A disease of the skin, common where sebaceous glands are numerous. Characteristic lesions include open blackheads and closed whiteheads, comedones, inflammatory papules, pustules, nodules and cysts.

Acoustic meatus: The external or internal canal of the ear.

Action potential: An electrical impulse consisting of a self-propagating series of polarizations and depolarizations transmitted across the plasma membranes of a nerve fibre during the transmission of a nerve impulse and muscle cell (fibre) during contraction or other activity. It is known as a nerve action potential when it relates to a neurone and a muscle action potential when it relates to a muscle cell (fibre).

Adenosine triphosphate (ATP): A compound consisting of the nucleotide adenosine attached to three phosphoric acid molecules, that serves to store energy, which is released when ATP is hydrolysed (reacts with water) to produce adenosine diphosphate.

Adipose tissue: Composed of fat-containing cells arranged in lobules.

Alae: Wing-like structure for the lateral aspect of the developing nose.

Alar (dorsal) columns: Pairs of columns of the spinal cord and brainstem, formed by grey matter of the dorsal regions of the neural tube; cells give rise to association neurones.

Allantois: A tubular outgrowth of the endoderm of the yolk sac that extends with the allantoic vessels into the body stalk of the embryo. Allontoic vessels become the umbilical vessels and chorionic villi.

Allele: One, two or more alternative forms of a gene that occupy corresponding loci on homologous chromosomes.

Alopecia: Partial or complete lack of hair.

Alveolar processes: The portion of the maxilla or mandible that forms the dental arch and serves as a bony investment for the tooth.

Alveolus (of tooth): Bony socket of the tooth formed by mesenchyme of the dental sac; teeth are anchored to it by the periodontal ligament.

Ameloblasts: An epithelial cell from which tooth enamel forms.

Amnion: Appears on day 8 as fluid begins to collect between the epiblast cells; eventually fills with amniotic fluid for protection and provides space for the growth of the embryo and fetus.

Amniotic fluid: Dialysate of blood first secreted by the amniotic membrane.

Amorphous: Describing an object that lacks definite visible shape or form.

Ampulla: A rounded sac-like dilatation of a duct, canal or any tubular structure.

Anastomose: To open a channel or passage between two vessels or cavities; gives rise to the conduction system and the abdomen.

Angioblast: Vessel-forming cells that can arise from any kind of mesoderm except prechordal plate mesoderm from which blood vessels and cells arise.

Angioblastic cords: Short blind-ended cords formed as angiocysts amalgamate.

Angioblastic plexuses: Formed as angioblastic cords amalgamate into complex, interconnected, vascular networks.

Angiocysts: Vesicles formed by angioblasts during the process of vasculogenesis.

Angiogenesis: The development of blood vessels in the embryo, whereby pre-existing vessels lengthen or branch by sprouting.

Antigens: Substances, usually proteins, that the body recognizes as foreign and that can evoke an immune response.

Apocrine: A type of gland in which the secretory products gather at the free end of the secreting cell and are pinched off, along with some cytoplasm, to become the secretion as in mammary glands.

Aponeurosis: A strong flat sheet of fibrous connective tissue that serves as a tendon to attach muscles to bone, or as a fascia to bind muscles together or to other tissues at their origin or insertion.

Apoptosis: Programmed cell death; a normal type of cell death that removes unwanted cells during embryological development, regulating the number of cells in tissues and eliminating many potential dangers, such as cancerous cells. During apoptosis the DNA fragments, the nucleus condenses, mitochondria cease to function and the cytoplasm shrinks, but the plasma membrane remains intact. Phagocytes engulf and digest the apoptotic cells, but an inflammatory response does not occur.

Appositional: Growth due to the surface deposition of material, as in the growth in diameter of cartilage and bone.

Aqueous humour: The watery fluid, similar in composition to cerebrospinal fluid, that fills the anterior chamber of the eye.

Arrector pili muscle: Smooth muscle within the papillary layer of the dermis, attached to the dermal root sheath of the hair follicle. Elevates the hair shaft producing 'goose-bumps'.

Atelectasis: Collapse of alveoli, preventing gaseous exchange (Greek *ateles* = incomplete, *ektasis* = expansion).

Atopy: Inheredited tendency to experience allergic reaction when exposed to an antigen.

Autosome: Any chromosome that is not a sex chromosome and that appears as a homologous pair in the somatic cells.

Auxology: The study of growth and development.

Axon: Processes that usually conduct impulses away from the neural cell body; usually synapse with another neurone or with an affector organ.

Basal (ventral) columns: Pair of columns of the spinal cord and brainstem formed by grey matter of the ventral regions of the neural tube. Cells give rise to somatic motor neurones.

Basilar membrane: A membrane in the cochlea of the internal ear that separates the cochlear duct from the scala tympani, and on which the spiral organ (organ of Corti) rests.

Blastocyst: The embryonic form that follows the morula in human development.

Blastomere: Any of the cells formed from the mitotic division of a fertilized ovum.

Bowman's capsule: Cup-shaped end of a renal tubule or nephron enclosing a glomerulus.

Brush border: Microvilli on the free surface of certain epithelial cells, particularly the absorptive surfaces of the small intestine and proximal convoluted tubules of the kidney.

Bursa: A fibrous sac between certain tendons and the bones beneath them. Acts as a cushion that allows the tendon to move over the bone as it contracts.

Calvaria: Dermal bones that constitute the cranial vault, skull cap or roof of the skull.

Cardiac index: Cardiac output corrected for body size; the term used for cardiac output in children.

Cardiac output: The amount of blood ejected from the heart per minute.

Cardiogenic: Originating in the heart muscle.

Carotene: A red or orange organic compound found in carrots, sweet potatoes, egg yolk and leafy vegetables.

Cartilage: Dense avascular connective tissue containing chondrocytes surrounded by an extracellular matrix.

Caudal: Signifying a position towards the distal end of the body.

Caudal and cranial neuropores: Openings produced by the initial formation of the neural tube. As the neural tube closes, both neuropores become progressively smaller, closing on day 24 and day 26.

Cementoenamel junction: Region at the neck of the tooth root that marks the boundary between the cementum of the root and the enamel of the crown.

Central nervous system (CNS): The portion of the nervous system that consists of the brain and spinal cord.

Central sulcus: A groove within the cerebrum that separates frontal and parietal lobes.

Centromere: The constricted region of a chromosome that joins chromatids to each other and attaches to spindle fibres in mitosis and meiosis.

Cephalic: Suffix meaning related to the head.

Cerebellum: Higher centre formed by alar plates of the metencephalon that controls balance, posture and the smooth execution of movements.

Cerebral cortex: The multilayered stratum of grey matter within the cerebrum.

Cerebral hemispheres: The bubble-like out-pouchings of the telencephalon that is the most evolutionary advanced part of the brain.

Cerebrospinal fluid: Produced by the choroid plexuses of the lateral, third and fourth ventricles.

Cerumen: A wax-like secretion produced by the ceruminous glands.

Ceruminous gland: A modified sweat gland in the external auditory meatus that secretes ear wax (cerumen).

Chemical: A substance composed of chemical elements or a substance produced by or used in chemical processes.

Chemotaxis: Movement away from or towards a chemical stimulus; phagocytic activity influenced by chemical factors.

Chiasm: The crossing over of two lines or tracts, as of the optic nerves at the optic chiasm.

Chiasma: A visible connection between homologous chromosomes during the first meiotic division in gametogenesis.

Chondroitin sulfate: An amorphous matrix material found outside connective tissue cells.

Chorda tympani: A strong filament such as a nerve or tendon.

Chorion: Outermost fetal membrane consisting of three kinds of tissue: syncytiotrophoblast, cytotrophoblast and the extraembryonic somato-pleuric mesoderm.

Choroid: A thin, highly vascular, layer of the eye between the retina and the sclera.

Chromatids: One of the two identical thread-like filaments of a chromosome.

Chromosome: Thread-like structures in the nucleus of a cell that function in the transmission of genetic material.

Chyme: The viscous, semi-fluid contents of the stomach during digestion.

Ciliary body: The thickened part of the vascular tunic of the eye that joins the iris with the anterior portion of the choroid.

Cleavage: The rapid mitotic divisions that follow fertilization of a secondary oocyte and result in the increased number of progressively smaller cells called blastomeres.

Cloaca: The end of the hindgut before the developmental division into rectum, bladder and primitive genital structures.

Cochlea: The auditory portion of the inner ear.

Coel: Combining form meaning 'colon' denoting relationship to a cavity or space.

Collagen: A fibrous, insoluble protein consisting of bundles of tiny reticular fibrils that combine to form a white, glistening, inelastic fibre that represents 30% of body protein.

Colostrum: A thin cloudy fluid secreted by the mammary glands for a few days before or after delivery of the infant, before the true milk is produced.

Conception: The beginning of pregnancy, usually taken to be the instant that a spermatozoon enters the ovum and forms a viable zygote.

Concha: A body structure that is shell shaped, as the cavity in the external ear that surrounds the external auditory canal meatus.

Congenital: Present at birth, as a congenital anomaly or birth defect.

Congenital athymia: Absence of the thymus gland at birth.

Connective tissue: One of the most abundant of the four basic tissue types in the body that performs the functions of binding and supporting. It consists of relatively few cells in a generous matrix.

Copula: Any connective part or structure; a median ventral elevation on the embryonic tongue formed by the union of the second pharyngeal arches, it represents the future root of the tongue.

Cord: A long, rounded, flexible structure.

Cornea: The convex, transparent, anterior part of the eye, comprising one-sixth of the outermost tunic of the eye bulb.

Cranial: Relating to the head, or signifying a position towards the upper part of the body.

Cranial nerve: One of 12 nerves that leave the brain, pass through foramina in the skull, and supply sensory and motor neurones to the head, neck, part of the trunk, and viscera of the thorax and abdomen. Each is designated by a Roman numeral and a name.

Cuticle: A sheath of a hair follicle; the thin edge of cornified epithelium at the base of a nail, or the eponychium.

Cyanosis: A bluish discoloration of the skin and mucous membranes caused by an excess of deoxygenated haemoglobin in the blood, or a structural defect in the haemoglobin molecule.

Cytokines: Low molecular weight proteins involved in cell to cell communications, coordinating antibody and T-cell immune interactions.

Cytoplasm: All of the substance of a cell, except for the nucleus and the cell wall.

Cytotrophoblast: The cells of the trophoblast that retain their cell membranes and enclose the blastocyst cavity.

Decidua: The epithelial tissue of the endometrium lining the uterus. It envelops the conceptus during gestation and is shed in the puerperium.

Deciduous: Falling off, or shedding.

Dental papilla: A small mass of mesenchymal tissue in the enamel organ that differentiates into dentin and dental pulp during tooth development.

Deoxyribonucleic acid (DNA): A large, double-stranded, helical molecule that is a carrier of genetic information.

Dermatome: The mesodermal layer in the early embryo that gives rise to the dermal layers of the skin.

Dermis: A layer of dense, irregular connective tissue lying deep within the epidermis.

Dermoid: Pertaining to the skin.

Desiccation: Drying out.

Desmosome: A small, circular, dense area within the intracellular bridge that forms the site of adhesion between certain epithelial cells.

Desquamation: A normal process in which the cornified layer of the epidermis is sloughed in fine scales.

Detrusor muscle: A muscle that pushes down.

Diaphysis: The shaft of a long bone consisting of a tube of compact bone enclosing the medullary canal.

Diastole: The phase of the cardiac cycle wherein the heart is at rest between contractions, during which time the two ventricles are dilated by the blood flowing into them from the aorta.

Diploid: Having two complete cells of homologous chromosomes, such as are normally found in somatic and primordial germ cells before maturation.

Diurnal: Happening daily, as with patterns of sleeping and waking.

Dorsal: Suffix meaning the back of something, or the back.

Dorsal mesogastrium: Where the mesentery of the gut attaches to the dorsal (the back) aspect in the developing embryo.

Dorsoventral: Pertaining to the axis that passes through the back of the body.

Ductus arteriosus: A fetal blood vessel joining the aorta and pulmonary artery.

Ductus venosus: A fetal blood channel through the embryonic liver joining the umbilical vein and the inferior vena cava.

Ectoderm: The outermost layer of the three primary cell layers of the embryo.

Eczema: Superficial dermatitis of unknown origin.

Elastic connective tissue: A type of connective tissue containing elastic fibres.

Embryo: The young of any organism in an early stage of development; in humans, the developing organism from fertilization to the end of the eighth week.

Embryogenesis: The process in sexual reproduction by which an embryo forms from the fertilization of the ovum.

Enamel: The hard white substance that forms the outermost covering of the clinical and anatomical crown of the tooth.

Endocardium: Lining of the heart tube derived from the lateral endocardial tubes.

Endocrine gland: A gland that secretes hormones into the blood or lymph that have a specific effect on tissues in another part of the body; a ductless gland.

Endoderm: The innermost of the cell layers that develop from the embryonic disc of the inner cell mass of the blastocyst. The endoderm comprises the lining of the cavities and passages of the body, and the covering of most of the internal organs.

Endolymph: The pale fluid in the membranous labyrinth of the internal ear.

Endolymphatic duct: A labyrinthine passage joining an endolymphatic sac with the utricle and saccule.

Enteroendocrine cell: A cell of the gastrointestinal tract that secretes the hormones gastrin, cholecystokinin and secretin.

Epicardium: Or visceral pericardium; outer tunic of thin serous membrane.

Epidermis: The superficial thinner layer of the skin, composed of keratinized stratified squamous epithelium.

Epigenesis: The belief that more complex structures develop from simpler ones by the interaction between the organism and the environment; the combined term 'probabilistic epigenesis' is based on the key assumption that there is always a bidirectional or reciprocal relationship between structure, function and/or behaviour.

Epiglottis: Thin cartilaginous structure that separates the oesophagus and larynx–trachea, stopping food from entering the lungs during swallowing (Greek *epi* + *glossa* = tongue).

Epiphyseal plate: A thin layer of cartilage between the epiphysis, a secondary bone-forming centre, and the bone shaft.

Epiphysis: The enlarged proximal and distal ends of a long bone.

Eponychium: Thin layer of epidermis covering the nail plate.

Exocoelomic cavity: Formed as cells at the periphery of the hypoblast proliferate and migrate out into the cytotrophoblast to line the blastocyst cavity.

Fetal haemoglobin: Haemoglobin F; the major haemoglobin present in the blood of the fetus and neonate.

Fetus: The human organism in utero after the embryonic period; the fetal period extends from the beginning of the ninth week until birth.

Fingerprints: The distinctive patterns of loops and whorls that represent the fine ridges marking the skin; an image left on a smooth surface by the pad of the distal phalanx.

Follicle: (1) A small secretory sac. (2) A fluid- or colloid-filled ball of cells found in some glands (e.g. the thyroid and ovary).

Fontanelle: A space covered by a tough membrane between the bones of an infant's cranium.

Foramen ovale: An opening in the septum of the fetal heart that provides a communication between both of the atria and closes at birth.

Freckle: A brown or tan molecule on the skin that results from exposure to sunlight.

Gamete: A mature male or female germ cell that is capable of functioning in the process of fertilization, and which contains the haploid number of chromosomes of the organism.

Gametogenesis: The origin and maturation of gametes that occurs through the process of meiosis.

Gastrin: A polypeptide hormone, secreted by the pylorus, that stimulates the flow of gastric juice and contributes to the stimulus for bile and pancreatic enzyme secretion.

Gastrulation: Formation of the three germ layers in the human embryo, characterized by an extensive series of coordinated morphogenetic movements within the blastocyst. The primitive body plan of the organism is established.

Gene: The biological unit of inheritance.

Genetics: The study of genes and genetics.

Germ cell: A sexual reproductive cell in any stage of development from the primordial embryonic form to the mature gamete.

Germinative layer: Layer of the mature epidermis derived from the basal proliferating layer of surface ectoderm; contains stem cells that differentiate into the keratinized cells of overlying layers that proliferate to replenish its own stem cells.

Gestation: The period from fertilization of the ovum to birth.

Gingiva: The gum tissue of the mouth.

Glomerular capsule: Also known as Bowman's capsule.

Glomerulus: A small convoluted mass of capillaries encased within Bowman's capsule. An integral part of the nephron, where the waste products being carried in blood pass through the glomerular membrane into the nephron.

Glossopharyngeal nerve: Either of a pair of nerves essential to the sense of taste.

Glossopharyngeal: Pertaining to the tongue and pharynx (Greek *glossa* = tongue, *pharynx* = throat).

Glossoptosis: Posteriorly placed tongue; the retraction or downward displacement of the tongue.

Gluten-dependent enteropathy: Disorder of the intestines characterized by an intolerance for the insoluble protein gluten, derived from wheat and other grains.

Gonad: A gamete-producing gland such as an ovary or testis.

Gonadotrophic hormone: A hormone secreted by the hypothalamus. It stimulates the release of the luteinizing hormone (LH) and follicle stimulating hormone (FSH) from the anterior pituitary gland.

Grey matter: Areas in the central nervous system and ganglia containing neuronal cell bodies, dendrites, unmyelinated axons, axon terminals and neuroglia, but little or no myelin; Nissl bodies impart a grey colour.

Gubernaculum: The primitive round ligament in the embryo that determines the descent of the gonads in both sexes.

Haematocrit: Measure of the packed cell volume of red blood cells expressed as a percentage of total blood volume.

Haematopoietic stem cells: Actively dividing cells that give rise to blood cells.

Haemopoiesis: The formation and development of blood cells.

Haemopoietic centre: Related to the process of formation and development of the various types of blood cell.

Haploid: Having only one complete set of non-homologous chromosomes.

Hepatocyte: A parenchymal liver cell that performs all functions ascribed to the liver.

Histocompatibility complex: A group of genes found in the plasma membrane of proteins that help to identify the cell as self or as foreign.

Holocrine: Pertaining to a gland whose only function is to secrete, or whose secretions consist of disintegrated cells of the gland itself.

Homologous: Pertaining to corresponding attributes; similar in structure.

Hormone: A complex chemical substance produced either in one part or in an organ of the body that initiates or regulates the activity or group of cells in another.

Hyaline cartilage: A type of elastic connective tissue composed of specialist cells in translucent pearly blue matrix; hyaline cartilage thinly covers the articulating ends of bones.

Hyaloid: Pertaining to or resembling hyaline.

Hyaluronic acid: A mucopolysaccharide formed by the polymerization of acetylglucosamine and glucuronic acid; occurs in the vitreous humour, synovial fluid and various tissues. Forms a gel in intercellular spaces.

Hypo: Prefix meaning under, below, beneath, deficient.

Hypoblast: The lower layer of the bilaminar embryonic disc in the human embryo, which gives rise to the ectoderm.

Hypobranchial: Pertaining to the body structures of the face, neck and throat areas.

Hypocalcaemia: Below normal level of calcium in the serum (blood).

Hypoglossal nerve: Either of a pair of nerves essential for swallowing and moving the tongue.

Hypothalamus: An inferoventral swelling of the diencephalon that helps to regulate endocrine activity of the pituitary gland and many autonomic responses; also functions in relation to the limbic system that regulates emotion and sleep–waking mechanisms.

Ileocaecal junction: Pertaining to both ileum and caecum, and the region where they are joined.

Immunoglobulin: A protein that functions as an antibody, destroying antigens in the serum and secretions of the body; includes five subsets: IgA, IgD, IgE, IgG and IgM.

Inflammation: The protective response of body tissue to irritation or injury.

Inheritance: The acquisition of body traits by transmission of genetic information from parent to child.

Inner cell mass (embryoblast): Blastomeres arising from the first cells to divide during early cleavages, that segregate within the centre of the morula and differentiate into the embryo (outer cells differentiate into placental membranes).

Integumentary: Relating to the skin.

Intercalated discs: Dense bands that run between myocardial cells both transversely and longitudinally in stepped configuration. They contain intercellular junctions that link adjacent cells electrically and mechanically.

Interstitial fluid: An extracellular fluid that fills the spaces between most cells of the body and provides a substantial portion of the liquid environment of the body.

Invagination: Found when one part of a structure telescopes into another.

In vitro: Out of body.

Iris: An annular, coloured membrane shaped like a disc and suspended in aqueous humour between the cornea and the crystalline lens of the eye, enclosing a circular pupil.

Islets of Langerhans: Clusters of cells within the pancreas that secrete insulin, glucagon, somatostatin and pancreatic polypeptide; also known as the pancreatic islet.

Isthmus: A narrow connection, passage or constriction between the larger parts of an organ or anatomical structure such as the isthmus of the thyroid gland.

Lacrimal gland: Secretory cells located in the superior anterolateral portion of each orbit, that secrete tears into excretory ducts that open on to the surface of the conjunctiva.

Lacteal: Refers to the tiny vessels in the villi of the small intestine.

Lactiferous ducts: Glands that secrete or convey milk.

Langerhans' cell: A stellate dendritic cell found mostly in the stratum spinosum of the epidermis; believed also to have function related to immunity.

Lanugo hairs: The soft downy hair covering a normal fetus.

Laryngeal webbing: A common congenital malformation; thin layer of tissue over the vocal cords that may cause hoarseness, aphonia or stridor.

Laryngopharynx: Area of throat that extends from the hyoid bone to the oesophagus.

Lateral: Pertaining to the side.

Lens: The crystalline lens of the eye.

Lens capsule: The clear, thin, elastic capsule that surrounds the lens of the eye.

Leucocytotoxic: Toxic to leucocytes (white blood cells).

Leydig cells: Cells of the interstitial tissue of the testes that secrete testosterone.

Ligament: One of the predominantly white, shiny, flexible bands of fibrous tissue binding joints together and connecting articular bones and cartilage to facilitate movement.

Linguinal: Pertaining to or resembling the tongue.

Lysis: Destruction or dissolution of a cell or molecule by a specific agent.

Mammary gland: Glandular tissue that forms a radius of lobes containing alveoli; each lobe has a system of ducts for the passage of milk.

Mammary ridges: Epidermal thickenings that extend from the axilla to the inguinal region.

Mandible: A large U-shaped bone constituting the lower jaw.

Masticate: To chew.

Mastoid: Pertaining to the mastoid process of the temporal bone.

Maxilla: One of a pair of large bones that forms the upper jaw and teeth.

Meconium: Material that collects in the intestine of the fetus and forms the first stools of the newborn.

Medulla oblongata: The most caudal region of the rhombencephalon. This part of the brain acts as a relay station between higher centres and the spinal cord, regulating respiration, heartbeat, reflex movements and several other functions.

Meiosis: A type of cell division that occurs during production of gametes, involving two successive nuclear divisions that result in daughter cells with the haploid number of chromosomes.

Melanin: A black or dark brown pigment that occurs naturally in the hair, skin, iris and choroid of the eye.

Melanoblast: An epithelial tissue cell containing black granules; develops into a melanocyte from the neural crest-derived cells that migrate into various parts of the body during the early stages of embryonic life. It then becomes a mature melanocyte capable of forming melanin.

Merkel cells: Contain keratin and form desmosomes with adjacent keratinocytes.

Mesenchyme: A diffuse network of tissue derived from the embryonic mesoderm.

Mesoderm: The middle layer of the three cell layers of the developing embryo; lies between the ectoderm and the endoderm.

Mesogastrium: A mesentery of the embryonic stomach.

Mesonephric duct: Also called the wolffian duct. A duct that in the male gives rise to the ducts of the reproductive tract; in the female it persists as Gartner's duct.

Microcephaly: A congenital anomaly characterized by abnormal smallness of the head in relation to the rest of the body, and by an underdeveloped brain.

Micrognathia: Underdevelopment of the jaw, especially the mandible, giving a small jaw.

Micturition reflex: A normal reaction to a rise in pressure within the bladder.

Mitochondrion: A rod-like, thread-like or granular organelle that functions in aerobic respiration and occurs in varying numbers in all eukaryotic cells, except mature erythrocytes.

Mitosis: A type of cell division that occurs in somatic cells and results in the formation of two genetically identical daughter cells containing the diploid number of chromosomes characteristic of the species.

Molecule: The smallest unit that exhibits the properties of an element or compound. A molecule is composed of two or more atoms that are covalently bonded.

Morphogenesis: The development and differentiation of the structure and form of the organism, specifically relating to changes that occur in the cells and tissues during embryonic development.

Morula: A solid, spherical mass of cells resulting from the cleavage of the fertilized ovum in the early stages of embryonic development.

Motor neurones: Develop within the grey matter of the ventral grey columns of the spinal cord and brainstem.

Mutation: The process or an instance of change or alteration. An unusual change in a gene occurring spontaneously or by induction. The change affects the expression of the gene.

Myelin sheath: The lamellar covering of nerve axons of the peripheral nervous system produced by Schwann cells.

Myocardium: Cardiac muscle that arises from splanchnopleuric mesoderm.

Myogenic: Forming or giving rise to muscle tissue.

Nail: A hard plate composed largely of keratin that develops from the epidermis of the skin to form a protective covering on the surface of the distal phalanges of the fingers and toes.

Neonatal period: The period of time covering the first 28 days after birth.

Nephrogenic cord: Either of the paired longitudinal ridges of tissue that lie along the dorsal surface of the coelom in the early developing embryo. Formed from the fusion of the nephrotome tissue and gives rise to the structures making up the embryonic urogenital system.

Neural canal: A lumen formed within the neural tube during the process of neurulation;

becomes the central canal of the spinal cord and the ventricles of the brain.

Neural cord: A solid midline structure formed from the caudal eminence during the process of secondary neurulation; fuses with the caudal end of the neural tube.

Neural groove: The longitudinal midline groove that bisects the neural plate into presumptive right and left neural folds.

Neural plate: Begins to form on day 18 of gestation in the epiblast along the midsagittal axis cranial to the primitive streak.

Neuroectoderm: Neural epithelium arising from the ectoderm within the neural plate.

Neurulation: The process of folding of the neural plate and closure of the cranial and caudal neuropores to form the neural tube.

Nipple: A pigmented projection on the surface of the breast that is the location of the openings of the lactiferous ducts for milk.

Notochord: A flexible rod of mesodermal tissue that lies where the future vertebral column will develop and plays a role in induction.

Notochordal process: One of the first mesodermal structures to arise by gastrulation as cells surround the primitive pit.

Nucleic acid: These are huge organic molecules that contain carbon, hydrogen, oxygen, nitrogen and phosphorus. Nucleic acids are of two varieties, deoxyribonucleic acid and ribonucleic acid.

Nucleus pulposus: The central region of the intervertebral disc arising directly from the notochord. The original tissue may be replaced by cells of the annulus fibrosus in early childhood.

Odontogenesis: The origin and formation of the developing teeth.

Oesophagus: The musculomembranous canal extending from cricoid cartilage to the cardiac sphincter, and along which food passes from the oropharynx to the stomach.

Olfactory: Pertaining to smell.

Omentum: An extension of the peritoneum that enfolds one or more organs adjacent to the stomach.

Oncofetal: Relating to tumour-associated substances present in fetal tissue.

Oögenesis: The formation of female gametes or ova.

Optic cups: A two-layered embryonic cavity that develops in early embryonic life. The optic cup is completed by week 7 of gestation, with the closure of the choroidal fissure.

Optic nerve: Composed of axons of ganglion cells in the anterior layer of the neural retina that pass from the eyeball at the optic disc as the optic nerve; convey visual sensation from the retina to the lateral geniculate bodies.

Orbit: The bony pyramid-shaped cavity of the skull that holds the eyeball.

Organ: A structure composed of two or more different types of tissue with a specific function and usually a recognizable shape.

Organ of Corti: The true organ of hearing; a spiral structure within the cochlea containing hair cells that are stimulated by sound vibrations.

Organism: An entity capable of carrying on life functions; one individual. All organisms are composed of cells.

Organogenesis: The formation and differentiation of organs during embryonic development.

Oropharynx: Area of the throat extending from the mouth and nasal cavities to the hyoid bone, where the laryngopharynx begins.

Ossicles: The small bones of the ear including the malleus, incus and stapes.

Ossification: The development of bone.

Osteoblast: A bone-forming cell that is derived from the embryonic mesenchyme. Osteoblasts synthesize the collagen and glycoproteins to form the osteoid matrix of bone.

Osteoclast: A large multinucleated bone cell with a large amount of acidophilic cytoplasm that functions to absorb and remove osseous tissue.

Osteogenesis: The origin and development of bone tissue.

Otic: Pertaining to the ear.

Oxidation: (1) Process by which the oxygen content of a compound is increased. (2) Reaction in which the positive valence of a compound or radical is increased by the loss of electrons.

Oxyphil: A cell of the parathyroid gland; can occur singly or in small groups, increasing with age.

Paramesonephric duct: Also called the müllerian duct; one of a pair of ducts that develop into the uterus and uterine tubes.

Paranasal sinuses: Any one of the air cavities in various bones around the nose.

Parenchymal cell: Any cell that is a functional element of an organ.

Pathogen: Any microorganism capable of producing disease.

Periderm: The outermost layer of flattened epidermis on an embryo or fetus during the first 6 months of gestation.

Periosteum: A thick fibrovascular membrane covering bone, except at the extremities. The membrane is thick and markedly vascular over young bones, but thinner and less vascular in later life.

Peristalsis: The coordinated, rhythmic, serial contraction of smooth muscle that forces food through the digestive tract. A worm-like movement consisting of a wave of contraction.

Phagocytosis: Process by which a cell engulfs another cell, debris or microorganism in order to destroy it.

Pharyngeal arches: Paired structures in the human embryo; evolved from branchial arches 1, 2, 3, 4 and 6 of primitive fishes to form facial and pharyngeal structures.

Philtrum: A central groove in the upper lip.

Pituitary gland: Formed from the roof of the stomadeum (Rathke's pouch).

Placenta: A fetomaternal organ derived from the maternal decidua basalis and the fetal chorion; provides a mechanism for exchanging nutrients, carbon monoxide and wastes between the fetal and maternal circulations.

Polypeptide: A long chain of amino acids joined by peptide bonds.

Prenatal: Before birth; occupying or existing before birth.

Primitive streak: A dense area on the central posterior region of the embryonic disc. The seam-like elongation indicates the cephalocaudal axis along which the embryo develops.

Primordium (pl. primordia): The first recognizable stage in embryonic development and differentiation of a particular organ, tissue or structure.

Primordial: Characteristic of the most underdeveloped or earliest state, especially of those cells or tissues that are formed in the early stage of embryonic development.

Prothymocytes: Cells derived from haematopoietic stem cells that continue to differentiate into thymocytes.

Puberty: The period of life at which the ability to reproduce begins.

Pulp cavity: The space in a tooth bounded by the dentin and containing the pulp cavity. It is divided into the pulp chamber and the pulp cavity.

Rete: A network, especially of arteries or veins.

Retina: A ten-layered, delicate nervous tissue membrane of the eye continuous with the optic nerve.

Ribonucleic acid (RNA): A nucleic acid, found in both the nucleus and the cytoplasm of cells, that plays several roles in the translation of the genetic code and the assembly of proteins.

Root canal: The space occupied by the nerves, blood vessels and lymphatic vessels in the tooth.

Root of the tooth: The region deep to the boundary of the cementoenamel junction;

embedded within the alveolus and covered with cementum.

Saccular: Pertaining to a pouch, or shaped like a sac.

Sclera: The tough, inelastic, white, opaque membrane covering the posterior five-sixths of the eye bulb. It maintains the size and form of the bulb and attaches to muscles that move the bulb.

Sclerotome: The part of the segmented mesoderm layer in the developing embryo that originates from the somites and gives rise to skeletal tissue of the body.

Sebaceous gland: An exocrine gland in the dermis of the skin, almost always associated with a hair follicle that secretes sebum; also called an oil gland.

Sebum: An oily secretion of the sebaceous glands of the skin, composed of keratin, fat and cellular debris. Combined with sweat, sebum forms a moist, oily, acidic film that is mildly antibacterial and antifungal, and protects the skin against drying out.

Semi-circular duct: One of the three ducts that make up the membranous labyrinth of the inner ear.

Sensitive period: Period in which an organ or organ system is sensitive to the effects of teratogens.

Sertoli cell: One of the supporting elongated cells of the seminiferous tubules of the testes. Its function is to nourish the developing spermatocytes.

Sialomucin layer: Highly charged coating of syncytiotrophoblast cells that provides protection from immune surveillance.

Situs inversus: Partial or total transposition of body organs to the side.

Skeletal muscle: A tissue specialized for contraction composed of striated muscle fibres, supported by connective tissue and attached to bone by a tendon or an aponeurosis, and stimulated by somatic motor neurones.

Skin: The external covering of the body that consists of a superficial thinner epidermis and a deep thicker dermis, that is anchored to the subcutaneous layer.

Smooth muscle: A tissue specialized for contraction composed of smooth muscle fibres, located on the hollow internal organs and innervated by autonomic motor neurones.

Somatic cell: Any of the cells of body tissue that have the diploid number of chromosomes, as distinguished from germ cells, which contain the haploid number.

Somite: Any of the paired segmented masses of mesodermal tissue that form along the length of the neural tube during early embryonic development.

Sphincter of the hepatopancreatic ampulla: Also known as the sphincter of Oddi; a circular muscle at the opening of the common bile and main pancreatic ducts in the duodenum.

Splanchnic: Suffix meaning 'viscera, entrails'.

Splanchnopleure: A layer of tissue in the early embryo formed by the union of the endoderm and the splanchnic mesoderm. It gives rise to the embryonic gut and the visceral organs and continues to the external embryo as the yolk sac and allantois.

Squames: Flat, thin, non-nucleated dead cells.

Squamous epithelium: A sheet of flattened scale-like cells attached at the edges.

SRY: Symbol for the 'maleness' gene found on the sex-determining region of the Y chromosome. The gene is believed to function as a master control switch that can turn other genes off or on.

Stratified keratinized squamous epithelium: Closely packed sheets of epithelial cells arranged in layers over the external surface of the body and lining most hollow structures.

Stratum corneum: The horny outermost layer of skin composed of dead flat cells converted to keratin that continually flake away.

Stratum germinativum: The deepest of the five layers of the epidermis, composed of cuboid-shaped cells.

Stridor: Abnormally high-pitched or musical sound caused by obstruction in the trachea or larynx, often heard on inspiration.

Stromal tissue: Connective tissue that forms a framework.

Sudoriferous gland: An apocrine, eccrine or exocrine gland in the dermis that produces perspiration; also called a sweat gland.

Sulcus: Shallow depression or furrow on the surface of an organ.

Sutures: (1) A border of a joint such as the bones of the cranium. (2) A surgical stitch.

Symphysis: A line of union, especially between a cartilaginous joint, in which adjacent bony surfaces are firmly united by fibrocartilage.

Syncytiotrophoblast: The expanding peripheral syncytial layer produced by mitosis of cells within the cytotrophoblast at the embryonic pole of the blastocyst, beginning on day 6 of gestation.

Synovial joint: A freely moveable joint in which contiguous bony surfaces are covered by articular cartilage and are connected by a fibrous connective capsule lined with synovial membrane.

Systole: The period of contraction of the heart, atrial and ventricular.

Teeth: Accessory structures of digestion, composed of calcified connective tissue and embedded in bony sockets of the mandible and maxilla that cut, shred, crush and grind food.

Teething: The physiological process of the eruption of the deciduous teeth through the gums.

Tendon: Any one of the white glistening bands of dense fibrous connective tissue that attach muscle to bone. Tendons are strong, flexible and inelastic, and occur in various lengths and thicknesses.

Terminal: Near to or approaching the end.

Totipotent: The ability of a cell, particularly a zygote, to differentiate into any number of specialized cells and form a new organism, or regenerate a body part.

Trachea: Tube made up of C-shaped cartilage and membrane that carries air to the lungs and extends from the larynx at the level of the sixth cervical vertebrae to the level of the fifth thoracic vertebrae, where it divides into two bronchi (Greek *tracheia* = rough artery).

Transforming growth factor (TGF) β: One of a group of proteins that, when inoculated into normal cells, cause a disorderly increase in the number of cells in the culture.

Triglyceride: A simple fat compound consisting of three molecules of fatty acid.

Trimester: One of the three periods of approximately 3 months into which a pregnancy is divided.

Trophoblast: The outermost layer of tissue that forms the wall of the blastocyst in placental mammals during the early stages of embryonic development.

Trophoblastic: Describes the outermost layer of tissue that forms the wall of the blastocyst of placental mammals in early development of the embryo.

Tuberculum: Module or rounded elevation.

Tunica albuginea: A tissue covering of white collagenous fibre such as the sclerotic coat of the eyeballs and the testes.

Tympanic membrane: A thin, semi-transparent membrane in the middle ear that transmits sound vibrations to the inner ear by means of the auditory vesicles.

Tyrosinase: An amino acid synthesized in the body from the essential amino acid phenylalanine. Tyrosine is found in most proteins and is a precursor of melanin and several hormones.

Umbilical cord: The long rope-like structure containing the umbilical arteries and veins; connects the fetus to the placenta.

Uncinate: Having hooks or barbs.

Ureters: A pair of tubes about 30 cm long that carry urine from the kidneys to the urinary bladder.

Utricle: The larger of the two membranous pouches in the vestibule of the membranous labyrinth of the inner ear.

Vagus nerve: Either of the largest pair of cranial nerves mainly responsible for parasympathetic control over the heart and many other internal organs, including the thoracic and abdominal viscera.

Vas deferens: The extension of the epididymis of the testes that ascends from the scrotum into the abdominal cavity and joins the seminal vesicle to form the ejaculatory duct.

Vasculogenesis: Formation of blood vessels form throughout the entire embryo as endoderm induces overlying splanchnopleuric mesoderm to form networks of vasculature characteristic of each specific region; angioblasts form angiocysts, which coalesce to form angioblastic cords and then angioblastic plexuses.

Ventral: (1) Refers to the stomach or abdominal region. (2) Towards the front; anterior.

Villus: One of many tiny projections, barely visible to the naked eye, clustered over the entire mucous surface of the small intestine. The villi are covered with epithelium that diffuses and transports fluids and nutrients.

Virus: A minute parasitic entity, much smaller than a bacterium, that has no independent metabolic activity; can replicate only within a cell of a living plant or animal host.

Visceral: Pertaining to the internal organs of the abdominal cavity.

Vittelline duct: The narrow channel connecting the yolk sac with the intestine.

White matter: Aggregations or bundles of myelinated and unmyelinated axons located in the brain and spinal cord.

Xiphoid: (1) Sword shaped. (2) The inferior portion of the sternum that is named the xiphoid process.

Yolk sac: An extraembryonic membrane composed of the extracoelomic membrane and hypoblast. It transfers nutrients to the embryo; contains primordial germ cells that migrate into the gonads to form primitive germ cells; forms part of the gut; and helps to prevent desiccation of the embryo.

Zona pellucida: Clear glycoprotein layer between a secondary oöcyte and the surrounding granulosa cells of the corona radiata.

Zygote: The combined cell produced by the union of the pronuclei of the egg and sperm, at the completion of the first cleavage.

Chapter 1

The child: a framework for development

Carol A. Chamley

CHAPTER OUTCOMES

This chapter will enable the reader to:

- Define the terms anatomy, physiology and embryology, and explain how these underpin the biological development of the child
- Outline the major phases of embryological and fetal development
- Define the terms growth, development, differentiation and maturation
- Describe the function of the fetomaternal organ (placenta)
- Define the term congenital, and explain potential causes of congenital abnormalities
- Explore the main principles of the 'nature versus nurture' debate
- Explain the reasons why human beings have an extended period of biological development.

CHAPTER OVERVIEW

The aim of this chapter is to outline the biological processes of child development, describing the biophysiological relationship between anatomy, physiology, embryology, genetics and the environment. The prenatal period of human development is one of the most fascinating, yet least understood. During prenatal development we witness the most rapid and complex processes of development, from the unicellular embryo to the birth of a unique human being.

Therefore, the study of developmental anatomy and physiology of children helps us to understand the development of body structures, anatomical and physiological relationships, and how the human organism has the potential to grow, differentiate and mature into adulthood, with embryology exemplifying key developmental issues. Clinical Notes address areas of clinical relevance and potential interest to the reader, and Self Assessment exercises assist the reader in reflecting upon the chapter and guiding the relationship between theory and practice.

INTRODUCTION

Have you ever seen a toddler trying to feed her/himself something gooey and messy, like a chocolate pudding, and wondered: if our physical development is nothing more than the unfolding of a pre-ordained plan, as we often assume it is; why then is it necessary to study it (Bee & Boyd 2004)?

Developmental anatomy and physiology describe the sequence of biological events from the fertilization of a secondary oocyte (germ cell or gamete) to the development of a highly complex mature organism. The prenatal period of development is one of the most fascinating yet least understood periods of human development. It is only over the last 20 years with advancing science and technology that the complexities of human development have been unravelled. The end of the prenatal period is marked by a beginning: the birth of the new-born infant. However, in most societies the infant is given a birth age of zero, as if denoting that nothing of much significance occurred before birth. Yet the prenatal period embraces the most rapid and complex phases of human development (Hepper 2002).

The study of prenatal stages of development, especially those developments occurring in the embryonic period, help us to understand normal body structures, anatomical relationships, and how tissues, organs and systems differentiate and mature into adult structures. Furthermore, embryology helps to explain the causes of potential health-related problems, particularly congenital abnormalities, and how these abnormalities may affect the child and his or her family during childhood and beyond. Therefore, embryology illuminates and exemplifies anatomy and physiology, explaining how we begin life and what biological factors determine our potential to develop into mature adults.

Three branches of science—anatomy, physiology and embryology—provide the foundations for understanding the biophysical development of children:

Anatomy is the science of body structures and parts, and the relationships among these structures.
Physiology is the science relating to how the body functions.
Embryology is the science concerned with the origins and development of the human organism from a unicellular embryo or zygote to the birth of a unique human being.

ORGANIZATION OF THE BODY

During embryological development the human body is organized into a hierarchy of structures that reflect the different levels of structural organization and associated complexity in physiological function:

Chemical level This includes the smallest units of matter—atoms—that combine to form molecules.

Cellular level Molecules combine to form cells of which there are millions in the fully developed human body.

Tissue level Tissues are groups of cells that work together to perform certain physiological functions.

Organ level Organs are structures that are composed of two or more different tissue types that, through the process of biological development, eventually assume a recognizable shape (e.g. heart, brain, liver) and specific functions. Organs develop through the embryological process of organogenesis.

Systems level Systems are composed of organs that are related and share a common function. However, one organ may be part of one or more systems; for example, the pancreas contributes to the digestive and endocrine systems.

Organismal level An organism is a living individual; in the human organism all parts of the body function together. The developing child grows and matures over a period of many years.

HUMAN INHERITANCE: GENETICS

Child development begins before the child is born and is directed by the action of many genetic mechanisms controlled in strict chronological order. *Inheritance* is the passage of hereditary traits from one generation to the next, and is a branch of biology referred to as genetics.

Genes not only influence individual differences, but also govern the anatomical differences between all human beings. Evolutionary processes have facilitated small changes (mutations) coupled with selective forces in the human organism that have determined our present anatomical form and body shape. Furthermore, these genetic processes influence and determine the timing and sequence of anatomical and physiological activities, and the rate at which the human organism grows and matures. This accounts for the relatively long period of time that the human organism takes to develop compared with other species.

The nuclei of all human cells, except for the gametes or germ cells (ovum and sperm), contain 23 pairs of chromosomes; the diploid (*dipl* = double; *oid* = form) number $2n$. There are two types of chromosome: 22 of the chromosome pairs are referred to as autosomes, and the chromosomes that determine the sex of an infant are referred to as the sex chromosomes (X and Y chromosomes). One chromosome in

Fig. 1.1
A A human chromosome: the deoxyribonucleic acid (DNA) is tightly wound up inside.
B DNA molecules are arranged like a twisted ladder into a spiral inside a protein-coated strand.
C The process of mitosis.

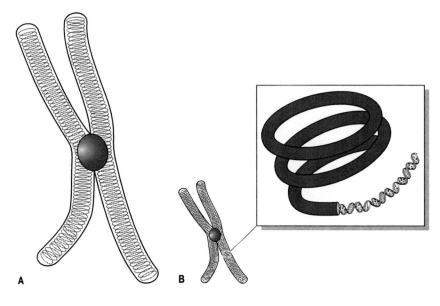

A

B

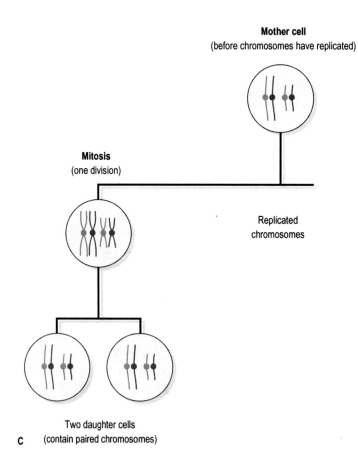

Mother cell
(before chromosomes have replicated)

Mitosis
(one division)

Replicated
chromosomes

Two daughter cells
C (contain paired chromosomes)

Fig. 1.1 (*Continued*)
D The process of meiosis.

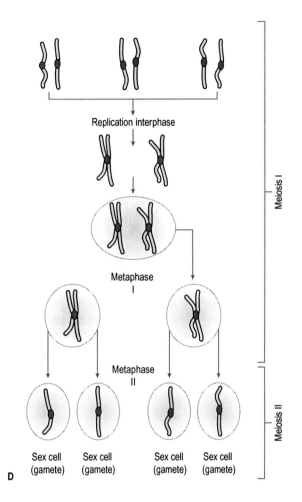

Replication interphase

Metaphase I

Metaphase II

Sex cell (gamete)   Sex cell (gamete)   Sex cell (gamete)   Sex cell (gamete)

Meiosis I

Meiosis II

D

each pair comes from the mother and the other from the father. The two chromosomes that make up a pair are referred to as *homologous* (*homo* = same). Furthermore, each homologue (one of the two chromosomes that makes up the same pair) contains genes that control the same traits. Alternative forms of a gene that code for the same trait, and are at the same location on the homologous chromosome, are called *alleles*. A *mutation* (*muta* = change) is a permanent inherited change in the allele that produces a different variant of the same trait.

Chromosomes (Fig. 1.1A) contain a long piece of *deoxyribonucleic acid* (DNA), which is a coiled, double-stranded molecule. The DNA molecule consists of two outer filaments with cross-pieces between them, rather like a ladder twisted into a spiral. A chromosome is approximately 0.004 mm long and contains a single piece of DNA that is 4 cm long. The DNA is therefore about 10 000 times longer than the chromosome, so has to coil and twist in order to assume the structure of the chromosome (Fig. 1.1B). Nucleic acids were first discovered in the nuclei of cells. They contain organic molecules, namely carbon, hydrogen, oxygen, nitrogen and phosphorus. There are two varieties of nucleic acid: DNA forms the inherited material inside each cell. Each gene is a segment of a DNA molecule, and our genes determine our hereditary traits. *Ribonucleic acid* (RNA) is the second type of nucleic acid, and is responsible for relaying instructions from the cell to guide the individual cell's synthesis of protein from amino acids. The DNA codes for all polypeptides (subunits of proteins) and all biochemical reactions in the body are catalysed by enzymes, which are also proteins. In this way genes control the body's metabolism, growth and development.

A child's *genotype* refers to the genes that he or she posseses. The term *phenotype* describes the physical characteristics determined by the genes.

Most patterns of inheritance are complex. Whenever given traits are governed by a single gene, as is true of 1000 individual physical characteristics, they follow well understood rules, with alleles for dominant and recessive traits. However, in polygenic inheritance many genes influence the phenotype.

CELL DIVISION

There are two methods of cell division: mitosis and meiosis.

MITOSIS

Mitosis is the process whereby somatic cells divide (Fig. 1.1C). Cells prepare for cell division by replicating their chromosomes; therefore a cell at this stage has double the amount of DNA. Each chromosome contracts into a dense body and splits lengthways to produce two identical daughter chromosomes. At this stage one new chromosome from each of the cell's 46 chromosomes locates to each of the daughter nuclei that are forming. The original cell divides and nuclei are formed in each of the two daughter cells, so that each new cell has the correct number of 46 chromosomes.

MEIOSIS

All gametes are formed by a process of meiosis (*mei* = lessening; *osis* = condition of) (Fig. 1.1D), which occurs in two successive phases:

Phase I The processes involved in this phase include halving the number of chromosomes in the gametes. The gametes contain a single set of 23 chromosomes and are referred to as haploid (*hapl* = single) cells, but the process of fertilization restores the diploid number.

Phase II As a result of replication, each chromosome consists of two genetically identical chromatids that are attached at their centromeres.

The process of meiosis is also responsible for independent assortment; that is, one chromosome from each pair will have been inherited from the father (paternal) and one from the mother (maternal). When the homologues separate during *anaphase*, a mixture of the maternal and paternal chromosomes end up in the gametes. During *prophase*, a process called 'crossing over', or genetic recombination, occurs: homologous chromosomes become joined together in a number of places (chiasmata), followed by breakage at these points and leading to the 'crossing over' of genes from one chromatid to the other.

MITOCHONDRIAL INHERITANCE

In mitochondrial inheritance children inherit genes that are carried in the mitochondria, which are found in the fluid that surrounds the nucleus of the ovum before it is fertilized. However, this type of inheritance can contribute to several types of anomaly, such as certain types of blindness.

SEX CHROMOSOMES AND SEX DETERMINATION

One of the smallest of the 23 pairs of chromosomes determines an individual's biological sex, referred to as the sex chromosomes. The physical appearance of these chromosomes is different in males and females.

Females have two X chromosomes and males have one X and a smaller Y chromosome. The Y chromosome has 231 genes—less than 10% of the 2968 genes present on chromosome 1, the largest chromosome in the body. Oocytes have no Y chromosome and produce only X-containing gametes. When the secondary oocyte is fertilized by an X-bearing sperm, the offspring is normally female (XX). However, when the oocyte is fertilized by a Y-bearing sperm, a male offspring (XY) is produced. Therefore, sex is determined by the father's chromosomes.

Both male and female embryos develop in an identical manner up until approximately 7 weeks' gestation, when one or more of the genes trigger a cascade of biological activities that eventually lead to sex differentiation.

CHROMOSOMAL ABNORMALITIES

Mistakes, or mutations, in the process of meiosis result in the production of gametes with altered structures or an alteration in the number of chromosomes. The consequence of these mutations is that all the cells produced from these gametes will carry forward the mutation(s) and will be unable to code for the correct proteins.

TWINS

Fraternal twins develop from two ova that have been produced and fertilized by separate sperm. Twins of this type may also be referred to as dizygotic twins; they are no more alike genetically than any other sibling. *Monozygotic twins* (identical twins) are produced when a single fertilized ovum divides in the normal way. However, for reasons that are unclear, the ovum separates further into two parts and each part develops into separate individuals, who have identical genetic pedigrees, because they both originate from the original fertilized single ovum.

CLINICAL NOTES	THE HUMAN GENOME PROJECT

The human genome contains in the order of 50 000 to 100 000 structured genes per haploid set. Many disease-causing genes have now been identified through scientific endeavours such as the Human Genome Project. It is expected that most genetic diseases will be mapped and sequenced during the early part of the twenty-first century, and it is possible that many congenital anomalies of unknown origin will be identified and consequently treatments made available. *Genome imprinting* is an epigenetic process whereby the female and male germlines confer a sex-specific mark on a chromosome subregion, implying that only the maternal or paternal allele of a gene is active. Thus, the sex of the transmitting parent influences the expression or non-expression of certain genetic traits in the child.

NATURE VERSUS NURTURE

One of the oldest and most contested arguments in relation to specific age-related developmental changes involves the nature versus nurture debate. Also referred to as heredity versus environment, or nativism versus empiricism, this is one of the oldest and most central theoretical issues within the disciplines of psychology and philosophy. The focus of the argument relates to the question: 'What is the best possible explanation for how development takes place?'. This debate is concerned with two theoretical positions regarding the relative roles and contributions of biology and the environment. *Nature* refers to the contribution that our genetic inheritance has upon our development. *Nurture* refers to the notion that the environment is primarily responsible for development (Keenan 2002). Many theories seek to explain human behaviour in terms of either inherited factors or experience. However, both ideals are mutually inclusive, and all organisms are a product of their genetic endowment and interaction with their environment.

In genetic terms, a specific genotype predisposes an organism to certain developmental outcomes, but the environment determines the outputs from the outcomes. Flanagan (1996) describes the *Canalization Principle*, which suggests that an individual's genes channel development along predetermined pathways that may be difficult for the environment to alter.

Historically, idealists and rationalists—principally Plato and Descartes—represented the nature side of the debate, believing that some knowledge is inborn, or innate. However, this was counter-argued by empiricists, such as John Locke, who represented the nurture side of the debate, claiming that the mind is an empty slate—a tabula rasa. From this perspective, developmental change is the result of external environmental forces affecting the child, whose only internal characteristic is the capacity to respond (Bee 1997, Bee & Boyd 2004).

Competing perspectives sought to explain development as an interaction between internal and external forces. Stanley Hall borrowed the Darwinian theory of evolution, believing that the milestones of childhood were orchestrated by an inborn developmental plan, and that developmentalists should identify norms or averages at which milestones should be achieved (Bee & Boyd 2004).

Contemporary views relating to the nature versus nurture debate have become much more complex. Rutter (2002) claims that every facet of a child's development is a product of interactive forces between nature and nurture. A view is now upheld by many theorists who contend that certain aspects of a child's development are incremental developments over many years, whereas other aspects are ongoing and continuous.

OVERVIEW OF EMBRYOLOGY AND FETAL DEVELOPMENT

Prenatal development is the period of time from fertilization to birth, and includes both embryological and fetal development. The period of *gestation* is sometimes cited as 280 days, or 40 weeks. Although development begins at fertilization, the stages and duration of a pregnancy are calculated from the date of the last menstrual period (LMP), which is approximately 14 days before conception. Therefore, the gestational age overestimates the actual fertilization by a period of 2 weeks (Moore & Persaud 1998).

The weeks are divided into three *trimesters* identified by specific changes that occur within the developing organism. The first trimester is the most critical and is characterized by the appearance of rudimentary organs and systems. It is also the period in which the developing organism is most vulnerable to the effects of drugs, viruses and radiation. The second trimester is characterized by organs and systems completing their initial development; by the end of this stage the organism assumes distinctly human features. The third trimester is characterized by a period of rapid fetal growth and development, and many of the developing systems are becoming functional in preparation for postnatal life.

THE EMBRYONIC PERIOD

This period refers to the early stages of human development, commencing with the germinal stage, which begins at conception and terminates when the zygote (pre-embryo) is implanted into the wall of the uterus. The embryonic period extends to the end of the eighth week when all the major structures are present, but only the heart and circulation are functional. During this period the conceptus is referred to as an embryo (*bryo* = grow).

THE FETAL PERIOD

The fetal period extends from the beginning of the ninth week, and marks the period when the developing organism is referred to as the fetus (offspring or young one). This period of development is not so dramatic or frenetic as the embryonic period when cells, tissues, organs and systems are all developing. However, development is quite rapid during the third and fourth gestational months.

OVERVIEW OF EMBRYONIC DEVELOPMENT

The first week of human development is characterized by significant developmental events that include:

- fertilization
- cleavage of the zygote
- blastocyst formation
- implantation.

FERTILIZATION

Fertilization is a complex sequence of coordinated events that involves the male sperm fusing with the female ooycte to form a specialized totipotent cell, or zygote—a unicellular embryo that heralds the beginning of the embryonic period (Fig. 1.2A). It is estimated that of the 200 million sperm introduced into the vagina less than 1% (2 million) reach the cervix of the female uterus, and only 200 reach the secondary oocyte (Tortora & Grabowski 2003). Fertilization usually occurs in the ampulla of the fallopian (uterine) tube and occurs 12–24 hours after ovulation. Hence sperm can remain viable for up to 48 hours, although the oocyte is viable for only 24 hours.

Fertilization occurs when the sperm penetrates the outer granulosa cells, the corona radiata (ko-RO-na = crown; rade-A-ta = shining), followed by the penetration of the glycoprotein layer, the zona pellucida (ZO-na = zone; pe-LOO-si-da = allowing a passage of light). Once the sperm and oocyte have fused together a zone reaction occurs and the fertilized oocyte becomes impermeable to penetration by other sperm. The unicellular embryo or zygote (Fig. 1.2B) is genetically unique because half of the chromosomes are derived from the mother and the other half are from the father. Therefore, the zygote contains a new and unique combination of chromosomes (Moore & Persaud 1998).

CLEAVAGE OF THE ZYGOTE

Cleavage consists of repeated mitotic divisions resulting in an increase in the number of cells, referred to as blastomeres (*blasto* = germ or sprout; *meres* = parts) (Fig. 1.2C). With successive changes a solid sphere of cells is produced, and by the end of the third day 16 cells are present. At this point the developing organism is referred to as a morula (mulberry) (Fig. 1.2D) because it resembles the fruit of the mulberry tree. At this stage of development the morula enters the uterus.

BLASTOCYST FORMATION

As the morula enters the uterus it draws in uterine fluid and forms fluid-filled spaces, which fuse to form a large central fluid-filled blastocyst cavity; the morula is now referred to as a blastocyst (Fig. 1.2E). There is further rearrangement of the blastomeres that results in the formation of two distinct structures:

- the *inner cell mass*, which is located internally and develops the process of embryogenesis
- the *trophoblast* (*troph* = develop or nourish), which develops into the embryonic portion of the placenta.

The early embryo has an amorphous, scanty, intercellular matrix containing a viscous substance that gives the early embryo a gel-like

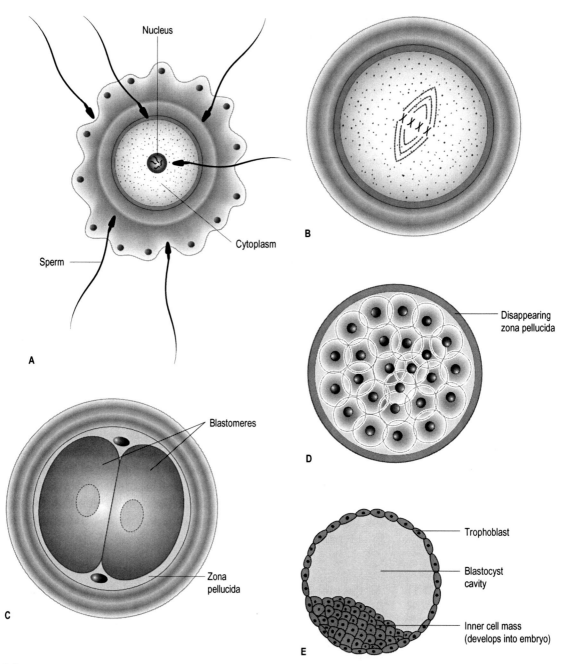

Fig. 1.2
A Fertilization of the ovum.
B Zygote.
C Blastomere.
D Morula.
E Blastocyst.

consistency, enabling it to hold large quantities of fluid. Other substances present within the intercellular matrix include hyaluronic acid, which is a polysaccharide that retains water tenaciously and becomes increasingly more viscous the more calcium that is present, and chondroitin sulphate, which is a firmer gel than the hyaluronic acid.

Approximately 5 days after fertilization the blastocyst hatches from the zona pellucida and begins the process of implantation.

IMPLANTATION

Approximately 6 days after fertilization the blastocyst attaches itself to the dorsal wall of the uterus (Fig. 1.3A). Following implantation the endometrium is known as the decidua (falling off). The spongy layer of the decidua is eventually shed (as the basal layer remains) and replaced by a new endometrium after birth.

DEVELOPMENT OF THE TROPHOBLAST

The embryonic period begins once implantation is complete and the trophoblast (the superficial covering of the blastocyst) has in the order of 150 cells (Tanner 1990). Subsequently, the outer layer of the blastocyst begins to specialize into two membranes, each of which forms critical support structures for the developing embryo. These are the syncytiotrophoblast and the cytotrophoblast (Fig. 1.3B). These two layers become part of the chorion, which is one of the fetal membranes. Approximately 8 days after fertilization, the cells of the inner cell mass further differentiate into the hypoblast, the primitive endoderm which is a single layer of columnar cells, and the epiblast, the primitive ectoderm which is composed of a double layer of cuboidal cells. Together these two layers form a flat disc known as the bilaminar (two layered) embryonic disc. In addition, a small cavity develops in the epiblast, eventually enlarging to form the amniotic (amnio = lamb) cavity (Fig. 1.3C). As the embryo grows and develops, the amnion eventually envelops the whole embryo completing the amniotic cavity, which eventually fills with amniotic fluid.

AMNIOTIC FLUID

Amniotic fluid plays a major role in fetal growth and development. Initially, some fluid is secreted by the amniotic cells, but most of the fluid is derived from maternal interstitial fluid by a process of diffusion across the amniochorionic membrane from the decidua parietalis. Secretions from the fetal respiratory tract also affect the fluid content of the amniotic fluid, and the water content of the amniotic fluid changes every 3 hours.

During week 11 of gestation, the fetus contributes to the amniotic fluid by excreting urine, and late in fetal life approximately 0.5 litres of urine are added daily. The volume of amniotic fluid gradually

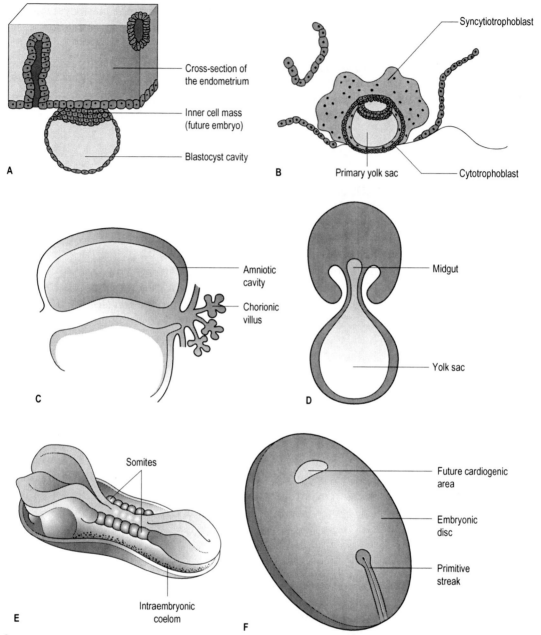

Fig. 1.3
A Implantation.
B Formation of syncytiotrophoblast and cytotrophoblast.
C Amniotic cavity.
D The yolk sac.
E Intraembryonic coelom.
F Development of the primitive streak.

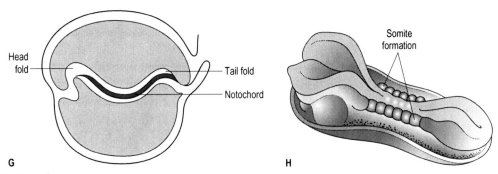

Fig. 1.3 (*Continued*)
G Development of the notochord.
H Somite formation.

increases, reaching 30 mL at 10 weeks, 350 mL at 20 weeks and 700–1000 mL by 37 weeks' gestation, after which the volume decreases (Moore & Persaud 1998). Amniotic fluid also helps to regulate body temperature, prevents desiccation and adhesion formation between the skin of the developing embryo and fetus, and acts as a shock absorber.

DEVELOPMENT OF THE EXOCELOMIC MEMBRANE

Also developing on day 8 is the exocelomic (*exo* = outside; *koilos* = space) membrane, the formation of which is complete by day 9. Together with the hypoblast, the exocelomic membrane forms the yolk sac (Fig. 1.3D), which is empty and decreases in size as development progresses. Approximately 12 days after fertilization, extraembryonic mesoderm develops, the cells of which are derived from the yolk sac and form a connective tissue, known as mesenchyme, around the amniotic yolk sac that eventually forms a single larger cavity known as the extraembryonic coelom (se-lom) (Fig. 1.3E). The extraembryonic mesoderm together with the two layers of the trophoblast (syncytiotrophoblast and cytotrophoblast) constitute the chorion (membrane), which eventually becomes the principal embryonic part of the placenta.

The third week of embryonic development marks a 6-week period of intensive embryonic development and differentiation. During weeks 4 to 8, the primary germ layers are established and provide the framework for organ development, organogenesis.

GASTRULATION

Gastrulation is a major developmental event occurring 15 days after fertilization. During this process the two-dimensional bilaminar embryonic disc transforms into a two-dimensional trilaminar (three-layered) disc consisting of three germ layers:

- *ectoderm* (*ecto* = outside)
- *mesoderm* (*meso* = middle)
- *endoderm* (*endo* = inside; *derm* = skin).

These primary germ layers constitute the major tissues of the embryo and therefore lay the foundations, or form the scaffolding, from which all major embryonic tissues and organs develop.

The first indication of gastrulation is the formation of the *primitive streak* (Fig. 1.3F). This clearly establishes the anatomical regions of the head and tail ends of the embryo. At the head end of the embryo, the epiblast cells form a mound known as the *primitive node* (knot). As the embryo continues to grow and develop, the endoderm contributes to the epithelial lining of the gastrointestinal tract, respiratory tract and several other structures. The mesoderm gives rise to the muscles, bones, peritoneum and other connective tissues. The ectoderm develops into the epidermis of the skin and developing nervous system.

DEVELOPMENT OF THE NOTOCHORD

The notochord is a flexible rod of mesodermal tissue forming in the region of the future vertebral column; it has a vital role in the process of cell and tissue induction. Approximately 16 days after fertilization, the notochordal process begins to form and develop, and by days 22 to 24 the notochordal process becomes a solid cylindrical mass of cells, known as the notochord (*noto* = back; *chord* = cord) (Fig. 1.3G). The process of induction is whereby one cell or tissue (inducing cell or tissue) chemically stimulates an adjacent unspecialized cell or tissue (responding cell or tissue) into a specialized cell or tissue. During weeks 4 to 7 of gestation, anatomically the vertebral column develops around the notochord, which begins to degenerate where it is incorporated into the vertebral bodies. Rudiments of the embryonic notochord persist and form the *nucleus pulposus* of the intervertebral discs, so that the notochord persists into adulthood in the form of these structures.

The notochord is also responsible for inducing ectodermal cells to form the neural plate. This is the first indication of the developing nervous system, a process that begins on day 18 of gestation. As the notochord and the neural tube form, the intraembryonic mesoderm cells proliferate to form a thick longitudinal column of paraxial mesoderm. In turn, the paraxial mesoderm soon segments into a series of paired, cube-shaped structures called somites (little bodies) (Fig. 1.3H). By the end of the fifth week of gestation, 42 to 44 pairs of somites are present, and correlate to the approximate age of the embryo. Each somite differentiates into three regions:

- a myotome
- a dermatome
- a sclerotome.

The *myotome* develops into skeletal muscles of the neck, trunk and the limbs. The *dermatome* forms connective tissue. The *sclerotome* gives rise to the vertebrae.

HUMAN DEVELOPMENT

Weeks 4 to 8 of gestation mark a significant period in embryonic development as all major organs and systems develop through the complex process of organogenesis. These processes also require the presence of blood vessels to supply the developing organs with oxygen and nutrients. Recent studies suggest that the blood vessels play a significant role in organogenesis even before blood flows through the vessels. It has been proposed that the endothelial cells of the blood vessels trigger a developmental signal, either chemically or by direct cell-to-cell interaction, that appears necessary to engage complex processes inherent in organ formation (Tortora & Grabowski 2003).

CLINICAL NOTES   HOMEOBOX GENES

Homeobox-containing (HOX) genes now appear important in controlling pattern formation during embryonic development. Homeobox genes are a group of genes found in all vertebrates. They have highly conserved sequences and order, and are involved in early embryonic development, specifying identity and spatial arrangements of body segments. Protein products of these genes bind to DNA and form transcriptional factors that regulate gene expression (Moore & Persaud 1998).

As the early embryo grows and develops, and the organs take shape and form, so the shape and proportions of the embryo change dramatically. This is coupled with processes that involve folding of the embryo, an important series of complex anatomical events that establish body form. These processes involve folding of the flat trilaminar embryonic disc into a cylindrical embryo. Folding of the embryo occurs in both the median and horizontal planes, and results from the rapid growth of the embryo, particularly the brain and spinal cord. Folding at the cranial and caudal ends of the embryo occurs simultaneously, and folding of the ends of the embryo ventrally produces head and tail folds. As a result, the cranial and caudal regions of the embryo grow apart ventrally and the embryo elongates in both cranial and caudal directions.

A greater biological challenge to the developing embryo is the growth of the left and right sides of the body and the maintenance of symmetry. It is still unclear how the developing body grows, ensuring that the two sides of the body are symmetrical in shape, size and proportions. It is, however, recognized that there are normal variations in symmetry that have no biological or medical significance. Equally, asymmetry can in some cases be pathological when associated with disease or abnormal growth and development of the child.

THE UMBILICAL CORD (UMBILICUS)

The umbilical cord is the structure that attaches the embryo and fetus to the placenta. It is composed of several important features, including blood vessels. Anatomically the attachment is usually near to the centre of the fetal surface of the placenta, but may be found at any point. After birth, the umbilical cord is clamped and the placenta discarded after careful examination. The umbilical stump eventually shrivels, leaving the structure commonly referred to as the belly-button. Because of the different growth patterns between the upper and lower body, the umbilicus at birth is 1–2 cm below the midpoint of the body. However, by the age of 1 year the umbilicus normally assumes the anatomically correct location at the midpoint of the body. In the adult the umbilicus is normally anatomically higher still.

THE ROLE OF THE PLACENTA

The placenta is a fetomaternal organ because it originates from both fetal and maternal tissues (Fig. 1.4). Early in week 12, two distinctive

Fig. 1.4
The placenta.

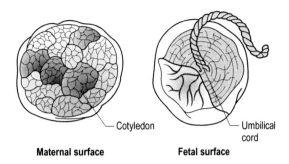

Maternal surface   Fetal surface

elements can be identified: the fetal portion formed by the villous chorion, and the maternal portion formed by the decidua basalis. The two portions are held together by stem villi, or anchoring villi, so named because they are anchored to the decidua basalis by the cytotrophoblastic shell. Together, the placenta and the umbilical cord (umbilicus) act as a transport system for various substances that pass between the fetus and the mother.

The primary functions of the placenta relate to:

- respiration, as the placenta acts as embryonic or fetal lungs
- nutrition
- excretion
- hormone production
- protection of the developing infant.

The placenta and fetal membranes are expelled from the uterus as the afterbirth following delivery of the infant.

SENSITIVE PERIODS OF DEVELOPMENT

Critical periods, or periods of special vulnerability (Bee & Boyd 2004, Tanner 1989, 1990), are those periods in the course of development when developing cells, tissues, organs or systems are vulnerable to the actions of agents or teratogens. The most critical periods of development are when cell division, cell differentiation and morphogenesis are at their peak. It is during the period between 4 and 8 weeks of gestation that exposure of the embryo to teratogens such as maternal disease, drugs, viral agents, exposure to ionizing agents, nicotine, alcohol, subnutrition, certain chemicals and maternal age can all have a deleterious effect upon the developing embryo (Fig. 1.5). Consequently, exposure to teratogenic agents during the first 14 days

after fertilization normally kills the embryo, and major malformations are more common in early embryos. Severely abnormal
embryos are spontaneously aborted during the first 6–8 weeks of gestation. The timing and extent of exposure are crucial factors; at one
extreme the abnormal embryo may be spontaneously aborted, or the
fetus stillborn, or the infant may be born with dysmorphogenesis

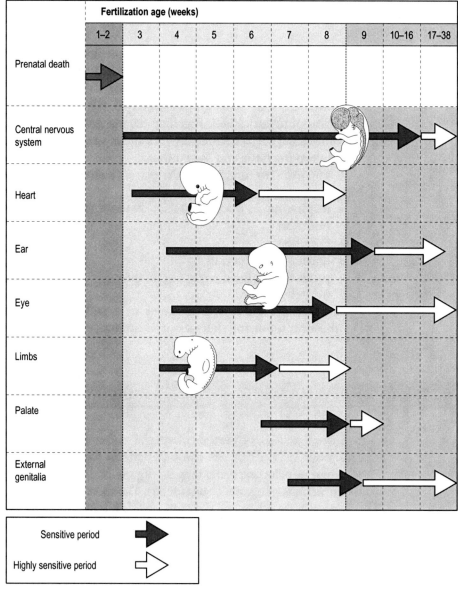

Fig. 1.5
Sensitive periods of development.

(*dys* = abnormal), physical or learning disabilities, genetic aberrations or congenital anomalies.

A congenital (*congenitus* = born with) abnormality is a structural abnormality of any type; however, not all anomalies are sinister as anatomical variations are relatively common. However, congenital abnormalities of clinical significance have one or more of the following features:

- *malformation*—which is a primary defect of an organ(s) or tissues
- *disruption*—to structure, form or function
- *deformation*—damage caused by external factors influencing a previously normal structure
- *dysplasia*—changes in the shape, size and organization of cells as a result of chronic irritation or inflammation.

It has been proposed that the genotype of the developing organism determines whether the teratogenic agent can potentially disrupt the growth and development of the embryo (Moore & Persaud 1998). Abnormalities may be single or multiple, simple or complex, overt or covert in their presentation. Abnormal numbers of chromosomes (aneuploidy) may also be associated with congenital abnormalities. The anomaly may result from defective chromosomes or chromatid separation (*non-disjunction*) during the first or second meiotic division during gametogenesis. Furthermore, the loss of one member of a chromosome pair (*monosomy*) appears to be lethal in the human species if it involves an autosome. There may also be gains in chromosomal configurations; Down syndrome is an example of *trisomy*, referred to as trisomy 21, denoting three number 21 chromosomes. There are also many examples of anomalies associated with the sex chromosomes. Turner syndrome is characterized by the presence of one sex chromosome (XO), and trisomy of the sex chromosomes can result in Klinefelter syndrome (XXY, XYY or XXX).

Most of the common abnormalities are probably the result of a complex interaction between the environment and the genes of the developing embryo, referred to as multifactorial inheritance. It is reasonable to suggest that any insult to gene activity at a critical period of development could potentiate developmental defects.

CLINICAL NOTES   FETAL ORIGINS HYPOTHESIS

The fetal origins hypothesis (Barker 1992, Nathanielsz 1999) suggests that the environment experienced by the fetus serves to programme the functional capacity of the individual organs, and has an effect on the child's health postnatally. Therefore, the prenatal environment may determine the lifelong functional capacity of individual organs (Slater & Lewis 2002).

PHASES OF EMBRYONIC DEVELOPMENT

Human development is divided into three interrelated phases: growth, morphogenesis and differentiation:

Growth The first phase of development relates to embryonic growth of structure, involving cell division and elaboration of cell products.

Morphogenesis The second phase relates to the development of form. This includes mass cell movement facilitating the cells to interact with one another biologically during the formation of tissues and organs (organogenesis).

Differentiation The third phase relates to the maturation of physiological processes. Therefore, completion of this stage results in the formation of tissues, organs and systems that have the potential to function.

The embryonic period of growth and development is finalized when organogenesis is complete.

OVERVIEW OF FETAL DEVELOPMENT

The period of fetal development commences at the beginning of week 9 of gestation and ends with the onset of the birth of the infant. The developing infant is now referred to as a fetus; the change in name signifies that the developing organism has now acquired human characteristics (Fig. 1.6A). The normal fetus grows and develops in length and weight, weighing in the order of 500 g at 23 weeks gestation, 1000 g at 27 weeks gestation, 1500 g at 30 weeks gestation, 2000 g at 33 weeks gestation and approximately 3000–3500 g at 37 weeks gestation (Candy et al 2001). Therefore, weight gain and length are incremental and the newborn infant may attain a length of approximately 50 cm and a birthweight of 3.5 kg. On average, male infants are 100 g heavier than female infants, and slightly larger (Thompson & Meggit 1997).

During the fetal period of growth and development, tissues and organs developed during the embryonic period grow and differentiate; very few new structures appear. Anatomically organs and systems have assumed their correct positions, and physiologically there is functioning in some systems. The rate of fetal growth and development is rapid, especially between weeks 9 and 16. The rate is also dependent upon an adequate supply of oxygen and nutrients from a healthy placenta.

At the end of the fetal period the fetus will normally have quadrupled in bodyweight; the fetal head will have changed shape and dimensions from being half the length of the fetal body at the beginning of the fetal period to only one-quarter the length of the body at

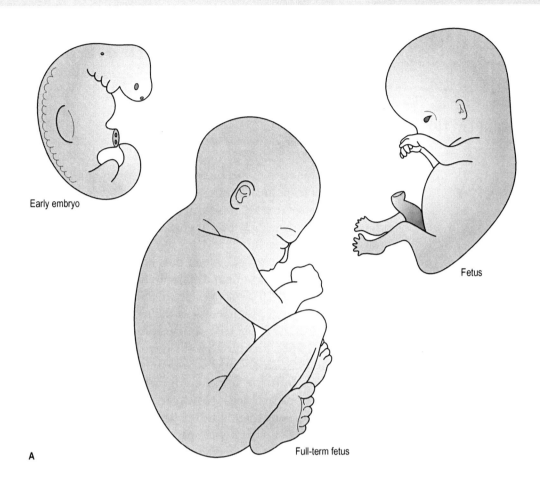

Early embryo

Fetus

Full-term fetus

A

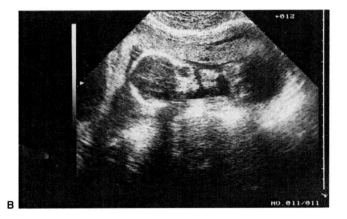

B

Fig. 1.6
A The fetus.
B Ultrasound scan of fetus.

the end of the fetal period. During the same period the fetal limbs increase in length from one-eighth to one-half the length of the fetus (Tortora & Grabowski 2003).

BEHAVIOUR OF THE FETUS

Normally the fetus remains busy and active throughout intrauterine life. The fetus responds to sounds from 22 to 24 weeks gestation, and research suggests that the fetus can distinguish between familiar and novel stimuli by week 32 or 33 of gestation (Sandman et al 1997). The internal environment inhabited by the fetus is noisy, with sounds from the mother's heartbeat, blood flow and digestive system all permeating the fetal environment. Fetal movements can normally be felt from a period of 18–20 weeks gestation, although movements are felt earlier in subsequent pregnancies as the mother recognizes the earliest flutterings of the fetus. Ultrasonography facilitates observation of the fetus (Fig. 1.6B), and movements have been observed as early as 8 weeks gestation. These early movements are slow, and originate in nerve impulses from the spinal cord, mainly causing passive movements of the arms and legs. However, over the following weeks a whole variety of movements and behaviours begin to emerge; by 15 weeks the fetus is moving in the order of 20 000 times a day, and by 20 weeks the fetus has developed an individual repertoire of movements (Slater & Lewis 2002).

BEHAVIOURAL STATES

Four behavioural states have been identified in the fetus (Slater & Lewis 2002), demonstrating a greater degree of integration within the various parts of the central nervous system. These behavioural states relate predominantly to periods of activity, rest and sleep:

Quiet sleep The fetus is quiet and sleeping, exhibiting the occasional startle. There are no eye movements and the heart rate is steady and stable.

Active sleep This state is characterized by frequent gross movements of the fetus; the eyes are moving and the heart rate is subject to alterations associated with fetal movements.

Quiet awake During this state no gross movements are observed, although eye movements are observed and the heart is stable with no accelerations.

Active awake The fetus is extremely active, continually busy with many gross movements of the limbs and body. The eyes are moving and busy, and the heart rate is unstable and prone to periods of acceleration and deceleration.

It is recognized that each fetus has its own individual and distinctive pattern of movements, behaviours and a daily routine combining activity, rest sleep and wake cycles; some of these activities continue into postnatal life.

CHILD DEVELOPMENT AND MATURATION

During a gestational period of approximately 280 days, the amorphous cytoplasmic ball of cells, fertilized from a single oocyte no bigger than a full stop on this page, grows and develops into a unique human being. The newborn infant emerges from an entirely aquatic, dependent existence with the potential for sustaining an independent life outside of the uterus, through structures and complex processes that were developed during the embryological and fetal periods of development. Human beings all share a biological pattern through conception, infancy and growth into adulthood (Boushel et al 2000). The process of growth and development is made up of a series of alternating periods of rapid growth accompanied by disruption, or disequilibrium, and periods of consolidation (Bee & Boyd 2004). This pattern of development is referred to as the *tempo of growth* (Tanner 1989, 1990). Therefore, child development concentrates on the developmental period between conception and adolescence (Keenan 2002) (Table 1.1), and development occurs in different domains including biological, psychosocial, cognitive, emotional and spiritual.

Table 1.1 Definitions of developmental periods during childhood.
(Adapted from Wong 1999.)

Period	Timeframe
Prenatal period	Conception to birth
Germinal stage	Conception to 2 weeks
Embryonic stage	2–8 weeks
Fetal stage	8–40 weeks
Infancy period	Birth to 12 months
Neonatal period	Birth to 28 days
Infancy	1–12 months
Early childhood	
Toddler	1–3 years
Preschooler	3–6 years
Middle childhood (school age)	6–10 years
Later childhood	11–19 years
Prepubertal	10–13 years
Adolescence	13–18/19 years

Growth and development are usually referred to as a unit, expressing the sum of numerous changes that take place during the lifetime of the individual. The entire course is dynamic, synthesizing growth, development, differentiation and maturation (Wong 1999).

Growth

Growth may be defined as the progressive development of a living organism, or any of its parts, from the earliest stages of development through to maturity (Sinclair & Dangerfield 1998).

Development

Development relates to patterns of change that commence at conception and continue throughout the lifespan. This includes advancement from simple to more advanced stages of complexity, thereby extending the individual's capacity (Bee & Boyd 2004).

Differentiation

Differentiation is the process by which early cells and biological structures are systematically modified and altered to achieve specific characteristics and competence (Tortora & Grabowski 2003, Wong 1999).

Maturation

This term is used to refer to those aspects of development that are genetically predetermined and will unfold independently of experience (Slater & Lewis 2002). Furthermore, maturational patterns have three qualities (Bee 1997, Bee & Boyd 2004):

1. They are *universal*, appearing in all children, across all cultural and societal boundaries.
2. They are *sequential*, involving the same characteristics.
3. They are relatively *impervious* to environmental influences.

Development is multidimensional and multidirectional. *Multidimensional* relates to the fact that development cannot be easily assigned to a single criterion. The principle of *multidirectionality* relates to the idea that there is no single normal pathway that development must take. Therefore, the outcomes of growth and development are achieved in a wide variety of ways.

Bee & Boyd (2004) claim that there are three fundamental aspects that inform our understanding of children:

- the way in which children are the same but different
- the effect of internal and external influences on these changes
- the quantitative and qualitative nature of development.

Fundamentally, all children are alike across all cultures and follow the same pattern of development and maturation. These processes have been shaped and moulded by evolutionary processes; however, inheritance and the environment shape who we are and our potential throughout life. There are definite and predictable patterns of growth and development that are orderly and progressive. These patterns are fundamental to the human species, albeit the physical elements of growth and development are more overt, observable and measurable.

Furthermore, children have distinctive periods of developmental change as they progress from one stage of development to the next.

PHASES OF GROWTH

There are fundamentally four phases of growth over the lifespan (Sinclair & Dangerfield 1998, Tanner 1989, 1990):

1. In the early embryo, development is subordinated to growth, with little differentiation of function.
2. During the second phase there is a balance between growth and differentiated functional activity. This phase continues throughout childhood.
3. The third phase intervenes at maturity and the attainment of adulthood. In this phase the goal is functional activity.
4. The final phase occurs into old age.

As the child grows and develops, the body becomes larger and more complex. External characteristics change but this is accompanied by alterations in the structure and function of internal tissues, organs and biological systems that also reflect the acquisition of physiological competence. Growth and developmental processes are simultaneous and mutually dependent upon one another, involving influences that are exerted by the neuromuscular and endocrine systems, nutritional status, genetics and environmental forces.

Growth and development follow a universal pattern basic to the human species. Directional trends or gradients reflect the physical development and maturation of the neuromuscular system and these trends follow two primary directions: cephalocaudal and proximodistal (Fig. 1.7):

Cephalocaudal direction (head to tail) The cephalic end of the organism is large and complex compared to the lower portion of the body, which is smaller and simple.
Proximodistal direction (near to far) This trend reflects development from the midline to the periphery.

Fundamentally, these trends are symmetrical and bilateral, and through the process of biological development and differentiation the early embryonic cells with their vague undifferentiated structures and functions progress to form a highly complex organism—the child—a framework for growth, development and maturation into adulthood.

The concept of development is both individual and collective. In the midst of change the individual child will carry forward certain core traits that link their past with their future development (*epigenesis*).

Fig. 1.7
Directional trends in growth.

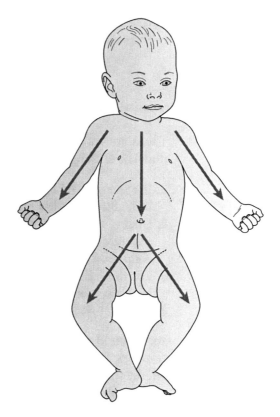

This element of continuity is vital and serves as a foundation for the child's future development.

GROWTH IN HEIGHT AND WEIGHT

HEIGHT

The human ovum measures approximately 100 μm in diameter, and is just visible to the naked eye. At birth the infant averages 50 cm in length, approximately 5000 times the length of the ovum. Further growth in length and height after birth into adulthood, an average of 175 cm, equates to three times the length of the newborn infant (Sinclair & Dangerfield 1998).

The process of growth (*auxology*) (Tanner 1989, 1990) is not uniform throughout life, and each anatomical region of the body has its own growth rate. The amount of growth achieved depends upon the time for which growth proceeds and the speed of growth per unit of time. Maximum growth occurs during the fetal period of development, when the fetus can achieve a maximum growth rate of 1.5 mm per day up to 4 months gestation. Thereafter growth slows down until birth. Lengthening of the body depends upon natural curvatures in the vertebral column as well as the width of the intervertebral discs.

During infancy, height increases by 2.5 cm per month during the first 6 months of life, settling to a slower, more gradual, pace during the second 6 months. Height increases by accelerations or spurts rather than in an incrementally paced pattern. In the first year of life the child's body length increases by approximately 50%. During toddlerhood a further 12–13 cm is added during the second year. Prediction of adult height is possible by the second birthday, by which time the child should have joined his or her genetic growth curve. This is a major determinant of height, and predictions become possible. Growth in height during toddlerhood is steplike rather than in a linear straight pattern, once again reflecting periods of growth spurts.

During middle childhood, growth in height is slow and at a steadier pace than in early childhood. On average the child aged between 6 to 12 years may grow 5 cm per year, to gain 30–60 cm in height. Sex differences in height mean that boys tend to be slightly taller than girls. After initial accelerations in growth in height, growth settles into a steady pace until the period of adolescence.

The adolescent growth spurt normally commences between 10 and 11 years of age, although there is a wide variation in individuals and between the sexes. Biological processes that begin to 'kick start' the growth spurt are initially covert, and the exact mechanisms are still unclear. However, the adolescent growth spurt is considered to be controlled genetically. The pubertal growth spurt refers to the general increase in the growth of the skeleton, muscles and internal organs that peaks on average at 12 years of age for girls and at 14 years for boys. The increase in the size of muscles reflects increased amounts of contractile protein and of nuclei, and underlies the increase in strength. Other muscles, including the heart, demonstrate similar growth curves (Tanner 1989, 1990). Although accelerated growth in height occurs during adolescence, there are tremendous variations and individual differences; however, once growth begins it is normally progressive and predictable.

Human beings are the only mammals with an extended quiescent interval before the growth spurt. It has been suggested that the biological need to postpone puberty and concomitant processes facilitates the maturation of the complex human brain (Sinclair & Dangerfield 1998). This is what distinguishes human beings from lower animals.

WEIGHT

The infant's weight at birth is more variable than length and reflects the maternal environment more than any genetic propensity. Loss of bodyweight occurs rapidly after birth, and the newborn infant can lose in the order of 10% of bodyweight during the first 3–4 days of postnatal life. This is due to losses of excessive extracellular fluid and meconium, coupled with the establishment of a feeding regimen.

Birthweight is normally regained by the tenth postnatal day. The infant's birthweight, length and head circumference are plotted on standardized graphs and identify normal values for gestational age. Therefore, infants whose weight is appropriate for gestational age (between the 10th and 90th percentiles) can be presumed to have grown at a normal rate regardless of the length of gestation, which may be preterm, term or postterm (Wong 1999).

Weight gain during the first 6 months of life is dramatic. Infants gain in the order of 680 g per month until approximately 5–6 months of age, when birth weight doubles. However, weight gain during the second 6 months to 1 year of age triples, and by the end of the second year birthweight has quadrupled, settling down to a steady annual increase of approximately 2.25–2.75 kg per year. Weight gain during toddlerhood is slow, with the average gain approximately 1.8–2.7 kg per year. During middle childhood, weight gain is steady but the child may double in weight, increasing by 2–3 kg per year.

Adolescence marks changes with the accumulation of lean body mass, primarily muscle mass, that peaks for girls at menarche then gradually decelerates, but for boys continues during puberty resulting in a significant greater lean body mass. Fat mass for girls markedly increases early during puberty and continues to increase after menarche. Boys' fat mass is marked by a peak deceleration in accumulated fat, at the time of their growth spurt.

Peak velocity for spurts in weight gain lags behind the peak velocity for attainment in height by a period of about 3 months. Bodyweight does not normally attain adult values until after adult height attainment.

CHANGES IN SHAPE

As the child grows and develops, so this alters the shape and proportions of the body (Fig. 1.8). At all ages the dimensions of the head are in advance of those of the trunk, the trunk is in advance of the limbs, and more peripheral parts of the limbs are in advance of central parts of the limbs.

The first year of life marks a period of rapid growth dominated by lengthening of the trunk and accumulation of subcutaneous fat. When the child becomes more mobile and begins to walk, the centre of gravity is higher caused by the child's disproportionate bulk; most notably a large head, protuberant abdomen, everted feet and bowed legs. At birth the circumference of the skull averages the circumference of the chest, and the circumference of the abdomen is greater than that of both the skull and the thorax until 2 years of age. The large disproportionate abdomen is due to the large liver and small pelvis, which does not

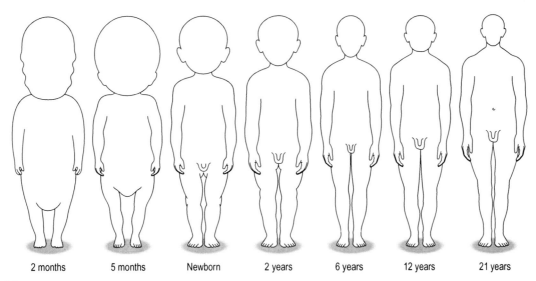

| 2 months | 5 months | Newborn | 2 years | 6 years | 12 years | 21 years |

Fig. 1.8
Changes in shape and proportion.

contain the organs found in the adult pelvis. However, rapid growth of the pelvis in early childhood facilitates the urinary bladder and intestines eventually assuming their normal anatomical positions and sinking down into a position that results in the gradual flattening of the abdomen (Sinclair & Dangerfield 1998, Wong 1999). Furthermore, because of the abdominal overcrowding, the thorax and shoulder girdle are displaced upwards towards the neck. With the changes to the growth of the pelvis and associated anatomical changes, this facilitates the upper structures to descend with the apparent lengthening of the child's neck.

As growth and development continue, the child becomes better proportioned, taking on a slimmer physical appearance as the legs lengthen and posture improves, with more efficient use of the arms and legs. After the first year of life up until puberty, the legs grow more rapidly than any other part of the body. During the pubertal growth spurt the feet and hands grow rapidly, making them appear disproportionately large in relation to the rest of the frame. This is followed by growth of the calf muscles and forearm, followed by the hips and chest, and finally the shoulders. The feet stop growing before almost all other parts of the skeleton.

FACIAL PROPORTIONS

At birth, the surface area of the head accounts for 20% of the whole body surface. During infancy the bones of the face grow faster than the cranial vault, reflecting the growth of the brain. During infancy the main growth of the jaws relates to accommodating the eruption of the teeth, and the development of the facial muscles that assist in mastication. All the primary deciduous teeth are lost during middle childhood, and this developmental period is referred to as the 'age of the loose teeth' (Wong 1999). The face grows first in width then in length, giving the impression that the face appears to emerge from underneath the skull.

PHYSIOLOGICAL MATURATION

Associated with growth and development of the child are a series of physiological and biochemical changes that occur in all organs and systems. The process of physiological maturation occurs over a period of many years, and many of these physiological and biochemical changes demonstrate a sex difference in timing that appears to be more closely associated with physiological maturation than chronological age. However, most physiological systems have reached relative maturity by the end of toddlerhood.

The skin functionally matures during the early part of childhood, with the epidermis and dermis becoming more tightly bound. Production of sebum is minimal, but the eccrine glands are functional during childhood and produce minimal amounts of sweat. The hair grows coarser, and usually darkens and assumes its genetically determined colour.

Thermoregulation is a critical adaptive response of the infant during the transition from intrauterine to postnatal life. Following the period of instability during the neonatal period, the mechanism of thermoregulation becomes more efficient as the system becomes physiologically more stable with maturity; the capillaries become more able to conserve core body temperature and the act of shivering serves its physiological purpose. This is coupled with the child learning to take some control over his or her temperature, by removing clothing if too hot and increasing the amount of clothing if too cold. Females maintain a slightly higher body temperature than males throughout life.

Development of the component parts of the brain correlate with progressive growth and intellectual capacity; for example, the Broca area of the brain relates to the development of speech. Maturation of the cortical area of the brain relates to control of the hands, feet, legs and sphincters (Wong 1999). The respiratory tract and associated structures continue to grow and mature during early childhood; however, structures within the ear and throat remain short and straight.

During early childhood blood protein values are low, although adult values are attained within a few years. The resting heart rate slows progressively from approximately 100 beats per minute at 2 years of age to nearer adult values. This correlates to the biological rule that the heart rate is inversely related to body size. Early during the period of toddlerhood digestive processes are maturing. In early childhood bile is dilute and the acidity of the gastric contents continues to increase; a major milestone in relation to the gastrointestinal tract is voluntary control of the elimination of faeces. Furthermore, due to complete myelination of the spinal cord, control of the anal and urethral sphincters is eventually achieved. The physiological ability to control sphincters normally occurs between 18 and 24 months of age. The glomerular filtration rate of the kidney reaches adult values by the age of 2–3 years. Bladder capacity increases by about 14–18 months of age, and the child can retain urine for up to 2 hours longer than previously.

Metabolism, that is all chemical and energy transformations, is affected by intrinsic and extrinsic factors. The basal metabolic rate (BMR), which reflects the rate of metabolism when the body is at rest, demonstrates significant changes throughout life. The BMR is highest in the newborn and during infancy, and is closely related to the proportion of surface area to body mass, declining rapidly between 6 and 20 years of age. In both sexes the proportion of surface area to body mass declines progressively with ensuing maturity. The rate of metabolism determines the calorific requirements of the child, and children's energy needs vary considerably at different ages and stages of development and maturation. Throughout life, water is crucial to survival and physiological functioning of the body; therefore, water requirements remain constant at approximately 1.5 ml per kcal (Wong 1999).

SELF ASSESSMENT

Answer the following questions in relation to your professional areas of practice:

A Developmental anatomy and physiology is the synthesis of four sciences:
 1.
 2.
 3.
 4.

B Outline the following stages of intrauterine growth and development:
 ● germinal stage
 ● embryonic stage
 ● fetal stage

C Define the following terms:
 ● growth
 ● development
 ● differentiation
 ● maturation

DEVELOPMENTAL ANATOMY AND PHYSIOLOGY WORDSEARCH

Using the following clues, identify the correct words from the maze of letters.

1. Unicellular embryo
2. Male gamete
3. Female gamete
4. One of two or more alternative forms of a gene that occupy corresponding loci on homologous chromosomes
5. Somatic cell division
6. The process of organ formation
7. The human organism in utero after the embryonic period
8. Fetomaternal organ
9. The process of growth
10. The structure that attaches the embryo and fetus to the placenta
11. Born with
12. One of the three 3-month periods into which pregnancy is divided.

F	H	C	A	L	L	E	L	E	B	O	O	P
O	C	O	N	G	E	N	I	T	A	L	G	K
D	E	D	D	R	Y	C	F	B	N	Z	O	M
O	R	G	A	N	O	G	E	N	E	S	I	S
U	T	X	C	C	V	L	T	F	Z	P	T	P
M	R	E	R	T	U	J	U	S	Y	E	L	L
B	I	A	E	I	M	C	S	B	G	R	I	A
I	M	I	S	D	C	S	C	W	O	M	K	C
L	E	A	W	O	O	C	B	R	T	O	V	E
I	S	A	Q	Z	D	F	I	V	E	X	Z	N
C	T	M	I	T	O	S	I	S	Z	E	C	T
U	E	I	O	S	W	C	O	U	D	X	M	A
S	R	A	U	X	O	L	O	G	Y	X	C	B

References

Barker D J 1992 Fetal and infant origins of adult disease. British Medical Association, London

Bee H 1997 The developing child, 8th edn. Harper Collins, New York

Bee H, Boyd D 2004 The developing child, 10th edn. Allyn and Bacon, Boston

Boushel M, Fawcett M, Selwyn J 2000 Focus on early childhood: principles and realities. Blackwell Science, London

Candy D, Davies G, Ross E 2001 Clinical paediatrics and child health. W B Saunders, London

Flanagan C 1996 Applying psychology to early child development. Hodder and Stoughton, London

Hepper P G 2002 Prenatal development. In: Slater A, Lewis M (eds) Introduction to infant development. Oxford University Press, Oxford, p 39

Keenan T 2002 An introduction to child development. Sage, London

Nathanielsz P W 1999 Life in the womb: the origins of health and disease. Promethan Press, New York

Moore K L, Persaud T V N 1998 Before we are born: essentials of embryology and birth defects, 2nd edn. W B Saunders, London

Rutter M 2002 Nature, nurture, and development: from evangelism through science towards policy and practice. Child Development 73:1–21

Sandman C, Wadhwa P, Hetrick W, Porto M, Peeke H 1997 Human fetal heart rate dishabituation between thirty and thirty-two weeks. Child Development 68:1031–1040

Sinclair D, Dangerfield P 1998 Human growth after birth, 6th edn. Oxford University Press, Oxford

Slater A, Lewis M 2002 Introduction to infant development. Oxford University Press, Oxford

Tanner J M 1989 Foetus into man: physical growth from conception to maturity, 2nd edn. Castlemead Publications, Hertford

Tanner J M 1990 Foetus into man: physical growth from conception to maturity, 2nd edn. Harvard University Press, Cambridge, MA

Thompson H, Meggit C 1997 Human growth and development for health and social care workers. Hodder and Stoughton, London

Tortora G J, Grabowski S R 2003 Principles of anatomy and physiology, 10th edn. John Wiley and Sons, New York

Wong D L 1999 Whaley and Wong's nursing care of children, 6th edn. Mosby, London

Bibliography

Abramsky L, Chapple J 1994 Prenatal diagnosis: the human side. Chapman and Hall, London

Becket C 2002 Human growth and development. Sage Publications, London

Frost M, Sharma A 2001 Mary Sheridan's from birth to five years: children's developmental progress. Routledge, London

Gilbert P 2000 A–Z of syndromes and inherited disorders, 3rd edn. Nelson Thornes, Cheltenham

MacGregor J 2000 Introduction to the anatomy and physiology of children. Routledge, London

Sweet B 1999 Mayes' midwifery, 12th edn. Baillière Tindall, London

Tortora G J, Grabowski S R 2003 Principles of anatomy and physiology, 10th edn. John Wiley & Sons, New York

Answers to the Wordsearch

1. Zygote
2. Sperm
3. Ovum
4. Chromatid
5. Mitosis
6. Organogenesis
7. Fetus
8. Placenta
9. Auxology
10. Umbilicus
11. Congenital
12. Trimester

Chapter 2

Development of the integumentary system

Carol A. Chamley

CHAPTER OUTCOMES

This chapter will enable the reader to:

- Define the term integumentary
- Describe the normal embryological and fetal development of the integumentary system
- List the major structures found in the skin
- Explain why the skin is the largest organ in the human body
- Describe the functions of the skin
- Explain the term skin appendages
- List the structure and functions of the skin appendages
- Explain the difference between white and brown fat.

CHAPTER OVERVIEW

The aim of this chapter is to explore the normal embryological and fetal development of the integumentary system, describing the development of the skin and appendages, which include hair, nails, glands and mammary glands. Teeth are normally included as part of this system; however, because of the central importance of normal dentition and good dental health in childhood, Chapter 12 is dedicated to this part of the integumentary system.

The chapter discusses the major components of the integumentary system, explaining the normal embryological and fetal anatomy and physiology, and outlining key elements relevant to the development and maturation of the system. Clinical Notes address issues of clinical relevance and potential interest to the reader, and Self Assessment exercises assist in reflecting upon the chapter and guiding the relationship between theory and practice.

INTRODUCTION

The integumentary (*inter* = whole; *gument* = body covering) system consists of the skin and appendages, which include hair, nails, glands, mammary glands and teeth. The skin is described as an organ because it consists of tissues that are joined together structurally to perform specific activities and functions. Anatomically and physiologically the human skin differs markedly in various regions of the body, and each region is specifically adapted to cope with special stresses. The growth of skin is able to regulate and adjusts itself to the variations in surface area of the body surface, most notably with weight loss or increase in weight and surface area. Regions of the body, for instance the soles of the feet, the eyelids and the back, vary in skin thickness and looseness, and in the type and quantities of appendages they contain.

The skin is described as the largest organ of the body, covering all of the body's external surfaces. It is a thin structure, approximately 1 mm thick at birth, increasing to about twice this thickness at maturity. Skin accounts for approximately 4% of total bodyweight in the newborn infant. It is one of the largest organs of the body in terms of weight and surface area, with the potential to occupy a surface area of approximately 2 square metres (3000 square inches) in adulthood. It is estimated that there are approximately 800 cm² of skin per kilogram bodyweight in the infant, compared with 300 cm² per kg in the adult. The skin is complex in structure and in terms of physiological functions that are essential for the survival of the human organism. It is also the principal seat of the sense of touch, and the more simple outer structure provides protection for deeper structures. At birth all the structures within the skin are present, but many of the functions of the integumentary system are immature.

EMBRYOLOGY

DEVELOPMENT OF THE SKIN

All tissues of the body develop from three basic germ layers:

- ectoderm
- mesoderm
- endoderm.

However, most tissues of the body are composed of a combination of these germ cells.

Essentially the skin is composed of two layers. The superficial thinner layer, the *epidermis* (*epi* = above), is the outermost surface layer of the skin, and the deeper thicker connective tissue layer, the *dermis*, is the innermost layer. These layers are derived from two different germ cells: ectoderm and mesoderm.

DEVELOPMENT OF THE EPIDERMIS

The outer layer of skin begins as a single layer of ectodermal cells and, as development progresses, the ectoderm becomes multi-layered, and regional differences in structure and function become apparent.

During the first and second trimesters, epidermal growth occurs in stages that culminate in increasing epidermal thickness. The *primordium* of the epidermis is the layer of surface ectodermal cells that proliferate and form a layer of *squamous epithelium*, the *periderm* and a basal *germinative* layer (Fig. 2.1). At this stage of development the epidermis is described as a *cellular mosaic*, with contributions from cells derived not only from the surface ectoderm, but also from precusor cells, including neural crest cells and mesenchyme. The cells of the periderm undergo a continuous process of keratinization and desquamation, and are replaced by cells arising from the basal layer. The exfoliated peridermal cells form part of the *vernix caseosa*, a white greasy substance that covers and protects the fetal skin from the constant exposure to amniotic fluid and urine during fetal life.

The basal germinative layer of the epidermis becomes the *stratum germinativum* (*germ* = sprout). By 11 weeks gestation, cells from the stratum germinativum have formed an intermediate layer. Replacement of peridermal cells continues until approximately 21 weeks gestation; thereafter the periderm disappears and the *stratum corneum* forms.

The proliferation of cells in the stratum germinativum produces *epidermal ridges*, which extend into the developing dermis. These ridges begin to appear in the developing embryo at approximately 10 weeks' gestation and are permanently established by week 17. The formation of epidermal ridges is closely associated with the earlier appearance of *volar pads* on the ventral surfaces of the fingers and toes. Volar pads first form on the palms of the hands at approximately 6.5 weeks, and appear 1 week later on the fingers. The volar pads begin to regress by the 10th week of gestation. Furthermore, the epidermal ridges produce grooves on the surface of the palms of the hands and the soles of the feet. The type and patterning of these ridges is determined genetically, and constitutes *fingerprints*.

Fig. 2.1
Development of the epidermis.

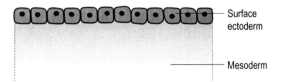

Surface ectoderm

Mesoderm

Late in the embryonic period, the *neural crest cells* migrate into the mesenchyme in the developing dermis and differentiate into *melanoblasts*. The differentiation of melanoblasts into *melanocytes* involves the formation of pigment granules. Melanocytes appear in the developing skin at 40–50 days gestation. The melanocytes begin to produce melanin before birth and distribute to the epidermal cells. The transformation of the surface ectoderm into a multilayered epidermis results from the continued interactions with the developing dermal layer.

The epidermis is the most superficial layer of skin composed of stratified keratinized squamous epithelium, and varies in thickness in different parts of the body. Blood vessels and nerve endings are present, and the deeper layers of the epidermis are bathed in *interstitial fluid* from the dermis; the interstitial fluid also provides oxygen and nutrients, and is drained away as lymph. There are several types of cell in the epidermis, extending from the deepest germinative layer to the surface stratum corneum. The cells on the surface are flat, thin, non-nucleated, dead cells, or *squames*, in which the cytoplasm has been replaced by fibrous protein keratin. These cells are constantly rubbed off and replaced by cells originating in the germinative layer and which have undergone change as they have progressed towards the surface of the skin. Complete replacement of the epidermis takes approximately 40 days.

The health of the epidermis depends upon three major processes:

- *Shedding*—a process of desquamation of keratinized cells from the skin surface
- Effective *keratinization* of the cells approaching the surface
- *Cell division*—a continual process in the deeper layers with newly formed cells being pushed to the surface.

Epidermal growth factor (EGF) is a protein hormone that functions as a growth factor and stimulates the growth of epidermal cells and fibroblasts.

DEVELOPMENT OF THE DERMIS

The dermis develops from mesenchyme, which is derived from the mesoderm underlying the surface ectoderm. Most of the mesenchyme that differentiates into the connective tissue of the dermis originates from the *somatic layer*, or lateral mesoderm, but some is derived from the dermatomes of the somites.

By week 11 of gestation, the mesenchymal cells have begun to produce collagenous and elastic connective tissue fibres. As the epidermal ridges form, the dermis projects into the epidermis, forming *dermal ridges*. Capillary loops develop in some of these ridges and provide some nourishment for the epidermis, and sensory nerve endings form in others. The developing afferent nerve fibres play an important role in the spatial and temporal sequence of dermal ridge formation.

The blood vessels in the dermis begin as simple endothelium-lined structures that differentiate from the mesenchyme. As new skin grows, new capillaries grow out from these simple vessels. Some of the capillaries acquire muscular coats through differentiation of myoblasts developing in the surrounding mesenchyme, and eventually evolve as arterioles and arteries. Other capillaries, through which a return flow of blood is established, acquire muscular coats and develop into venules and veins. Some of the transitory blood vessels disappear as new blood vessels form and become established, and by the end of the first trimester the major vascular organization of the fetal dermis is established. Lymph vessels form a network throughout the dermis.

The dermis is composed of connective tissue containing collagenous and elastic fibres. *Fibroblasts, macrophages* and *mast cells* are the main cells to be found in the dermis. Underlying its deepest layer there is areolar tissue and varying amounts of adipose tissue (fat). The main structures to be found in the dermis are:

- blood vessels
- lymph vessels
- sensory (somatic) nerve endings
- sweat glands and ducts
- hair
- arrector pili muscles
- sebaceous glands.

SENSORY NERVE ENDINGS

The skin is an important sensory organ through which the human organism receives information about the physical environment. Incoming stimuli activate different types of sensory receptor (Table 2.1), including touch, temperature, pressure and pain. Sensory receptors are widely distributed in the dermis; nerve impulses generated in the sensory receptors are conveyed to the spinal cord by sensory nerves (somatic cutaneous). They then pass to the sensory area within the cerebrum where the sensations are interpreted.

Table 2.1 Sensory receptors of the skin

Type of sensory receptor	Stimulus
Meissner's corpuscle	Light touch
Pacinian corpuscle	Deep pressure
Free nerve endings	Pain

At 17–20 weeks gestation the skin is covered in the greasy *vernix caseosa*, consisting of a mixture of fatty secretions from the fetal sebaceous glands and dead epidermal cells.

At 21 weeks gestation the skin is wrinkled and translucent; it appears pink-red in colour owing to the blood being visible in the capillaries. At birth, the two layers of the skin are loosely bound together and are very thin. Slight friction across the epidermis may cause separation of these layers, with blister formation. Furthermore, the *transitional zone* between the cornified and living layers of the epidermis forms an effective layer to prevent fluid from reaching the skin surface.

CLINICAL NOTES	ECZEMA (ATOPIC DERMATITIS)

Eczema, or eczematous inflammation of the skin, refers to a descriptive category of dermatological diseases, the cause of which is poorly understood (Candy et al 2001, Wong 1999). It can be regarded as an intrinsic type of hypersensitivity reaction in the skin, probably involving Type I and Type IV hypersensitivity reactions (Candy et al 2001). Eczema presents in three basic forms, according to the distribution and the age of the child:

1. *Infantile*—usually presents between 2 and 6 months of age, and generally undergoes spontaneous remission by the age of 3 years.
2. *Childhood*—may follow the infantile form, but manifests between the ages of 2 and 3 years.
3. *Preadolescent*—begins at approximately 12 years of age and may continue into early adulthood, or for an indefinite period.

GLANDS OF THE SKIN

Three types of gland are associated with the skin: sebaceous glands, sudoriferous (sweat) glands and ceruminous glands. Two of these, sebaceous and sweat glands, are derived from the epidermis and grow into the dermis.

SEBACEOUS GLANDS

Sebaceous glands (*sebace* = greasy), oil glands or holocrine glands are simple branched acinar glands and, with few exceptions, are connected to hair follicles. These glands develop as simple outgrowths on the side of the hair beginning as buds (Fig. 2.2A) that eventually develop and form glandular buds that branch repeatedly to form a system of solid ducts and alveoli. The central cell of the alveolus breaks down to form an oily secretion known as *sebum*, a mixture of

Fig. 2.2
A Development of the
sebaceous gland.
B Secreting portion of the
sebaceous gland: week 18
gestation.

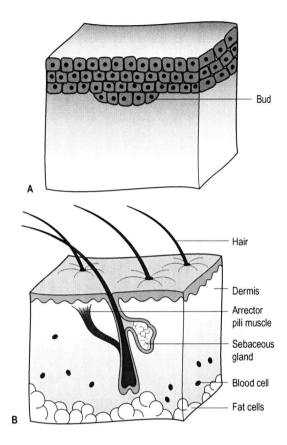

triglycerides, fats, cholesterol, proteins and inorganic salts. The secreting portion of the gland is situated in the dermis (Fig. 2.2B), and glands that are connected to hairs open into the necks of the hair follicle. Sebaceous glands not associated with hair follicles open directly onto the surface of the skin. Sebum coats the surface of hairs and helps to keep them from drying out and becoming brittle. Sebum also prevents excessive evaporation of water from the skin, keeping the skin soft and pliable, and inhibits the growth of bacteria.

SUDORIFEROUS GLANDS

Sudoriferous (sweat; *ferrous* = bearing) or sweat glands are the organs by which a large portion of aqueous and gaseous materials are excreted from the skin. The cells of the sweat glands release their excretions by *exocytosis*, and empty them into the hair follicles or on to the skin surface through pores. They are divided into two main types depending upon their structure, type of excretion and location. These are *eccrine* sweat glands and *apocrine* sweat glands.

Eccrine sweat glands

Eccrine glands (*eccrine* = secreting outwardly) are located in the skin throughout most of the body; they develop as epidermal downgrowths

Fig. 2.3
A Development of the sweat glands.
B Skin strata in the newborn.

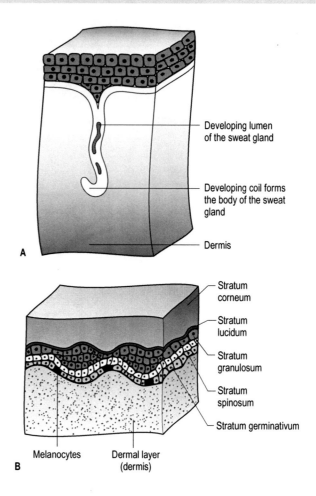

A

Developing lumen of the sweat gland

Developing coil forms the body of the sweat gland

Dermis

B

Stratum corneum

Stratum lucidum

Stratum granulosum

Stratum spinosum

Stratum germinativum

Melanocytes

Dermal layer (dermis)

into the underlying mesenchyme. As the buds elongate, they coil to form the *primordium* of the secretory component of the gland and the epithelial attachment of the developing gland, forming part of the primordium of the epidermis. Subsequently, the central cells of the primordial ducts degenerate, forming a *lumen* (Fig. 2.3A). The peripheral cells of the secretory part of the gland differentiate into secretory cells and myoepithelial cells, which are thought to be specialized smooth muscle cells that assist in the expulsion of sweat. Secretion from the eccrine glands consists of water, ions (Na^+, Cl^-; sodium and chloride ions), urea, uric acid, ammonia, amino acids, glucose and lactic acid. The onset of function is soon after birth, and the main functions of the eccrine glands are in the regulation of body temperature and waste removal. The density of eccrine glands is greater at birth than at any other time of life. No new glands are formed after birth and the sweat glands are equivalent in terms of size, structural maturity and position in the dermis of the full-term newborn and the adult. Sweat glands reach the level of adult functioning at approximately 2 years of age.

Eccrine sweat glands are widespread in the human skin and represent a major source of evaporative heat loss from the body. Sweat production and sweat excretion are complex phenomena, involving the transport of ions and protein secretion, as well as the activities of myoepithelial cells. Local microvasculature and the existence of local regulatory mechanisms are likely to contribute to these activities (Zancanaro et al 1999).

CLINICAL NOTES   **WATER LOSS THROUGH THE SKIN**

Water loss through the thin uncornified skin of infants less than 28 weeks gestation may be extremely high (Crawford & Morris 1995). These losses are increased if the infant is nursed under a radiant heater or phototherapy unit. Transepidermal loss is markedly increased in the preterm infant compared with the term infant. The preterm infant is also unable to sweat until a few weeks of age, compared to the term infant who can sweat from birth (Lissauer & Clayden 2001).

Apocrine sweat glands

These are simple, coiled, tubular glands. They develop as downgrowths from the stratum germinativum of the epidermis, which gives rise to hair follicles. Therefore, apocrine glands are another type of sweat gland that develop as an attachment to the hair follicle; the ducts of these glands open into the upper part of the hair follicles. Secretions from the apocrine glands are similar to those of the eccrine glands, although they are more viscous, containing lipids and proteins. The major onset of function is at puberty.

CLINICAL NOTES   **ACNE**

Acne is an inflammation of the sebaceous (oil) glands. The onset is usually during puberty. During this period of development and change, the sebaceous glands, under the influence of male sex hormones, androgens, grow in size and have an increased production of sebum. Acne occurs predominantly in the sebaceous glands, which are rapidly colonized by bacteria that survive upon the lipid-rich sebum. When this happens, the cystic sac of connective tissue cells can be destroyed and displace epidermal cells, which can then result in permanent scarring of the skin.

CERUMINOUS GLANDS

Ceruminous (wax) glands are modified sweat glands that produce a waxy secretion. The secretory portion of the ceruminous glands lies in the subcutaneous layer deep in the sebaceous gland. The combined secretions of the ceruminous and sebaceous glands are referred to as *cerumen*, or ear wax. The main function of cerumen is to provide protection for the ear with a sticky barrier.

MAMMARY GLANDS

Mammary (*mastos* or *mamma* = breast) are modified and highly specialized sudoriferous (sweat) glands whose main function is to produce milk.

Mammary buds begin to develop during week 6 of gestation as solid downgrowths of the epidermis that infiltrate the mesenchyme (Fig. 2.4A). The mammary buds begin developing from the thickened mammary ridges (lines), which appear during the fourth week of gestation. Each primary bud gives rise to secondary mammary buds that develop into the lactiferous ducts and their subsequent branches. This process continues until late gestation, and by full term 15 to 20 lactiferous buds are formed (Fig. 2.4B).

Fig. 2.4
A Development of the mammary glands.
B Structure of the mammary gland at birth.

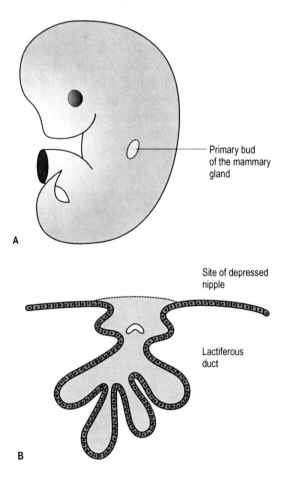

Primary bud of the mammary gland

A

Site of depressed nipple

Lactiferous duct

B

During the fetal period the epidermis at the site of origin of the mammary gland becomes depressed, forming a shallow, or *mammary pit*. The nipples form close to full term or into the neonatal period, as the mesenchyme proliferates below the downgrowths and elevates this area above the adjacent skin. The rudimentary mammary glands of the newborn of both sexes are identical. Some enlargement may be present and a secretion, referred to as 'witches' milk' (Moore & Persaud 1998), may be produced. The mammary glands remain underdeveloped until puberty, when the female breasts enlarge rapidly, mainly as a result of fat and connective tissue development.

BLOOD RESERVOIR

The skin's vascular blood supply is quite extensive and can hold large volumes of blood. When other body organs, such as vigorously working muscles, need a greater blood supply, the nervous system constricts the dermal blood vessels, thereby shunting more blood into the general circulation and making it available to the muscles and other body organs.

SURFACE AREA

An infant's relatively greater surface area allows greater quantities of fluid to be lost in insensible perspiration through the skin. It is estimated that the surface area of the premature neonate (an infant born before completion of the 37th gestational week) is proportionally five times greater than that of the term newborn. Furthermore, the surface area of the newborn is two to three times greater than that of the older child and adult (Wong 1999).

SKIN STRATA

THE EPIDERMIS

The epidermis is composed of four basic layers, or strata, except for areas where the skin is exposed to great friction, where there are five layers (see Fig. 2.3B).

Stratum basale (*basal* = base)

This layer may also be referred to as the stratum germinativum (*germ* = sprout) and is the deepest layer of the epidermis. It is composed of cuboidal or columnar keratinocytes.

Stratum spinosum
(*spinos* = thornlike)

This layer is composed of eight to ten layers of many-sided keratinocytes which fit closely together.

Stratum granulosum
(*granules* = little grains)

In the middle of the epidermis, the stratum granulosum consists of three to five layers of flattened keratinocytes that undergo apoptosis (orderly, genetically programmed cell death that removes unneeded cells during embryological development).

Stratum lucidum
(*lucid* = clear)

This layer is present only in the skin of the fingertips, the palms of the hands and the soles of the feet.

Stratum corneum
(horn/horny)

This layer consists of 25 to 30 layers of flattened dead keratinocytes. These cells are continuously shed and replaced by cells from the deeper layers.

THE DERMIS

The dermis is the deepest part of the skin, and is composed mainly of connective tissue, containing collagen and elastic fibres. The dermis is divided into two regions:

- papillary region
- reticular region.

The papillary region

This is the superficial section of the dermis, consisting of areolar connective tissue with elastic fibres. This region has papillae that contain capillaries, corpuscles of touch, and free nerve endings.

The reticular region

The deeper section of the dermis consists of dense, irregular connective tissue with bundles of collagen and coarse elastic fibres. The spaces between the fibres contain adipose cells, hair follicles, sebaceous glands and sudoriferous glands.

CELL TYPES

The epidermis is composed of stratified epithelium, and contains four principal cell types:

1. *Keratinocytes* (*keratino* = hornlike; *cytes* = cells).
2. *Melanocytes* (*melano* = black). Approximately 8% of epidermal cells are melanocytes and produce the pigment melanin.
3. *Langerhans cells*, which arise from red bone marrow and migrate to the epidermis. These cells participate in immune responses and are easily damaged by ultraviolet light.
4. *Merkel cells*, which are the least numerous of the epidermal cells and are located in the deepest layer of the epidermis.

| CLINICAL NOTES | PRESSURE SORES |

Contrary to popular belief, children can and do develop pressure sores for a variety of different reasons. Pressure sores, or decubitus ulcers, occur when the capillary blood flow in the skin is interrupted by pressure and the blood flows back into the tissues when the pressure is relieved. As the body attempts to reoxygenate the area, a bright red flush appears. This is known as reactive hyperaemia, and may be present for one-half to three-quarters as long as the time for which the pressure occluded the blood flow to the area. If the redness persists this may lead to skin breakdown with the potential for extensive damage below the surface of the skin. Pressure sores or decubitus ulcers occur in several stages:

Stage 1: Non-blanchable erythema of intact skin.
Stage 2: Partial-thickness skin loss involving epidermis and/or dermis. The ulcer is superficial and may present as an abrasion, blister or shallow crater.
Stage 3: Full-thickness skin loss involving damage or necrosis of subcutaneous tissue.
Stage 4: Full-thickness skin loss with extensive destruction and tissue necrosis with or without damage to muscle, bone and/or tendons.

Waterlow (1997) identified that extrinsic rather than intrinsic factors predispose the child to developing pressure sores; these include:

- pressure compression on a local point
- shearing of the skin
- friction
- moisture.

   Pressure sores can develop at any point on the body, but particular pressure points for children include the bony prominences, the sacrum, heels, ears, buttocks and the back of the head. Furthermore, Waterlow (1997) noted the risks inherent in plaster casts, splints, tubing and long lines. Special attention needs to be given to neonates because of the nature of their fragile immature skin. Heel pricks or strapping may cause bruising or torn skin, as neonates have slightly different damage patterns compared with older children.
   Waterlow (1997) recommends that each child should be assessed by means of a questionnaire combined with the use of infant and child body maps and full documentation. It is useful to assess the following:

- bodyweight
- continence
- skin condition
- mobility
- nutritional status
- hydration

- tissue hypoxia
- medication.

Risk assessment for each child should identify potential problems and interventions that may reduce risk. Huband & Trigg (2002) suggest that positioning of the infant or child is crucial, especially if mobility is compromised. Furthermore, if a child at risk is lying on something hard, such as the lead of a monitor, a pressure sore can develop. In addition, the back of a child's head is particularly at risk, but this is often forgotten.

FUNCTIONS OF THE SKIN

The physiological functions of the skin include (Tortora & Grabowski 2003, Waugh & Grant 2001):

- thermoregulation
- protection
- reception of stimuli
- immunity
- excretion and absorption
- synthesis of vitamin D.

THERMOREGULATION

Regulation of body temperature (thermoregulation) becomes more efficient during infancy with the skin more able to contract, and the muscles able to shiver in response to the cold. Shivering (thermogenesis) causes the muscles and the muscle fibres to contract generating metabolic heat throughout the child's body. Furthermore, increased amounts of adipose tissue during the first 6 months of life insulates the body against heat loss (Wong 1999). As the child continues to develop during toddlerhood, under moderate variations in temperature the child is better able to respond physiologically as the capillaries conserve body temperature and the process of shivering becomes an efficient source of thermoregulation. In response to elevated environmental temperature or strenuous exercise, the production of sweat assists in lowering body temperature through the process of evaporation from the surface of the skin. Conversely reduced environmental temperature decreases the production of sweat to conserve heat. When the child becomes active, during moderate amounts of activity or play the blood flow through the skin increases which in turn increases the amount of heat radiated from the skin. Young children produce heat rapidly and can become overheated, therefore clothing needs to be changed to accommodate climatic variations.

PROTECTION

The skin covers the body and provides protection in a variety of ways. It provides a physical barrier that protects the underlying tissues and structures from physical abrasion, bacterial infection, dehydration and ultraviolet (UV) radiation. Two types of cell carry out protective functions that are essentially immunological in nature. The *epidermal Langerhans cells* alert the immune system to the presence of pathogens, and *macrophages* in the dermis phagocytose bacteria and viruses.

RECEPTION OF STIMULI

The skin contains many nerve endings and receptors, including tactile discs in the epidermis, the corpuscles of touch in the dermis, and hair root plexuses around individual hair follicles. Sensations that arise in the skin include touch, pressure, vibrations, 'tickles', pain and warmth.

IMMUNITY

The intact skin and mucous membranes are the first defence against pathogens. These structures contain chemical and mechanical factors that are involved in combating the initial assault on the body by pathogens in an attempt to cause disease.

EXCRETION AND ABSORPTION

The skin has a minor role in excretion and absorption. Perspiration helps in regulating normal body temperature. Small amounts of water, salts and organic compounds are excreted from the skin.

SYNTHESIS OF VITAMIN D

The synthesis of vitamin D requires the activation of a precursor molecule present in the skin, and is activated by the exposure to ultraviolet radiation. This process involves enzymes in the liver and kidneys that modify the activated molecule. The end-result is the most active form of vitamin D, namely calcitriol. Calcitriol is essentially a hormone that aids the absorption of calcium and phosphorus from dietary foods, from the gastrointestinal tract into the blood.

BODY FAT

Adipose tissue is a loose connective tissue in which the cells, adipocytes (*adipo* = fat), are specialized for the storage of triglycerides. The cell fills with a single large triglyceride droplet, which displaces the cytoplasm and nucleus to the periphery of the cell.

Brown fat forms during weeks 17 to 20 of gestation and is the site of heat production, particularly in the newborn infant. This specialized adipose tissue produces heat by breaking down fatty acids to release energy in the form of heat. Brown fat is found predominantly at the nape of the neck, posterior to the sternum, and in the perirenal area. The 'brown hue' is attributed to the high content of cell mitochondria.

Heat generated by brown fat is distributed to other parts of the body by the blood, which is warmed as it flows through the layers of tissue. Brown fat is widely distributed around the body until 10 years of age (MacGregor 2000). The location of brown fat may explain the reason why the nape of the neck feels warmer than the rest of the body.

White fat increases to form approximately 3.5% of body fat from 26 to 29 weeks, and by full term the white fat content of the body is approximately 16% of bodyweight. The fetus adds approximately 14 g of fat per day during the last weeks of gestation.

Normal fat distribution during childhood follows a definite pattern. Although fat contributes substantially to bodyweight, it is not certain whether it 'grows' like other tissues. Therefore, fat is described as a labile tissue markedly affected by the nutritional status of the child. Furthermore, the amount and distribution of fat correlates with a genetically defined 'body build'.

CLINICAL NOTES | **COMPOSITION OF BODY FAT**

There is some evidence to suggest that there is an alteration in the biochemical composition of body fat with the discovery of alterations in levels of stearic and oleic acid. Evidence indicates that the proportion of stearic and oleic acid is declining, while the proportion of linoleic acid is rising. This has been attributed to dietary changes in relation to the consumption of vegetable and animal fats (Sinclair & Dangerfield 1998).

According to Tanner (1990), during the last 10 weeks of fetal development the fetus stores considerable amounts of energy in the form of fat. At approximately 26 weeks gestation, most of the fetal weight is due to the gradual buildup of protein stores as the main cells and anatomical structures are developing. However, it is during this period that the differentiation and laying down of the 'scaffolding' of fat tissue begins in earnest, occurring in a definite order of development:

- At 14 weeks' gestation the fat pad of the cheeks begin to develop and can be identified.
- At 20 weeks' gestation the fat tissue in the neck and trunk can be identified.
- At 22 weeks' gestation the fat in the lower limbs develops.

By 25 weeks of gestation all the body tissues appear to have assembled ready to receive the fat droplets that aggregate into the fat store. From that time until term, fat within the body of the fetus, both subcutaneous and deep stores, increases from 30 to 430 g. Furthermore, fat packages much more energy than protein or carbohydrate per unit volume, therefore this represents a larger reserve of energy available to the fetus, ready for the critical time after birth (Tanner 1989, 1990).

SKIN COLOUR

Three pigments contribute to skin colour:

- melanin
- carotene
- haemoglobin.

Of these, only melanin is made in the skin.

MELANIN

Melanin, a peptide (a very short protein molecule), ranges in colour from yellow, reddish brown to black. Its synthesis depends upon an enzyme in melanocytes called *tyrosinase*, and it passes from melanocyte to basal keratinocytes. The number of melanocytes present in the skin is relatively the same in all races. Cultural differences in skin colour reflect the amount of pigment that the melanocytes produce and disperse. Melanocytes of black and brown-skinned people produce much more and darker melanin than those of fair-skinned individuals. An inherited inability to produce melanin results in *albinism*. In albinism, the pigment is absent in the skin, hair and eyes. An individual affected by albinism is referred to as an albino. Freckles and pigmented moles are localized accumulations of melanin.

Melanocytes are stimulated when the skin is exposed to sunlight. Prolonged sun exposure causes a substantial melanin buildup, which is a protective response of the skin to protect the deoxyribonucleic acid (DNA) of viable skin cells from ultraviolet radiation. However, despite the protective effects of melanin, excessive skin exposure eventually damages the skin.

Because the amount of melanin is low at birth, newborn infants are lighter skinned than they will be as older children. This also means that infants are more susceptible to the harmful effects of the sun.

CLINICAL NOTES   MONGOLIAN PIGMENTATION ('BLUE SPOTS')

This condition results in areas of increased melanin deposition over the lower back and sacrum of the infant; however, it may be more extensive in its presentation. Mongolian pigmentation presents in newborn infants born to parents with increased melanin in their skin, irrespective of racial background.

These 'blue spots' gradually lighten as the child grows, and the remaining skin increases in pigmentation. These may be mistaken for bruises.

CAROTENE

Carotene is a yellow-orange pigmentation found in certain plant foods, such as carrots. It tends to accumulate in the stratum corneum and in fatty tissue of the *hypodermis*. Its colour is most obvious in the palms of the hands and the soles of the feet, where the stratum corneum is at its thickest.

HAEMOGLOBIN

The pinkish hue of fair skin reflects the crimson colour of oxygenated haemoglobin red blood cells circulating through the dermal capillaries. As caucasian skin contains only small amounts of melanin, the epidermis is nearly transparent enabling the haemoglobin's colour to show through.

When haemoglobin is poorly oxygenated, both the blood and the skin of light-skinned children appear 'blue'. This condition is called *cyanosis* (cyan = dark). In darker-skinned children the skin does not appear cyanotic because of the masking effects of melanin, but cyanosis manifests clinically in the nailbeds and the mucous membranes.

GROWTH AND DEVELOPMENT OF HAIR

Hairs are specialized epidermal derivatives arising as the result of inductive stimuli from the epidermis. Hair begins to develop early in fetal development, at approximately 7–12 weeks gestation; however, they do not become apparent or recognizable until approximately 20 weeks. Hairs are first recognized on the eyebrows, upper lip and chin.

The development of the hair follicle commences with the proliferation of the stratum germinativum of the epidermis and extends down into the dermis. The hair bud forms and becomes club-shaped, forming the hair bulb.

The epithelial cells of the hair bulb constitute the *germinal matrix*, which eventually produces the hair. The hair bulb is invaginated by the *mesenchymal hair papilla*. The peripheral cells of the developing hair follicle form the *epithelial root sheath*. As cells in the germal matrix develop and proliferate they are pushed upwards towards the surface, where they eventually become keratinized to form the hair shaft.

Each hair is composed of columns of dead keratinized cells bound together by extracellular proteins. The *shaft* is the superficial portion of the hair, most of which projects from the surface of the skin. The root and shaft consist of three concentric layers:

- inner medulla
- middle cortex
- cuticle (outermost layer).

Small bundles of smooth muscle fibres—arrector pili muscles—differentiate from the mesenchyme surrounding the hair follicle, and attach to the dermal root shaft of the hair follicle and the papillary layer of the dermis. Surrounding each hair follicle are dendrites of neurones that collectively form the hair root plexus, which is sensitive to touch. The hair root plexuses generate nerve impulses if the shaft of the hair is moved.

Lanugo (lana-wool or down) is the first growth of hair to appear; these hairs are fine, soft and lightly pigmented. They begin to appear by week 12 of gestation and are abundant by 17–20 weeks. These fine hairs assist functionally by holding the vernix caseosa on the skin, but are mostly shed before term, with the exception of hair found on the scalp, eyebrows and eyelashes. Slightly thicker hairs replace these downy hairs after a few months of life. A new growth of short fine hairs occurs over the rest of the infant's body.

Genetic and hormonal influences determine hair thickness and the pattern of distribution. Although the skin is similar in structure over most of the body, there are several variations related to:

- thickness of the epidermis
- strength
- flexibility
- degree of keratinization
- distribution and types of hair
- types of gland
- pigmentation
- vascularity
- innervation.

TYPES AND GROWTH OF HAIR

Millions of hairs are scattered over nearly all of the body. Only the lips, nipples, parts of the external genitalia and the thickly skinned areas of the palms of the hands and the soles of the feet totally lack hair. There are approximately 100000 hairs present on the scalp. Hairs come in various sizes and shapes, but as a rule are classified as *vellus* or *terminal*.

The body hair of children and adult females is of the fine vellus (vel'us, *vell* = wool, fleece) variety, commonly referred to as 'peach fuzz' (Tortora & Grabowski 2003). The coarser, often longer, hair of the scalp and eyebrows is terminal hair; which is darker hair. At puberty, terminal hairs appear in the axilla and pubic regions of both sexes, and on the face and the chest (and typically the arms and legs) of males. Hair growth and density are influenced by many important factors including genetic, nutritional and hormonal influences. Poor nutrition often equates with poor hair growth. Alternatively, some conditions that increase the local dermal flow, for example chronic physical irritation or inflammation, may enhance local hair growth. The rate of hair growth varies from one body region to another, and in relation to sex and age. However, the average growth is approximately 2 mm per week. Each follicle goes through growth cycles, which includes an active growth phase and a resting phase. Hair growth is cyclical with alternate periods of growth (*anagen*) and rest (*telogen*). The anagen phase is generally longer than the telogen phase, and the lifespan of hair seems to vary. The follicles of the scalp remain active for years (in the order of approximately 4 years) before becoming inactive for a few months. In adulthood, on average, 90 to 100 hairs are lost daily.

At birth all hairs are normally in the anagen phase; subsequent regenerative activity lacks synchrony resulting in an overall random pattern of growth and shedding. During the first few months of life this disruption of hair loss and regrowth may manifest as an overgrowth of hair or as temporary alopecia—the partial or complete lack of hair. On average, boys' hair grows faster than girls' hair, and in both sexes scalp hair growth is slower at the crown.

FUNCTIONS OF THE HAIR

Hair has limited protective functions; however, hair on the scalp protects the scalp from the harmful effects of the sun and injury, and helps to limit heat loss from the scalp (Tortora & Grabowski 2003). Eyebrows and eyelashes offer some protection to the eyes from particles, as does the presence of hairs in the nostrils and the external ear. Hairs also have a function in relation to touch. This relates to the touch receptors associated with the hair follicles (hair root plexus), which are activated when a hair is moved or even lightly touched.

DEVELOPMENT OF THE NAILS

Nails are plates of tightly packed, hard, keratinized epidermal cells. They consist of a nail body, free edge and a nail root. The

Fig. 2.5
Development of the nail.

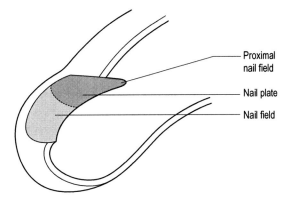

- Proximal nail field
- Nail plate
- Nail field

nail body is the part of the nail that is visible and appears pink due to the blood flow through the underlying capillaries. The *free edge* is the part of the nail that may extend past the distal end of the digit and appears white because of the absence of underlying capillaries. The *nail root* is the part of the nail that is buried in a fold of skin.

The *nail fields* of both the fingers and toes first appear at 10 weeks gestation as ectodermal thickenings on the tips of each digit. Later the nail fields migrate on to the dorsal surface, carrying their innervation from the ventral (flexor) surface. As the nail fields reach their dorsal position, the epidermis surrounding them folds on both sides and proximately. The nail plate, and future nail, appear as cells from the proximal nail fold, grow over the nail field and become keratinized to form the nail plate (Fig. 2.5). Initially the developing nail is covered by a superficial layer of epidermis, the *eponchium*. This later degenerates to expose the nail, except at its base where it persists to the cuticle.

Development of the fingernails precedes the toenails by an interval of 4 weeks. The fingernails reach the fingertips by 32 weeks gestation, and the toenails reach the toetips by 36 weeks gestation. In both cases the nails reach the tips of the digits by birth. If the nails have not reached the tips of the digits at birth, this is an indicator of prematurity.

FUNCTIONS OF THE NAILS

Nails offer protection against trauma to the ends of the digits, provide a means of 'scratching' parts of the body, and help to grasp and manipulate small objects (Tortora & Grabowski 2003).

SELF ASSESSMENT

Answer the following in relation to your area of professional practice:

- Write short notes on the normal embryological and fetal development of the integumentary system.
- Outline key features of normal growth, development and maturation of the integumentary system.
- Describe the major functions of the skin.
- Discuss the primary functions of hair and nails.
- Explain the structure, function and classifications of body fat.
- List six common conditions that may affect the integumentary system in childhood.

References

Candy D, Davies G, Ross E 2001 Clinical paediatrics and child health. W B Saunders, London

Crawford D, Morris M 1995 Neonatal nursing. Chapman and Hall, London

Department of Health 1994 Weaning and the weaning diet: report of the Weaning Group on the Weaning Diet, of the Committee on Medical Aspects of Food Policy (COMA). HMSO, London

Huband S, Trigg E 2002 Practices in children's nursing: guidelines for hospital and community. Churchill Livingstone, London

Lissauer T, Clayden G 2001 Illustrated textbook of paediatrics, 2nd edn. Mosby, London

MacGregor J 2000 Introduction to the anatomy and physiology of children. Routledge, London

Moore K L, Persaud T V N 1998 Before we are born: essentials of embryology and birth defects. W B Saunders, London

Sinclair D, Dangerfield P 1998 Human growth after birth, 6th edn. Oxford University Press, Oxford

Tanner J M 1989 Foetus into man: physical growth from conception to maturity, 2nd edn. Castlemead Publications, Hertford

Tanner J M 1990 Foetus into man: physical growth from conception to maturity, 2nd edn. Harvard University Press, Cambridge, MA

Tortora G J, Grabowski S R 2003 Principles of anatomy and physiology, 10th edn. John Wiley, New York

Waterlow J 1997 Pressure sore risk assessment in children. Paediatric Nursing 9(6):21–24

Waugh A, Grant A 2001 Ross and Wilson anatomy and physiology in health and illness, 9th edn. Churchill Livingstone, London

Wong D L 1999 Whaley and Wong's nursing care of children, 6th edn. Mosby, London

Zancanaro C, Merigo F, Crecimanno S, Osculati A, Osculati O 1999 Immunohistochemical evidence suggests intrinsic regulatory activity of human eccrine sweat glands. Journal of Anatomy 194:433–444

Bibliography

Bee H, Boyd D 2004 The developing child, 10th edn. Allyn and Bacon, Boston

Crawford D, Hickinson W 2002 An introduction to neonatal nursing, 2nd edn. Nelson Thornes, Cheltenham

Lissaur T, Clayden G 2001 Illustrated textbook of paediatrics, 2nd edn. Mosby, London

MacGregor J 2000 Introduction to the anatomy and physiology of children. Routledge, London

Matsumura G, England M A 1992 Embryology colouring book. Wolfe, London

Slater A, Lewis M 2002 Inroduction to infant development. Oxford University Press, Oxford

Tortora G J, Anagnostakos N P 1990 Principles of anatomy and physiology, 6th edn. HarperCollins, New York

Tortora G J, Grabowski S R 2003 Principles of anatomy and physiology, 10th edn. John Wiley, New York

Chapter 3

The musculoskeletal system

Carol A. Chamley

CHAPTER OUTCOMES

This chapter will enable the reader to:

- Discuss the normal embryological and fetal development of the musculoskeletal system, subsequent development and maturation
- Explain the anatomical differences between the axial and the appendicular skeleton
- Explore the anatomical relationships between the skull, sutures and fontanelles, explaining their structure and function during early development, and their subsequent maturation
- List the primary functions of the musculoskeletal system
- Describe the major hormonal influences on the developing skeleton.

CHAPTER OVERVIEW

The aim of this chapter is to explore the normal embryological and fetal development of the musculoskeletal system, describing the formation, structure and function of the skeleton, muscles, joints, tendons and ligaments.

The chapter discusses the major components of the musculoskeletal system, explaining the normal embryological and fetal anatomy and physiology. This includes development of bone and cartilage, centres of ossification, and the significance of the growth plates during childhood and maturity; the anatomical divisions of the skeleton, notably the axial skeleton, the appendicular skeleton with special attention to the development of the fetal and newborn skull, the structure and function of the sutures and fontanelles, and their significance in early development; the concomitant development of muscles, joints and attachments; and the contributions of hormones and calcium to the growth and development of a healthy skeleton.

Clinical Notes address issues of clinical relevance and potential interest to the reader, and Self Assessment exercises assist in reflecting upon the chapter and guiding the relationship between theory and practice.

INTRODUCTION

The musculoskeletal system is composed of several key structures, and each component of the system is essential for the mobility and movement associated with survival. The skeleton, or bony framework of the body, provides support and attachments for muscles, tendons and ligaments. The various bones of the body are connected together at different parts of their surfaces by articulations or joints. All movements that change the position of bony parts of the body occur at the joints. Although bones and joints provide leverage, they are not capable of moving the body themselves. Muscles are attached to bones by tendons and ligaments, which are strong fibrous bands. Motion is an essential function of the human body that results from the contraction and relaxation of muscles, and sensory and motor fibres from the central nervous system innervate muscles.

Skeletal age, or bone age appears to correlate more closely with other measures of physiologic maturity than chronological age or height. Furthermore, there are a number of developmental and medical reasons why it might be important to assess the maturity of the child. The most important of these measures is the assessment of bone that is also referred to as 'skeletal', 'anatomical' or 'radiological' age (Sinclair and Dangerfield 1998). During growth and development every bone undergoes a series of changes that can be observed radiologically. It is the timing and appearance of primary and secondary ossification centres that can be observed most notably because the calcium content of the ossification centres renders them radio-opaque. The wrist and the hand are the most commonly used sites as this region has a large number of ossification centres and is easily accessible with minimum risks to the child. However, carpal bones are not visible under two years of age and fusion generally occurs one or two years eariler in females than males (MacGregor 2000).

THE SKELETON

The total skeletal bone mass increases to a maximum in the third decade of life, after which time there is gradual diminution. Furthermore, because the skeleton is so accessible to investigation, more is known about the growth and development of the human skeleton than any other human tissue.

The adult human skeleton (*skeletos* = dried up) consists of 206 bones, most of which are paired on the right and left side of the body. However, infants and children are born with more than 300 bones, which are composed primarily of cartilage (Fig. 3.1). During childhood and

Fig. 3.1
Child's skeleton.

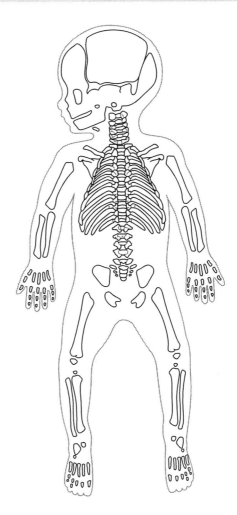

throughout the process of normal growth, development and maturation, certain parts of the skeleton begin to join together, or fuse, to form single bones, resulting in the composition and architecture of the normal adult skeleton with 206 bones. Bone is a strong and durable type of connective tissue consisting of:

- organic constituents including osteoid and bone cells (25%)
- inorganic constituents, mainly calcium phosphate (50%).

Bones are grouped into two principal divisions:

- axial skeleton
- appendicular skeleton (*appendic* = to hang on to).

The skeleton of a human embryo is composed of fibrous membranes and hyaline cartilage. The process by which bone is formed is referred to as *ossification* (*ossi* = bone; *-fication* = making), or *osteogenesis*.

Embryonic tissues provide the template for ossification that begins during week 6 or 7 of embryonic life and continues throughout adult life. Two types of bone formation occur. The first is *intramembranous* (*intra* = within) ossification, which is bone formation on or within loose fibrous connective tissue. The second type is *endochondral* (*endo* = within; *chondro* = cartilage) ossification, in which bone forms within the hyaline cartilage.

BONE FORMATION

Bone, or osseous tissue, contains a great deal of intercellular substance surrounding widely separated cells. Four types of cell are characteristic of bone tissue:

1. *Osteoprogenitor* (*osteo* = bone; *pro* = precursor; *gen* = produce)
2. *Osteoblast* (*blast* = germ or bud)
3. *Osteocyte* (*cyte* = cell)
4. *Osteoclast* (*clast* = break).

BONE DEVELOPMENT

INTRAMEMBRANOUS BONE FORMATION

During week 4 of gestation, embryonic connective tissue in the region of the future skeleton shows signs of differentiation (MacGregor 2000). Bones develop via two biological mechanisms: through either intramembranous or cartilaginous formation from mesenchymal cells, which form a template of future bone.

Intramembranous bone formation involves the mesenchymal cells becoming condensed and highly vascular; some of these cells develop into bone-forming cells, or osteoblasts. These cells deposit matrix or intercellular substances, notably osteoid tissue—the bone precursor, or pre-bone (Fig. 3.2). As this osteoid tissue is organized into bone, calcium and phosphate are deposited.

Fig. 3.2
Bone formation.

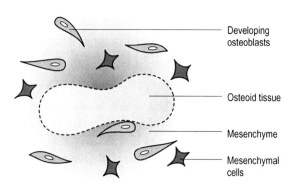

Developing osteoblasts

Osteoid tissue

Mesenchyme

Mesenchymal cells

As bone continues to form, osteoblasts become trapped and are then known as osteocytes. As the bony tissue continues to develop, a calcified matrix forms in the centre of each uncalcified matrix. Some of the osteoblasts continue to lay down new matrix around the perimeter of each 'island' of matrix. Initially new bone has no organized pattern, but spicules of bone eventually organize and coalesce into layers known as lamellae. Concentric lamellae develop around blood vessels, forming an osteon or haversian system.

Some of the osteoblasts remain at the periphery of the newly developing bone and eventually form 'plates' of compact (dense) bone, while the rest remains as 'spongy' bone. In the interstices of spongy bone the mesenchyme differentiates in the bone marrow.

During fetal development and postnatal life there is a continuous remodelling of bone that results from the simultaneous action of osteoclasts and osteoblasts.

CARTILAGE AND INTRACARTILAGE BONE FORMATION

Cartilage develops from the mesenchyme and first appears during week 5 of gestation. In some of the anatomical areas where cartilage is later to develop, the mesenchyme condenses to form chondrification centres. Cartilage-forming cells (chondroblasts) secrete collagenous fibrils and a 'ground' substance of matrix. Subsequently collagenous and/or elastic fibres are deposited in the matrix. There are three types of cartilage:

- hyaline articular cartilage
- fibrocartilage
- elastic cartilage.

Cartilage is composed of approximately 70% water, and the residual tissue is an aggregate of sulfate polysaccharides and collagen.

The periosteum of the bone, which is the membrane that covers bone consisting of connective tissue, osteogenic cells and osteoblasts, is essential for bone nutrition, growth and repair. This develops from the perichondrium, which is a thin layer of bone deposited under this layer. As the cartilage cells in the diaphysis enlarge, the matrix calcifies and the cells die.

By penetrating the periosteum, arteries invade the diaphysis and also break down the arrangement of the cartilage cells into spicules. Furthermore, some of the vascular connective tissue differentiates into the bone marrow.

Ossification continues towards the ends of the bones, known as the epiphysis, which is usually larger in diameter than the diaphysis (Tortora & Grabowski 2003). Therefore, lengthening of bone occurs at the diaphysio-epiphyseal junction (Matsumura & England 1992). Cartilage cells near to the diaphysis divide and enlarge, the matrix calcifies and is broken into spicules by the invading vascular tissue, and then bone cells are deposited on the spicules. Only two areas of a long bone remain cartilaginous: the articular cartilage and the epiphyseal plate cartilage that separates the diaphysis and the epiphysis.

The diameter of the bone is increased by the deposition of bone cells at the periosteal surface and reabsorption at the medullary surface of the bone.

DEVELOPMENT OF THE AXIAL SKELETON

The axial skeleton comprises:

- ribs
- sternum
- vertebral column
- skull.

During development of the axial skeleton, cells in the sclerotomes are rearranged. During week 4 of gestation, the sclerotomes surround the neural tube, that is the primordium of the spinal cord and the notochord (*noto* = the back; *chord* = a string), form the primordium of the vertebrae.

The positional change of the sclerotomal cells is effected by differential growth of surrounding structures and not by the active migration of sclerotomal cells (Moore & Persaud 1998).

DEVELOPMENT OF THE RIBS

The ribs develop from mesenchymal costal processes of the thoracic vertebrae. The ribs become cartilaginous during the embryonic period and ossify late in fetal life (Sinclair & Dangerfield 1998, Tortora & Grabowski 2003). The costovertebral joints replace the original site of union of the costal (*costa* = rib) processes with the vertebra. Twelve pairs of ribs develop, although there is some variation in structure.

A typical rib (ribs 3–9) comprises:

- head
- facets (two)
- interarticular crest
- neck
- tubercle
- body (shaft).

Seven pairs of ribs (true ribs) attach to the sternum through their own cartilage. Five pairs of ribs are referred to as 'false ribs' because their costal cartilage does not attach directly to the sternum. Two pairs of ribs (floating ribs) do not attach to the sternum.

The spaces in between the ribs are referred to as intercostal spaces, occupied by intercostal muscles, blood vessels and nerves.

In infancy, the cross-section of the barrel-shaped chest is seen as virtually circular in shape, and remains this shape for the first 2 years of life, with the ribs in a more or less horizontal position. Therefore, it is impossible for the infant to increase chest diameter by movement of the ribs. This means that the infant has to rely upon virtually complete diaphragmatic breathing, and, because the rib cage and sternum are anatomically located higher than in the adult, the abdominal cavity and contents are less well protected.

Secondary centres of ossification occur in the head of all ribs; however, all but the last two pairs fuse at approximately 25 years of age.

DEVELOPMENT OF THE STERNUM

The sternum, or breast bone (plate), begins development when a pair of mesenchymal vertical bands (sternal bars) develop ventrolaterally in the fetal body wall; chondrification occurs in these bars as they migrate medially. Furthermore, the bars fuse craniocaudally in the median plane to form cartilaginous models of the component parts of the sternum, namely:

- manubrium
- sternebrae
- xiphoid process—the smallest part of the sternum.

During infancy and childhood the xiphoid process consists of hyaline cartilage and does not ossify until approximately 40 years of age. The manubrium does not ossify until old age, when the sternum becomes a rigid structure and can potentially interfere with respiration.

DEVELOPMENT OF THE VERTEBRAL COLUMN

The vertebral column, spine or back bone is composed of a series of structures referred to as vertebrae. During childhood there are in the order of 33 vertebrae; however, in adulthood the sacral and coccygeal bones fuse together, so that the typical adult spine contains 26 bones.

During the fourth week of embryological development the sclerotomes appear as paired *condensations*. The sclerotome portion of each somite migrates into three general anatomical regions of the embryo. One group migrates into the fetal body wall, a second group migrates around the neural tube, and the third group migrates around the notochord (Fig. 3.3A).

The notochord eventually degenerates and disappears where it is surrounded by developing vertebral bodies (Fig. 3.3B). Within the embryonic vertebral discs the notochord expands to form the *nucleus pulposus* (*pulposus* = pulp-like), which becomes highly elastic and forms

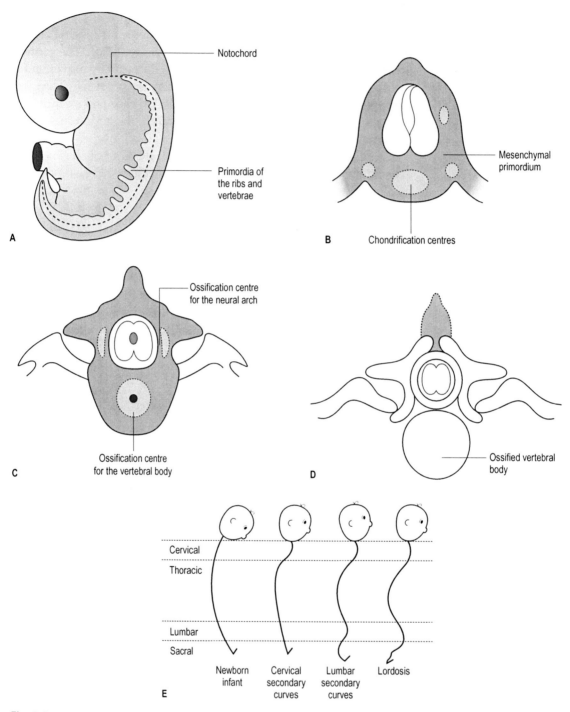

Fig. 3.3
A Development of the vertebral column.
B Primordia of the vertebrae.
C Ossification centres.
D Vertebra at term.
E Normal curvatures of the spine during childhood.

the soft and pulpy inner substance of the disc. The nucleus is later surrounded by fibres that form the *annulus fibrosus* (*annulus* = ring-like), an outer fibrous ring that, together with the nucleus pulposus, forms the intervertebral disc. Each vertebra is formed from two different sclerotome cells. The individual vertebrae increase in thickness by the deposition of bone in cartilage, and the presence of the *annular epiphysis* during childhood facilitates the increase in length of the body during the growth spurt in adolescence.

Ossification of a typical vertebra begins during the embryonic period and is evident in the vertebral arches during week 8 of gestation (Fig. 3.3C). The bony halves of the vertebral arch usually fuse between 3 and 5 years of age.

The intersegmental arteries become the intercostal arteries, located either side of the vertebral body, and the spinal nerves emerge between the mesenchymal vertebrae.

CLINICAL NOTES   **TUMOURS FROM THE NOTOCHORD**

Both benign and malignant tumours may arise from the notochord. Remnants of the notochord may persist and give rise to a chordoma. Approximately one-third of these are slow-growing malignant tumours developing at the base of the skull and infiltrating into the nasopharynx. They have the potential to infiltrate bone and become difficult to remove.

It is the growth of several elements of the vertebral column that determines overall adult height. The lumbar spine and sacrum are relatively small at birth compared to the thoracic and cervical vertebrae, which have to grow the most in order to attain their adult size (Fig. 3.3D).

The *intervertebral discs* account for one-quarter to one-third of the overall length of the vertebral column and therefore make a major contribution to the height of the individual. These are dynamic structures; changes in their fluid content occur between lying and standing (Sinclair & Dangerfield 1998), and account for diurnal alterations in height.

Accordingly, radiological investigations of the vertebral column have illustrated that the discs below the eighth thoracic vertebra do not increase significantly in vertebral diameter between the ages of 6 and 8 years, apart from an initial growth spurt at birth. However, the thickness of the disc below the fourth vertebra increases steadily up to the age of 2 years and follows a steady pattern of growth after this time (Sinclair & Dangerfield 1998).

NORMAL CURVES OF THE VERTEBRAL COLUMN

The prenatal posture is one of complete flexion as the fetus is confined within the uterus. The spine curves, with the head and the extremities bent in upon the fetus. The bones in the vertebral column of the newborn infant form two primary curves, one in the thoracic region and the other in the sacral region. Both of these curves are described as concave (forward) curvatures. The thoracic curve is stable, and movement is limited by thin intervertebral discs and oblique spinal processes (Whaley & Wong 1991).

As the infant gains head control, secondary curves appear in the cervical region of the spine. The cervical region is convex, and flexibility of the spine is afforded by thick intervertebral discs and the tension offered by the large muscles across the area.

As the infant develops and is able to sustain the sitting position, a further secondary curve appears in the lumbar region, which is convex and mobile. As the child acquires mobility and assumes the bipedal upright position, the weight of a large liver and a higher centre of gravity is compensated for by an exaggerated lordosis (Fig. 3.3E).

DEVELOPMENT OF THE SKULL

The fetal skull is ovoid or egg-shaped, and correlates to the shape of the developing brain. The shape of the fetal skull differs from that of an older child or adult because of the large size of the vault in relation to the face (Fig. 3.4).

Fig. 3.4
Fetal skull.

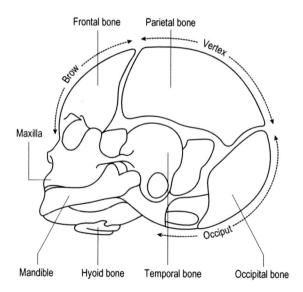

The skull is supported on the summit of the vertebral column and is composed of two sets of bones, cranial (*crani* = brain case) and *facial* bones, which are collectively described as flat bones. The cranium is composed of the two frontal bones, two parietal bones, two temporal bones, occipital bone, sphenoid and ethmoid bones. Facial bones form the face, and include two maxillae, two zygomatic bones, the mandible, two lacrimal bones, two palatine bones, two inferior nasal conchae and the vomer. The skull also forms several smaller cavities, including the nasal cavity and the eye sockets (orbits). The skull develops from embryonic mesenchyme and is divided into two major anatomical regions:

- *neurocranium*—a case to protect the brain
- *viscerocranium*—gives rise to the origins of the skeleton of the face.

Each of these regions has some membranous and some cartilaginous bones; the vault of the skull is membranous whereas the face and base of the skull are cartilaginous.

CARTILAGINOUS NEUROCRANIUM (CHONDROCRANIUM)

This consists of the cartilaginous base of the skull that develops by fusion of several cartilages. Endochondral ossification of the neurocranium forms the base of the skull.

The *parachordal cartilage* (basal plate) forms around the cranial end of the notochord, fusing with cartilage that originates from the sclerotome regions of the occipital somites. This mass of cartilage contributes to the base of the occipital bone, and *hypophyseal cartilage* forms around the developing pituitary gland.

MEMBRANOUS NEUROCRANIUM (CALVARIA)

The cranial vault develops when intramembranous ossification occurs in the mesenchyme at the sides and top of the brain. During intrauterine life the flat bones of the calvaria are separated by dense connective tissue membranes that form sutures.

SUTURES

The bones of the cranium are connected together by sutures (seam); these include:

- sagittal suture (interparietal)
- coronal suture (frontoparietal)
- lambdoidal suture (occipitoparietal)
- frontal suture.

The articulating surfaces, or edges, of the bones are roughened or uneven and are closely connected to one another with a small amount of fibrous tissue; the sutural ligament fastens them together. The edges of the bones are covered by a layer of osteoblasts and osteoclasts, and the growth of the skull takes place at the sutures. In the first instance growth is very rapid, but evens out to a steadier pace; as the bones grow in a lateral direction, additional bone is deposited on the outer surface of the vault by the process of apposition from the periosteum. At the same time, osteoblasts remove bone from inside the vault to ensure that the brain cavity grows in line with the marrow cavity of the bone. As the vault continues to grow a process of remodelling converts the original single layer of bone into a double layer of compact bone with a spongy layer in between. Soft areas (*craniotabes*) are sometimes found in the parietal bones near to the sagittal suture; however, they are usually of no particular consequence.

During the first few years of life the sutures of the vault interlock and form jagged serrated lines (Sinclair & Dangerfield 1998); later in life the sutures become obliterated by extension of ossification into the sutural joints, and eventually the individual bones of the skull become fused to one another. This begins at approximately 25–30 years of age on the inner surface of the skull, but does not manifest on the outer surface for some 10 years later. There is great variation in the time at which the sutures close. The frontal suture closes at approximately 8 years of age; however, partial obliteration of the sagittal suture occurs at about age 30 years, that of the coronal suture occurs at approximately 40 years, and that of the lamboidal suture at approximately 50 years.

| CLINICAL NOTES | CRANIOSYNOSTOSIS |

The premature closure of the skull sutures (craniosynostosis) gives rise to several deformities of the skull; the most severe result from premature prenatal closure. The aetiology is unclear, but genetic factors probably make a significant contribution. The abnormalities are more common in males than in females, and may be associated with other defects.

The type of deformity produced depends upon which of the cranial sutures close prematurely:

- *Scaphocephaly* is a long wedge-shaped skull produced as a result of the early closure of the sagittal suture and constitutes approximately half of the cases of craniosynostosis.
- *Oxycephaly* (turricephaly) produces a high tower-like skull resulting from the premature closure of the coronal suture, and constitutes 30% of cases.
- *Plagiocephaly* produces an asymmetrical twisted-shaped skull due to closure of the coronal or lambdoidal sutures on the left side of the skull (Moore & Persaud 1998, Wong 1999).

FONTANELLES

Before birth the bones of the skull are separated from one another by a membrane of connective tissue known as pulsating fontanelles (little

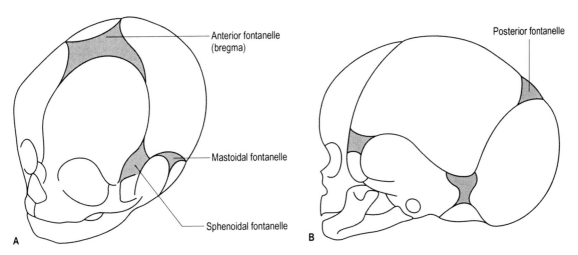

Fig. 3.5
A Fontanelles: anterior, mastoidal and sphenoid.
B Posterior fontanelle.

fountains) or 'soft spots', found mainly at the four angles of the parietal bones. The fontanelles include:

- The *anterior fontanelle* (or bregma). This is the largest fontanelle, located at the midline between the two parietal bones and the frontal bones (Fig. 3.5A). It is described as diamond or kite shaped with the longer tail pointing towards the face, which, if palpated on vaginal examination during labour, enables the position of the occiput at the opposite side to be identified. The anterior fontanelle tends to increase naturally in size during the first few months of life, and closes at approximately 18–24 months of life.

- The *posterior fontanelle*. This is located in the midline between the two parietal bones and the occipital bone (Fig. 3.5B). It is triangular in shape and generally smaller than the anterior fontanelle, closing approximately 2 months after birth.

- The *anterolateral fontanelles*. These are paired fontanelles situated laterally between the frontal, parietal and sphenoid bones. They are small in size and irregular in shape, closing about 3 months after birth.

THE NEWBORN SKULL

The skull of the newborn infant undergoes moulding during labour and vaginal delivery. It is round and the bones are thin, and the size of the skull is large in proportion to the rest of the skeleton. However, the face is small compared to the calvaria owing to:

- underdevelopment of the facial bones at birth
- virtual absence or rudimentary presence of the paranasal sinuses
- underdeveloped jaws.

In the normal newborn infant, the cranial sutures are separated by membranous seams several millimetres wide. For the first few hours until a couple of days after birth, the cranial bones are highly mobile, allowing the bones to mould and slide over one another. This also facilitates the cranial bones to accommodate the changing shape and character of the birth canal during vaginal delivery (Wong 1999).

POSTNATAL GROWTH OF THE SKULL

The presence of the sutures in the skull during childhood facilitates the growth of the brain, although the increase in the size of the skull is greatest during the first 2 years of life. As growth continues, the contours of the cranial vault change. After birth, growth of the skull occurs in a direction perpendicular to the line of the suture. The base of the skull and the face do not grow at the same rate as the vault of the skull and the orbit. The growth of the vault and orbit are more closely related to the growth and development of the nervous system, but the rest of the face and the base of the skull are more closely aligned to the growth of the muscles of mastication and the eruption of the teeth.

As teeth appear, the upper jaw increases in size by surface apposition; therefore, bone is removed from the inner aspects of the jaw to keep the proportions constant, and the bones of the face are evacuated by osteoblasts to form air sinuses that lighten the front of the skull. The mandible is very small at birth, consisting of two separate halves that fuse during the first year of life. Subsequently the main growth of the mandible relates to length. Furthermore, in preparation for the eruption of teeth, bone is absorbed from bone in the front of the ramus, altering the angle of the mandible from approximately 140° in the infant to 120° in the adult jaw.

The skull increases in capacity until approximately 16 years of age; after this the skull increases only slightly in size, mainly due to thickening of the bones. Rapid growth of the face coincides with dental eruption; however, these changes become more evident after the eruption of the permanent teeth. The changing shape of the face is also attributed to the enlargement of the frontal and facial regions, which is associated with the increase in size of the paranasal sinuses. The growth and development of the sinuses are not only important in altering the shape of the face, as they also contribute to adding resonance to the voice (Moore & Persaud 1998).

Vioarsdottir et al (2002) suggest that anatomically modern humans show considerable geographical variations in the form of the facial skeleton. During growth and development the facial skeleton changes dramatically in shape and size, but remains a functional unit throughout the course of its development. These authors conclude that population-specific facial morphologies develop principally through distinctions in facial shape that are probably already present at birth, and are further accentuated and modified to variable degrees during normal growth and development.

CLINICAL NOTES   **MICROCEPHALY AND ACRANIA**

Failure of the calvaria to grow and develop may manifest in several types of pathology.

Microcephaly
Infants born with this condition are born with a normally sized or slightly small calvaria. The fontanelles close during early infancy and the sutures close during the first year; however, the pathology is not attributed to the premature closure of the sutures.
Microcephaly is caused by the abnormal development of the central nervous system in which the brain and the skull fail to grow.

Acrania
In this condition the calvaria is absent and there may be extensive defects of the vertebral column. Acrania associated with meroanencephaly or anencephaly is incompatible with life.

DEVELOPMENT OF THE APPENDICULAR SKELETON

The appendicular (*appendic* = hang on to) skeleton consists of the bones that make up the upper and lower limbs, as well as the bones referred to as girdles that attach the limbs to the axial skeleton. The principal bones of the appendicular skeleton are:

- pectoral (shoulder) girdle
- pelvic (hip) girdle
- upper and lower limbs.

The pectoral or shoulder girdle attaches the bones of the upper extremities to the axial skeleton. These bones include:

- clavicles (collar bones)
- scapulae (shoulder blades)
- upper extremities
- humerus
- radius and ulna
- carpals, metacarpals and phalanges.

The pelvic (*pelv* = basin) girdle consists of two hip bones also referred to as coxal (*cox* = hip) bones. In the newborn, each of the two halves of the hip bone consists of three separate bones separated by cartilage that eventually fuse together. The principal bones of the pelvic girdle include:

- pelvic girdle (hip bones)
- ilium (flank)
- ischium (hip)
- pubis.

EMBRYOLOGY AND FETAL DEVELOPMENT OF THE APPENDICULAR SKELETON

The pectoral girdle and the arms appear before the pelvic girdle and the legs. During week 5 of gestation, mesenchymal bones form as condensations of mesenchyme in the limb buds.

The clavicle develops initially by a process of intramembranous ossification, later forming growth cartilages at both ends of the developing bone. Furthermore, the clavicle is the first bone in the appendicular skeleton to ossify during week 6 of embryological development. Ossification begins in the long bones by week 8 of gestation, and by 12 weeks of fetal development ossification centres have appeared in all the bones of the limbs (Fig. 3.6A). The centres develop towards the middle of the bone, referred to as the *diaphysis*. Early indication of ossification in the cartilaginous models of the long bones is visible near the centre of the future shaft. However, primary centres appear at different times in different bones, although most centres are apparent between weeks 7 and 12 (Matsumura & England 1992).

Within the lower limbs, the centres of bones at the knee are first to appear. The centres for the distal end of the femur and the proximal end of the tibia appear in weeks 34–38, and are usually present at birth. However, most secondary centres of ossification appear at birth, and the part of the bone ossified from this centre is known as the *epiphysis*.

FORMATION AND ROTATION OF THE LIMBS

Upper limb buds first appear during week 4 (day 26 or 27) of embryological development, and lower limb buds appear 1–2 days later. They appear as small elevations of the ventrolateral wall of the embryo (Fig. 3.6B). Each limb bud consists of a mass of mesenchyme covered by ectoderm; the mesenchyme is derived from the somatic layer of the lateral mesoderm.

The upper limb buds are located opposite spinal levels C5 to T1 (caudal cervical segment), and the lower limb buds are located opposite

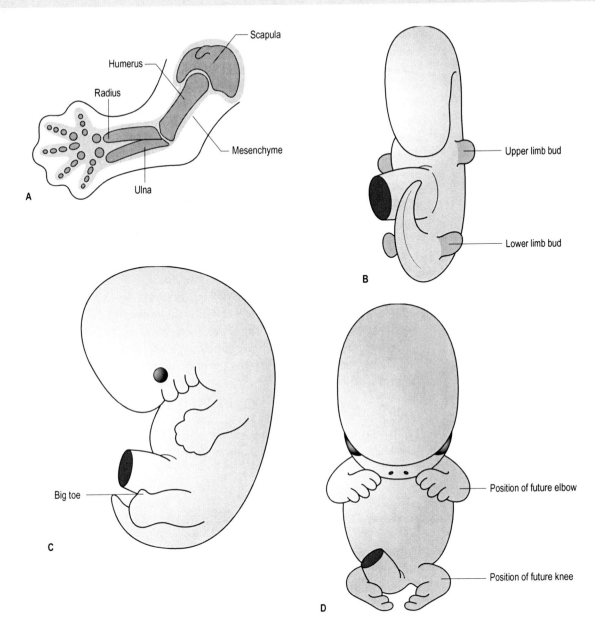

Fig. 3.6
A Development of the upper limb.
B Upper and lower limb buds.
C The normal anatomical position of the limbs, relative to the trunk.
D Hands resting on the thoracic region of the embryo.

L2 to S3 (lumbar sacral segment) by day 28 of gestation. However, during weeks 6 to 8 the limbs descend to their normal anatomical positions relative to the trunk (Fig. 3.6C).

Initially the limbs appear low on the trunk due to early development of the cranial half of the embryo, which has a more highly oxygenated blood supply.

The early stages of limb development are alike for both the upper and lower limbs, with the limb buds elongating by proliferation of the mesenchyme within them. The *apical ectodermal ridge* forms at the apex of each limb bud, and interaction between the mesenchyme and the apical ectodermal ridge is essential for normal limb development. There are also distinct differences between the development of the hands and feet, because of the physical differences between them in form and function.

Early in week 7, the limbs extend ventrally and the developing upper and lower limbs rotate in opposite directions and at different degrees. The upper limbs rotate laterally through 90° on their longitudinal axis. Thus the future elbows point dorsally and the extensor muscles lie on the lateral and posterior aspects of the limb (Moore & Persaud 1998), so that the hands come to rest on the thoracic region of the embryo (Fig. 3.6D).

The lower limbs rotate medially through almost 90°; the future knees face ventrally and the extensor muscles lie on the anterior aspect of the lower limbs. Synovial joints appear during weeks 8–9, which coincides with the functional differentiation of limb muscles and their innervation.

CLINICAL NOTES   ABNORMALITIES OF THE LIMBS

Abnormalities of the limbs occur at different stages of development. Suppression of limb bud development during the early part of week 4 results in *amelia*, which relates to the complete absence of a limb or limbs.

Disturbance or arrest of differentiation or growth of the limbs results in various types of *meromelia* (*meros* = part; *melos* = extremity), relating to partial absence of a limb or limbs. Absence of the long bones of a limb is referred to as *phocomelia*, but there may be a rudimentary or well developed hand or foot arising from the shoulder or hip respectively.

The classical examples of these abnormalities relate to the fetal anomalies caused by the drug thalidomide.

INNERVATION OF THE LIMBS

Motor axons arising from the developing spinal cord enter the limb buds in week 5 of gestation. The ventral rami of spinal nerves C5 to T1 invade the upper limbs, and L2 to S3 invade the lower limbs.

As the limbs elongate, the cutaneous distribution of spinal nerves migrates along the surface of the distal part of the limb. However, as the limbs grow and rotate, the dermatomes adjust to form the adult pattern of innervation.

When the limbs descend, they carry with them their nerves; this would explain the oblique course of nerves arising from the brachial and lumbosacral plexuses.

BLOOD SUPPLY TO THE LIMBS

The limb buds are supplied by branches of the intersegmental arteries. The primitive vascular system consists of a *primary axial artery* and its branches; however, the vascular pattern changes as the limbs develop, mainly by new blood vessels developing from existing vessels that eventually converge.

The primary axial artery forms the brachial artery in the arm and the common interosseous artery in the forearm. In the leg, the primary axial artery is represented by the profunda femoris artery in the thigh and by the anterior and posterior tibial arteries in the calf.

CLINICAL NOTES | **CONGENITAL LIMB MALFORMATIONS**

Congenital limb formations occur in 1:500 to 1:1000 live births, and include both gross reduction defects and more subtle alterations in the number, length and anatomy of digits. Formation of the limbs was a relatively late refinement of vertebrate development and it is therefore not surprising that many mutations that cause limb anomalies may also affect the development of other systems, referred to as pleiotrophy.

Congenital talipes equinovarus, often referred to as 'club foot', is a common but little studied developmental disorder of the lower limb. There is some evidence to suggest a genetic contribution to the condition, but its incidence varies with ethnic group, with a familial tendency in some cases. The only firm evidence is that the mildest form is associated with intrauterine posture (Miedzybrodzka 2003). Club foot is defined as fixation of the foot in adduction, supination and in varus; that is, the foot is inclined inwards, axially rotated outwards and pointing inwards (Miedzybrodzka 2003).

Furthermore, Meidzybrodzka (2003) describes congenital equinovarus as 'syndromic' when it occurs in association with other features as part of a genetic syndrome. Syndromic talipes may arise in association with many neurological and neuromuscular disorders, for example spina bifida or spinal atrophy. Equally, this condition can occur in isolation and is termed 'idiopathic'; this type of talipes is by far the commonest.

Club foot was depicted in Egyptian hieroglyphs and was described in around 400 BC by Hippocrates, who advised treatment with manipulation and bandages, claiming that the foot should be manipulated as if holding a wax model, not by force but gently. Modern treatment still uses manipulation, but the most effective method is the 'Ponseti' method, which can substantially reduce the need for surgery (Miedzybrodzka 2003).

DEVELOPMENT OF THE DIGITS

During week 6 of gestation, mesenchymal tissue in the hand plates condenses to form the outline and pattern of the digital rays. Subsequently, during week 7, similar condensations form rays in the foot plates.

The development of the digits is programmed by the mesenchyme developing into the mesenchymal primordia of the phalanges. The gaps between the digital rays are occupied by loose mesenchyme, which eventually breaks down. Interdigital cell death is an important element in digit morphogenesis, and helps to sculp the autopod by freeing the digit (Cecconi et al 1998, Linsden et al 2000). Separate digits are produced by the end of week 8 of gestation; however, the mechanisms involved in establishing digital and interdigital areas, thus anatomically spacing the digits, are not fully understood.

According to Sanz-Ezquerro & Tickle (2003), digital rays begin as continuous rods of cartilage that elongate to form interphalangeal joints, thus generating the precise number of phalanges. Both digit number and digit identity are controlled by signals from the polarizing region, a small group of mesenchymal cells at the posterior margin of the limb bud. However, development of the digital rays is relatively elastic and can lead to gains and losses in the number of digital phalanges.

CLINICAL NOTES	CLEFT HAND AND CLEFT FOOT

These are described as rare 'lobster-claw' deformities, in which one or more of the central digits are missing as a result of failure in the development of one or more of the digital rays. Typically, the hand or the foot is divided into two parts that oppose each other, like pincers or claws. The remaining digits are completely or partially fused.

OSSIFICATION

During the second month of development, ossification begins directly in the connective tissue of the embryo and is described as bone ossified in membrane (Sinclair & Dangerfield 1998). This includes the clavicle (ossified at 6 weeks gestation) and the bones of the vault of the skull; the remaining bones are ossified in cartilage.

Primary centres of ossification are the areas in which bone formation begins, and these centres appear at different timescales in different bones. After birth, the bones grow in length by the process of ossification, and growth is complete when the cartilage becomes completely ossified (Waugh & Grant 2001).

Skeletal maturity begins with the appearance of the centres of ossification in the embryo, and is complete when the last epiphysis, or growth plate, is firmly fused to the shaft of the bone (Table 3.1).

Table 3.1   Summary of skeletal development

Age	Anatomical development
Upper limbs	
Weeks 4–6 (gestation)	Limb buds develop
	Upper extremities with pronated forearms appear and begin to rotate externally
Week 7 (gestation)	Ten upper digit rays appear
	Continue to differentiate until weeks 12–13, when the hands appear
Week 12 (gestation)	Formation of the body's solid framework begins
	Systematically, each cartilage model becomes solid bone
	Primary centres of ossification appear in the diaphysis of most bones
	Secondary centres for ossification do not present until birth
Development of the vertebrae	
Weeks 3–5 (gestation)	Formation of vertebrae
Weeks 6–8 (gestation)	Segmentation and chondrification
First year to 3–6 years	Two halves of neural arch fuse, and further fusion to centrum.
11–13 years	Final height of vertebral column is reached in girls
14–16 years	Final height of vertebral column is reached in boys
25 years	Ossification complete
Development of the pelvis	
8 weeks (gestation)	Ilium appears
12 weeks (gestation)	Ischium appears
16 weeks (gestation)	Pubis appears
7 years	Ischial and pubic rami fuse
15 years	'Y'-shaped cartilaginous physis of the three bones, fuse soon after puberty
Development of the femur	
8 weeks (gestation)	Appearance of the centre of the shaft
9 months (term)	Appearance of the centre of the lower end of the femoral shaft
1 year	Centre appears in femoral head
3 years	Centre appears in greater trochanter
12 years	Centre appears in lesser trochanter
18 years	Centres fuse with femoral shaft
Development of the patella	
3 years	Centre appears in the patella
Puberty	Ossification is complete soon after puberty
Development of the tibia	
8 weeks (gestation)	Primary centre of tibial shaft appears
9 months	Upper epiphysis appears
2 years to puberty	Distal epiphysis ossifies; secondary centre of tibial tuberosity appears
18 years	Distal epiphysis joins the shaft
20 years	Upper epiphysis joins the shaft

table continues

Table 3.1 *Continued*

Age	Anatomical development
Development of the fibula	
8 weeks	Primary centre appears
2 years	Centre of the lower end of the fibula ossifies
4 years	Centre of the proximal end of the tibia ossifies
18 years	Lower end of fibula fuses with tibial shaft
20 years	Proximal end of the fibula fuses with shaft
Development of the bones of the foot	
6 months (gestation)	Ossification of calcaneus
7 months (gestation)	Ossification of talus
9 months (gestation)	Ossification of cuboid
Birth	Bones of the tarsus are ossified
First year	Lateral ossification of the cuneiforms
Third year	Medial ossification of the cuneiforms
Fourth year	Intermediate ossification of the cuneiforms
	Navicular ossifies
5 years	Metatarsal epiphysis (feet) ossify
18 years	Metatarsals fuse
Development of the clavicle	
Week 5 (gestation)	The first bone in the skeleton with two centres that rapidly fuse
Adolescence	Elongation of the sternal end
	Cartilaginous epiphysis appears and fuses several years later
Development of the scapula	
6–8 weeks (gestation)	Scapula forms by chondrification of mesenchyme followed by bony centres appearing in the glenoid angle
10 years to puberty	Appearance of the base of the coracoid appears and fuses with glenoid at puberty
Puberty to 25 years	Secondary centres appear at puberty in acromion, medial border, inferior angle and coracoid, fusing by the age of 25 years
Development of the humerus	
6–8 weeks (gestation)	At 6 weeks the humerus is cartilaginous; primary centre of ossification appears during week 8
Development of the radius	
6–8 weeks (gestation)	At 6 weeks, appears in cartilage; primary centre of ossification appears during week 8
2 years	Secondary centres appear
4 years	Radial head appears
18 years	Radial head fuses with the shaft
Development of the ulna	
6–8 weeks (gestation)	At 6 weeks, appears as cartilage; primary centres appear in the shaft at 8 weeks
6 years	Head of ulna ossifies at 6 years

Table 3.1 *Continued*

Age	Anatomical development
8–18 years	Olecranon epiphysis appears; fusion does not involve the articular surfaces
20 years	Head fuses with the shaft
Development of the hand	
In utero	Shafts of metacarpals and phalanges ossify
Year 1	Each carpal bone ossifies from one centre, the largest. Carpal ossifies in the first year of life
Year 2	Ossification of the hamate
Year 3	Ossification of triquetral
Year 4	Ossification of the lunate
Year 5	Ossification of the trapezium
Year 6	Ossification of the scaphoid
Year 7	Ossification of the trapezoid
Year 10	Ossification of the pisiform

Adapted from: http://www.orthoteers.co.uk./courses/index.htm

EPIPHYSEAL PLATES

During childhood, all bones grow in thickness by appositional or exogenous growth, and long bones lengthen by the addition of bone material on the diaphyseal side of the epiphyseal plate, which is a layer of cartilage in the metaphysis of bone (Tortora & Grabowski 2003). When the epiphyseal plates close and the growth of the epiphyseal cartilage cells arrest, bone eventually replaces the cartilage and the epiphyseal plates fade, leaving a bony structure which is then referred to as the epiphyseal line.

The epiphyseal plate comprises of four zones:

1. *Zone of resting cartilage.* This layer is nearest to the epiphysis and is referred to as 'resting' because the cells do not contribute to the bone growth.

2. *Zone of proliferating cartilage.* Larger chondrocytes in this zone are stacked like coins, and the cells replace those that die on the diaphyseal side of the epiphyseal plate (Tortora & Grabowski 2003).

3. *Zone of hypertrophic cartilage.* Larger chondrocytes stacked in columns accumulate glycogen in their cell cytoplasm. Lengthening of the diaphysis results from cells replicating in the zone of proliferating cartilage, coupled with the maturation of cells in the zone of hypertrophic cartilage.

4. *Zone of calcified cartilage.* This is the thinnest zone of the epiphyseal plate, consisting of dead chondrocytes as the matrix surrounding

them has calcified. Osteoblasts lay down bone matrix, eventually replacing the calcified cartilage, and the diaphyseal border of the epiphyseal plate becomes cemented to the diaphysis of the bone.

CLINICAL NOTES	SLIPPED FEMORAL CAPITAL EPIPHYSIS
	This occurs through a 'stress' fracture sustained through the femoral capital epiphyseal growth plate, and often occurs during the pubertal growth spurt before fusion of the epiphysis. The incidence is greater in males (1–4 : 100 000), is usually unilateral (although this may not always be the case) and may follow trauma. However, the epiphysis may slowly displace in obese or rapidly growing children (Candy et al 2001).

The growth of bone is not uniform within the same epiphyseal plate. It is suggested that this helps to maintain the stability of the bone by producing grooves and ridges on the surface of the bone, and it may also be responsible for producing a 'cupping' effect of some of the epiphysis (Sinclair & Dangerfield 1998). However, it remains unclear as to why one end of a bone should grow faster than the other end; for instance, the growing end of the femur lengthens twice as fast as that of the tibia (Sinclair & Dangerfield 1998).

The closure of the epiphysis terminates the growth of bone length (Table 3.1), and in most long bones closure is achieved by the age of 25 years.

Growth in bone thickness or diameter can occur only through the process of appositional growth. As new bone is deposited on the outer surface of the bone, the lining of the medullary canal is destroyed by osteoclasts, so that the medullary canal becomes enlarged as the bone increases in diameter.

MUSCLE FORMATION

The origin of embryonic skeletal muscle is well documented, but what is less clear is the development of muscles later in the perinatal period. In human beings, skeletal muscle forms in the embryo from paraxial mesoderm, which segments into somites on either side of the neural tube and notochord. Most of the muscular system is derived from embryonic mesoderm, with the exception of the muscles of the iris, which develop from neuroectoderm, and the arrector pili muscles attached to hairs. As the mesoderm develops, it becomes arranged in dense columns on either side of the developing nervous system. These columns of mesoderm undergo a process of segmentation into a series of block cells called *somites*.

The ventral portion of the somite, known as the *sclerotome*, contributes to the development of the cartilage and bone of the vertebral column and ribs. The dorsal portion of the somite, known as the *dermomyotome*, gives rise to the derm of the back and to the skeletal muscles of the body and limbs. The first pair of somites appear at 22 days gestation; by the end of week 5, 42 to 44 pairs of somites are formed. With the exception of the skeletal muscles of the head and limbs, skeletal muscles develop from the mesoderm of the somites. With very few somites in the region of the developing embryonic head, most of the skeletal muscles in the head develop from general mesoderm.

The first indication of *myogenesis* (*myo* = muscle), or muscle formation, is the elongation of the nuclei and cell bodies of the mesenchymal cells as they differentiate into myoblasts. These embryonic muscle cells fuse to form multinucleated muscle cells or muscle fibres. Small structures, *myofibrils* (the contracting element of the muscle), appear in the cytoplasm, and cross-striations develop soon afterwards, forming striated muscle cells. Similarly, a process occurs in the ventrolateral body walls where mesenchymal cells are derived from somatic layers of mesoderm. The somatic mesoderm layer gives rise to striated muscles of the body walls and the limbs.

At a molecular level, these events are preceded by a hierarchy of gene activity. Muscle growth during development results from the ongoing fusion of myoblasts and myotubes, which are multinucleated cylindrical structures. Myoblast cell differentiation into muscle fibres also depends upon the MyoD family: MyoD, Mrf4 and, particularly, myogenin (Buckingham et al 2003).

The first muscle fibres to develop are known as primary fibres, around which secondary fibres form at the time when innervation begins to be established. Furthermore, primary and secondary fibres demonstrate some differences in muscle gene expression. Primary fibres are described as 'slow fibres' and secondary fibres acquire the characteristics of 'fast fibres'. Most notably, muscle masses undergo extensive growth during the fetal and postnatal periods.

Most skeletal muscle develops before birth and almost all remaining muscles are formed by the end of the first year of life. Increase in the size of muscles is due to an increase in the diameter of the muscle fibres, and muscles increase in length and width in order to grow with the skeleton. Not all embryonic muscle fibres persist, as many fail to establish themselves as viable units of muscle, and ultimately perish.

The composition of muscles varies with age. During fetal development, muscle fibres contain a great deal more water and intercellular matrix. After birth, both of these structures reduce as the cells grow in size by accumulating cytoplasm. Muscle fibrils remain constant in their diameter; as the muscle grows, fibrils increase in length, growing at their ends.

The growth of the connective tissue element of a muscle is maximal in the vicinity of the junction of the tendon with the muscle. After birth, mitotic structures in the skeletal muscle do not appear within the structure of the muscle fibres, but in the undifferentiated cells outside them. These are described as 'satellite cells' and appear in early embryonic development, with their nuclei estimated to account for 5–10% of the total number present in the muscle. In order to reproduce they multiply and form muscle cells, which eventually fuse together to increase the length of the muscle fibre. It is suggested that there are two distinct types of satellite cell:

- those that continue to perpetuate the satellite cells
- those that produce new muscle cells.

Interestingly, there are sex differences in the number of muscle fibres found in the muscles of girls and boys. The number of muscle fibres found in the gluteal muscles of boys increases 14-fold between birth and maturity. However, in girls it is estimated that the increase is in the order of 10-fold. Furthermore, muscle fibres attain a maximum diameter in girls at approximately 10 years of age, but not until approximately 14 years in boys.

Maximal muscle strength is usually attained between 25 and 30 years of age; after this there is a gradual decline in the speed and power of muscles. The muscles of the upper body, especially those of the head, trunk and upper limbs, are relatively heavier in the infant due to the relatively poor development of the lower limbs. The respiratory muscles and the muscles associated with facial expression are well developed at term to facilitate vital functioning of breathing and suckling.

PHARYNGEAL ARCH MUSCLES

Myoblasts migrate from the pharyngeal arches to form the muscles of mastication, facial expression, larynx and pharynx.

OCULAR MUSCLES

The extrinsic eye muscles are thought to be derived from mesenchymal cells near the prechordal plate.

TONGUE MUSCLES

Originally there are four occipital (postotic) myotomes; however, the first pair disappear and myoblasts from the remaining myotomes form the muscles of the tongue.

MUSCLES OF THE LIMBS

The muscles of the limbs develop from the myogenic cells (myoblasts) surrounding the developing bone. The cells are formed from epithelium and are first located in the ventral part of the dermomyotome. Following mesenchymal–epithelial transformation, the cells migrate into the primordium of the limb.

SMOOTH MUSCLE

Smooth muscle develops when fibres differentiate from splanchnic mesenchyme surrounding the endoderm of the primordial gut and derivates. Smooth muscle in the walls of many blood vessels and lymphatic vessels arises from ectoderm. As smooth muscle fibres develop into sheets or bundles, they receive autonomic innervation.

CARDIAC MUSCLE

Cardiac muscle develops from splanchnic mesenchyme surrounding the developing heart tube and is recognizable in the fourth week of embryological development. Cardiac muscles arise from the differentiation and growth of single cells, and growth of cardiac muscle fibres constitutes the formation of new myofilaments. Late in the embryonic period, specialized bundles of fibres develop, with few myofibrils. These are typical cardiac cells known as Purkinje fibres, which form the conducting system of the heart.

TENDONS

The apparent stimulus for tendon development is potentiated by the pull of the muscle rudiment on undifferentiated connective tissue. *Tendinification* is the replacement of muscle by tendons, and appears to be the result of limitation of movement in some instances. Regeneration of tendon tissue is relatively achievable, but full functional recovery is unusual in a tendon that has been completely severed. This may be attributed to the cut or severed ends uniting with each other and with the local connective tissue, thereby limiting movement.

LIGAMENTS

Ligaments consist of bands of various shapes and forms that serve to bind or connect together the articular extremities of bones. Ligaments are composed of bundles of either yellow elastic or white fibrous tissue (which gives a white shiny, silvery appearance) packed parallel or closely interlocked with one another. Ligaments are pliable and flexible, and facilitate freedom of movement. Equally, ligaments are strong, tough and inextensile.

ARTICULATIONS OR JOINTS

An articulation, or joint, is the point of contact between bones. Movement at joints is also determined by the structure of the articulating bones, the flexibility of the connective tissue, ligaments and joint capsule that binds the joint together, and the position of ligaments, muscles and tendons. Functional joints are classified as *synarthroses* (immovable joints), *amphiarthroses* (slightly movable joints) and *diarthroses* (freely moveable joints).

Structurally, joints are classified according to the presence or absence of a synovial cavity (a space between the articulating bones) and the kind of connective tissue that binds the bones together.

Joints begin to develop during week 6 of gestation, and by the end of the eighth week they resemble adult joints (Moore & Persaud 1998) (Fig. 3.7). Joints are classified as:

- fibrous
- cartilaginous
- synovial.

FIBROUS JOINTS

During the development of this type of joint the interzonal mesenchyme between the developing bones differentiates into dense fibrous tissue. Fibrous joints lack a synovial cavity and articulating bones are held together very closely together by fibrous connecting tissue which permits little or no movement.

SUTURES   A suture (*sutur* = seam) is a fibrous joint composed of a thin layer of dense fibrous connective tissue. The irregular interlocking edges of the sutures give them added strength, thereby reducing the risk of fracturing. The cranial sutures can be divided into three subsets:

- the *vertex* of the skull
- the *sides* of the skull
- the *base* of the skull.

Sutures present during infancy and childhood are replaced by bone in adulthood. As a rule, the sagittal and coronal sutures are the first to become ossified, and it is probable that the sutures facilitate the growth

Fig. 3.7
Development of a joint.

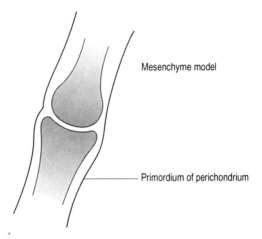

Mesenchyme model

Primordium of perichondrium

of bones. This type of suture is referred to as a synostotic, or bony, joint in which there is complete fusion of bone across the suture line, for example the frontal (metopic) suture between the left and right sides of the frontal bones that fuse during infancy.

CARTILAGINOUS JOINTS

During the development of cartilaginous joints, the interzonal mesenchyme between the developing bones differentiates into hyaline cartilage. Here the articulating bones are tightly connected by cartilage that facilitates little or no movement. The two major types of cartilaginous joints are:

- synchondroses
- symphyses.

Synchondroses (*chondro* = cartilage) are cartilaginous joints in which the connecting material is hyaline cartilage. The most common type of synchrondrosis is the epiphyseal plate that connects the epiphysis and diaphysis of a growing bone and is immovable. Eventually the hyaline cartilage is replaced by bone, when growth ceases.

CLINICAL NOTES | **GROWTH PLATES**

There coexist two types of growth plate:

- *physis*—a growth plate primarily responsive to loading forces
- *apophysis*—a growth plate primarily responsive to traction (tensile) loading forces. However, the apophysis is unique in that the normal physeal cell columns of hypertrophic cartilage are replaced by fibrocartilage with the typical tensile stress patterns.

If a growth plate is fractured, it is the hypertrophic zone that fails, leaving the germinal and dividing zones intact and attached to their blood supply.

SYMPHYSIS

A symphysis (growing together) is a cartilaginous joint in which the ends of the articulating bones are covered with hyaline cartilage. These joints are slightly movable as in the symphysis pubis, and are referred as *amphiarthroses* (*amphi* = on both sides).

SYNOVIAL JOINTS

This is by far the commonest type of joint. During development, the inter-zonal mesenchyme between the developing bones differentiates periph-erally to form the capsule and ligaments. Centrally it disappears, and the resulting 'space' becomes the synovium. Where the synovium lines the fibrous capsule and the articular surfaces, it forms the synovial mem-brane. Furthermore, as a result of joint movements the mesenchymal cells subsequently disappear from the surface of the articular cartilages.

CLINICAL NOTES

FLEXIBILITY OF THE FEET

The foot of a normal full-term infant is proportionately longer and thinner than that of an older child. The joints of the ankle and the foot are very supple and the feet of newborn infants can be held in 'abnormal' positions; the foot can be dorsiflexed so that the top of the foot touches the tibia anteriorly, and plantar flexed so that the dorsum of the forefoot is parallel with the tibia. However, these positional configurations are temporary and resolve spontaneously. The normal foot of the toddler is chubby and wider than that of an older child, and the fat pad on the medial aspect of the foot creates a fullness so that the foot appears flat.

NERVE AND BLOOD SUPPLY

The nerves that supply a joint are the same as those that supply the skeletal muscles that move the joint.

Arteries in the vicinity of a synovial joint send out many branches that penetrate the ligaments and the articular capsule to deliver oxygen and nutrients. The articulating portions of the synovial joint receive nourishment from the synovial fluid, whereas all other joint tissues are supplied by blood capillaries.

BURSAE AND TENDON SHEATHS

Movement of the human body can precipitate friction between the moving parts. Sac-like structures, referred to as bursae (purses), are strategically placed in order to reduce friction. In addition to bursae,

Fig. 3.8
Position of the branchial arches.

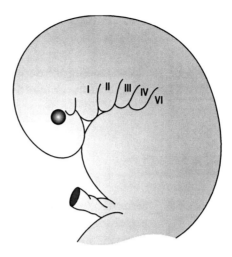

tendon (*tendere* = to stretch out) sheaths are tube-like bursae that wrap around tendons where there may be considerable friction.

BRANCHIAL APPARATUS

In the early embryo a series of arches, pouches, grooves and membranes develops in the pharyngeal region of the head and neck. These structures are referred to as the *branchial apparatus* and superficially resemble gills. There are six of these structures, numbered I–VI in a craniocephalic order; however, only the first four are visible externally.

The mesenchyme from each arch originates from the lateral mesoderm and neural crest cells that have migrated into the arch. The mesenchyme will form cartilage, bone, muscle and blood vessels. The neural crest cells will give rise to some skeletal structures.

BRANCHIAL ARCH SKELETON

Except for branchial arch V, mesenchyme and neural crest cells condense to form a cartilaginous bar known as the branchial arch cartilage (Fig. 3.8).

Branchial arch I

Referred to as Meckel's cartilage, branchial arch I provides the scaffolding for the intermembranous development of the mandible, and the dorsal end forms two of the three middle ear bones—the malleus and the incus.

Branchial arch II

Reichert's cartilage is formed from the dorsal component of the second branchial arch. Following ossification it will form the stapes and the styloid process of the temporal bone.

Branchial arch III	This cartilage will form the inferior portion of the greater cornu and body of the hyoid bone.
Branchial arches IV and VI	These cartilages fuse together and form all the cartilages of the larynx, except for the epiglottis.

BRANCHIAL ARCH MUSCLES

Branchial arch I	Muscles derived from arch 1 include muscles of mastication, the mylohyoid, the anterior part of the digastric muscle, the tensor tympani and the tensor veli palatini.
Branchial arch II	The muscles derived from this arch include the facial muscles (of expression), the stapedius, the stylohyoid and the posterior part of the digastric muscle.
Branchial arch III	The muscles derived from this arch are the stylopharyngeus.
Branchial arches IV and VI	The muscles formed from these arches are the striated muscles of the oesophagus, constrictors of the pharynx, intrinsic laryngeal muscle, levator veli palatini and the cricothyroid muscles.

FUNCTIONS OF THE SKELETON

Bone tissue and the bony framework of the skeleton perform several important functions:

1. The bony architecture of the body provides a *structural framework* that also supports soft tissues.
2. The skeleton provides *attachments* for muscles and tendons.
3. The skeleton provides *protection* for the internal organs of the body.
4. The skeleton assists in *movement* facilitated by the body as a whole, and/or by parts of the body, by the formation of joints that are moved by muscles.
5. The skeleton forms the *anatomical boundaries* of the cranium, and thoracic and pelvic cavities.
6. *Mineral homeostasis* is provided by bone storage of several minerals, including calcium and phosphorus.
7. The skeleton produces *blood cells* from the red bone marrow; this includes the production of red and white blood cells, and platelets

produced through a process of haemopoiesis (*haem* = blood; *poiesis* = making).

8. *Triglycerides* stored in the adipose cells of yellow bone marrow are important chemical energy reserves.

9. In childhood, the skeleton provides the framework for *growth, development and maturity*. The achievement of neuromuscular milestones changes posture from a quadrupedal organism to a mobile biped.

GROWTH HORMONES

Human growth hormone is a protein that causes most body cells to increase in size and divide; however, although blood plasma levels peak and trough they remain relatively constant throughout life (MacGregor 2000).

The polypeptide growth hormone (human growth hormone, or hGH) exists in two forms and is produced by the anterior lobe of the pituitary gland. The differences in form relate to the molecular weight: one form of hHG is heavier with a molecular weight of 22 000 Da, the smaller form being 20 000 Da. Human growth hormone does not appear to be essential for growth of the fetus, but the concentration of hGH in the umbilical cord at birth is high and subsequent daily output does not appear to vary with age (Sinclair & Dangerfield 1998).

THE ACTIONS OF GROWTH HORMONE

The actions of hGH include (MacGregor 2000):

- cellular uptake of amino acids from the blood and subsequent incorporation into proteins
- uptake of sulfur required for the synthesis of chondroitin sulfate into the cartilage matrix
- mobilization of fats from adipose tissue for transport to cells, thus increasing the blood levels of fatty acids
- decrease in the rate of glucose uptake and metabolism to maintain homeostasis of blood glucose levels.

There are some wide variations in the concentration of hGH at any given time. The release of hGH is influenced by the hypothalamus, which produces a growth-releasing hormone mediated by somatostatin. It is estimated that during sleep 20–40% of the total 24-hour output occurs in the first 90 minutes of sleep. Several bursts of activity may occur during the day, sometimes lasting for 2 hours and influenced by exercise or the intake of food (Sinclair & Dangerfield 1998).

Independently, thyrotrophic hormone affects growth by stimulating the thyroid gland to secrete *thyroxine* and *tri-iodothyronine*, both of which stimulate general metabolism and are important for growth and development. The parathyroid glands secrete *parathyroid hormone*, which draws calcium from the skeleton to maintain constant levels of calcium in the blood plasma. *Calcitonin* opposes the action of parathyroid hormone by inhibiting the drainage of calcium from the skeleton, particularly during periods of active growth.

At puberty, *sex steroids* are released in large quantities including:

- oestrogen
- androgens.

The *adrenal glands* in both sexes produce androgens, and other tissues within the body convert androgens to oestrogens. These hormones are responsible for the increase in osteoblast activity and synthesis of bone matrix, and for the sudden growth spurt common during adolescence. Oestrogens are responsible for promoting the noticeable growth changes in the female pelvis (i.e. widening of the pelvis). In both sexes, the sex hormones, especially oestrogen, are responsible for shutting down growth in the epiphyseal plates and arresting bony growth. Equally, lengthwise growth completes earlier in females than in males, mainly due to higher levels of circulating oestrogens in females (Tortora & Grabowski 2003).

MAINTAINING A HEALTHY SKELETON

The optimization of bone mass during childhood and adolescence is recognized as an important strategy to help reduce skeletal problems and pathology in later life. Important elements that influence bone health include normal amounts of phosphorus, sodium, potassium and other minerals, including vitamins C and K. However, certain trace elements such as zinc, copper and magnesium are essential co-factors in bone metabolism, although their contribution to bone health is uncertain.

CALCIUM AND BONE HEALTH

Calcium is essential for bone formation, and 99% of calcium in the human organism resides in the skeleton. It is deposited as an impure hydroxyapatite, together with a small amount of non-apatitic calcium phosphate.

The skeleton accumulates approximately 975 g of calcium from the diet between birth and adulthood. The bone mineral content and bone mineral density increase in infancy and peak in early childhood.

Table 3.2 Dietary reference values for calcium (United Kingdom)

Age	RNI calcium (mg/day)	LRNI (mg/day)
0–6 months	525	240
7–12 months	525	240
1–3 years	350	200
4–6 years	450	275
7–10 years	550	325
11–18 years (female)	800	450
11–18 years (male)	1000	480

(L)RNI, (Lower) Reference Nutrient Intake. Source: The Dairy Council 1998.

However, the exact age at which the peak in bone mass is attained is unclear.

It is also possible that the timing of peak bone mass is different for different parts of the skeleton. By the end of the second decade, most postpubertal young women will have accrued most of their bone mass, with the peak mass for the hip and trabecular of the spine.

Milk and milk products are a major source of calcium, supplying in the order of 50% of calcium. However, it is estimated that calcium intake is adequate for only 1% of children under the age of 4 years, and for only 2% of children aged over 4 years, with calcium levels below the Lower Reference Nutrient Intake (LRNI) (Department of Health 1994).

The dietary reference values for calcium were established in 1991 (Table 3.2), and were co-endorsed by the Committee on Medical Aspects of Food and Nutrition (COMA) (Department of Health 1994). The Reference Nutrient Intake (RNI) is the amount of a nutrient judged to be present in sufficient amounts for approximately 97% of the population. The LRNI is the amount of a nutrient judged to be enough for a minority of the population (3%). Therefore, those individuals eating less than the LRNI would be at risk of being deficient in that nutrient.

VITAMIN D AND SKELETAL HEALTH

Vitamin D plays a pivotal role in calcium homeostasis and bone metabolism. There are two recognized forms of vitamin D, which include:

- *cholecalciferol*—synthesized through the action of sunlight on the skin
- *ergocalciferol*—found in plants.

OPTIMIZING GOOD BONE HEALTH

A healthy skeleton and good bone health is multifaceted. Peak bone mass and bone density are mutually inclusive factors and are broadly attributed to genetic and environmental factors. However, it is recommended that a healthy lifestyle at all ages protects bone health, and, although the variance attributed to genetic factors is in the order of 40–80%, environmental factors are modifiable even from an early age.

SELF ASSESSMENT

Answer the following in relation to your professional area of practice:

- Briefly describe the normal development of bone and cartilage.
- Compare and contrast the structure and functions of the axial and appendicular skeleton.
- Name and list the structures of the skull.
- Outline the primary functions of the fontanelles.
- Define the term 'ossification'.
- Outline the functions of the 'growth plates'.
- Name and list four different types of muscle.
- Describe the influences that hormones exert upon the musculoskeletal system.

References

Buckingham M, Bajard L, Chang T et al 2003 The formation of skeletal muscle: from somite to limb. Journal of Anatomy 202:59–68

Candy D, Davies G, Ross E 2001 Clinical paediatrics and child health. W B Saunders, London

Cecconi F, Alvarez-Bolando G, Meyer B I, Gross P 1998 Apafi (CED-4-homolog) regulates programmed cell death in mammalian development. Cell 94:727–737

Department of Health 1994 Weaning and the weaning diet: report of the Working Group on Weaning Diet of the Committee on Medical Aspects of Food Policy (COMA). HMSO, London

Linsden T, Ross A J, King A, Zong W X, Rathmell J C, Shiels H A 2000 The combined functions of proapoptic Bcl-2 family members Bak and Bax are essential for normal development of multiple tissues. Molecular Cell 6:1389–1399

MacGregor J 2000 Introduction to the anatomy and physiology of children. Routledge, London

Matsumura G, England M A 1992 Embryology colouring book. Wolfe, London

Miedzybrodzka Z 2003 Congenital talipes equinovarus (clubfoot): a disorder of the foot but not the hand. Journal of Anatomy 202:37–42

Moore K L, Persaud T V N 1998 Before we are born: essentials of embryology and birth defects. W B Saunders, London

Sanz-Ezquerro J J, Tickle C 2003 Digital development and morphogenesis. Journal of Anatomy 202: 51–58

The Dairy Council 1998 Quarterly Review. The Dairy Council, London

Sinclair D, Dangerfield P 1998 Human growth after birth, 6th edn. Oxford University Press, Oxford

Tortora G J, Grabowski S R 2003 Principles of anatomy and physiology, 10th edn. John Wiley, New York

Vioarsdottir U S, O'Higgin P O, Stringer C 2002 A geometric geomorphic study of regional differences in the ontogeny of the human facial skeleton. Journal of Anatomy 201:211–229

Waugh A, Grant A 2001 Ross and Wilson anatomy and physiology in health and illness, 9th edn. Churchill Livingstone, London

Whaley L F, Wong D 1991 Nursing care of infants and children, 4th edn. Mosby, London

Wong D L 1999 Whaley and Wong's nursing care of children, 6th edn. Mosby, London

Bibliography

Bee H, Boyd D 2004 The developing child, 10th edn. Allyn and Bacon, Boston

Bonjour J P, Theintz G, Buchi B, Slosman D, Rizzoli R 1991 Critical years and stages of puberty for spinal and femoral bone mass accumulation during adolescence. Journal of Endocrinology and Metabolism 73:555–563

Buckingham M, Bajard L, Chang T et al 2003 The formation of skeletal muscle: from somite to limb. Journal of Anatomy 202:59–68

Department of Health (1994) Weaning and weaning diet: report of the Working Group on Weaning Diet of the Committee on Medical Aspects of Food Policy (COMA). HMSO, London

Miedzybrodzka Z 2003 Congenital talipes equinovarus (clubfoot): a disorder of the foot but not the hand. Journal of Anatomy 202:37–42

Sanz-Ezquerro J J, Tickle C 2003 Digital development and morphogenesis. Journal of Anatomy 202:51–58

Sweet B 1999 Mayes' midwifery, 12th edn. Baillière Tindall, London

Wilkie A O 2003 Why study human limb malformations? Journal of Anatomy 202:27–35

Young R W 2003 Evolution of the human hand: the role of throwing and clubbing. Journal of Anatomy 202:165–174

Chapter 4

Development of the control systems

Carol A. Chamley

CHAPTER OUTCOMES

This chapter will enable the reader to:

- List the component parts of the central nervous system, peripheral nervous system and autonomic nervous system
- Name the major elements of a neurone
- Draw and label a typical neurone
- List the 12 cranial nerves
- List the glands that form the endocrine system
- Explain the differences between endocrine glands and exocrine glands
- Describe the functions of the nervous system and the endocrine system.

CHAPTER OVERVIEW

The aim of this chapter is to consider the normal embryonic and fetal development of the control systems of the body, describing the formation and development of the nervous system and the endocrine system. These are complex systems that share and coordinate the maintenance of homeostasis; therefore both systems share mutually inclusive roles in sustaining life.

This chapter discusses the major components of both systems, explaining the normal embryological and fetal developments, structure and functions, and drawing the reader's attention to key perspectives in relation to the development and maturation of these systems as the child grows and matures.

Clinical Notes address issues of clinical relevance and potential interest to the reader, and Self Assessment exercises assist in reflecting upon the chapter and guiding the relationship between theory and practice.

INTRODUCTION

With a cumulative mass of 2 kg, approximately 3% of total bodyweight, the nervous system is the most complex of all the body systems. Nervous control between the child and the environment is mediated through the interactions of the nervous system. Any disturbance in this system can produce alterations in the way in which the system receives, integrates and responds to stimuli entering the system. Moreover, children are constantly changing and developing in response to the development and maturation of body systems, and the achievement of neurodevelopmental milestones represents the transition from immature primitive reflexes to mature activity (Wong 1999).

Together, the nervous and endocrine systems share and coordinate the maintenance of homeostasis, the objective being to maintain controlled conditions to sustain life. The nervous system regulates activities by responding rapidly to stimuli. The endocrine system responds more slowly, although no less effectively, by releasing hormones (Tortora & Grabowski 2003).

The nervous system is a highly organized network of billions of neurones and even more neuroglia (*neuro* = nerve; *glia* = glue), or glial cells. The nervous system is composed of three intimately connected and functioning elements:

- central nervous system (CNS)
- peripheral nervous system (PNS)
- autonomic nervous system (ANS).

In contrast to many other body tissues that grow rapidly after birth, proportionately the nervous system grows more rapidly before birth, with two critical bursts of activity occurring during fetal development. Between weeks 15 and 20 of gestation there is a dramatic increase in the number of neurones produced, followed by a second dramatic increase that begins at week 30 of gestation extending to the age of 1 year (Wong 1999).

ORIGINS OF THE NERVOUS SYSTEM

The nervous system develops from the neural plate during week 3 (day 18) of embryological development. The neural plate is a thickened 'slipper-shaped' tissue formed when the ectoderm, cephalic to the primitive knot, is induced by the notochord, and the mesoderm differentiates into neuroectoderm or the neural plate. These activities indicate the origins of the nervous system (Fig. 4.1).

Fig. 4.1
Early neurulation: neural plate.

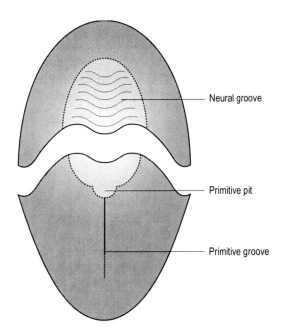

Neural groove

Primitive pit

Primitive groove

Formation of the neural tube (*neurulation*) begins at 22–23 days gestation, in the origins of the fourth to sixth pairs of somites. At this stage the site of the future brain is represented at the cranial two-thirds of the neural plate and tube as far as the fourth pair of somites. The caudal one-third of the neural plate and tube represents the future spinal cord.

Fusion of the neural folds proceeds in a cranial to caudal direction until the two ends of the tube remain open. The rostral and caudal *neuropores* and the lumen of the neural tube communicate freely with the amniotic cavity. The neuropores close and as the tube forms, the integrity of the overlying ectoderm is re-established. The rostral or anterior neuropore closes on gestation day 25, followed by the closure of the caudal or posterior neuropore 2 days later. The closure of the neuropores also coincides with the establishment of the vascular system of the neural tube (Moore & Persaud 1998).

As the neural folds fuse to form the neural tube, a specialized group of neuroectodermal cells lying between the tube and overlying ectoderm, known as the *neural crest*, separates from them both. Under the influence of several embryonic factors, the neural crest cells migrate throughout the developing body. This gives rise to many derivatives including pigment cells, the spinal ganglia, Schwann cells and derivatives of the germ layers including the ectoderm, endoderm and mesoderm. The three germ layers are the primordia of all embryonic tissues and organs.

DEVELOPMENT OF THE CENTRAL NERVOUS SYSTEM

THE BRAIN

The brain consists of four major parts (Table 4.1):

- brainstem
- cerebellum
- diencephalon
- cerebrum.

The brainstem is continuous with the spinal cord and is composed of the medulla oblongata, pons and midbrain. Posterior to the cerebellum (little brain) and superior to the brainstem is the *diencephalon* (*di* = through; *encephalon* = brain). This part of the brain consists of the thalamus and hypothalamus, including the epithalamus and subthalamus. Supported superior to the diencephalon and brainstem is the largest part of the brain, the *cerebrum*. This part of the brain eventually occupies the anterior and middle cranial fossae, and a deep cleft divides the brain into right and left cerebral hemispheres (Waugh & Grant 2001). Each hemisphere is divided into lobes that

Table 4.1 Summary of parts of the brain, and primary functions

Part of brain	Primary function
Diencephalon	
Epithalamus	Consists of pineal gland that secretes melatonin
Thalamus	Transfers all sensory input to the cerebral cortex
Subthalamus	Contains nervous tissue and communicates with basal ganglia, helping to control body movements
Cerebellum	Regulates posture and balance; motor coordination
Cerebrum	Responsible for sensory impulses
	Motor areas control muscular functions
	Basal ganglia coordinate gross automatic muscle movements
Brainstem	
Medulla oblongata	Relays motor and sensory impulses between other parts of brain and spinal cord
	Responsible for vital functions, including cardiac, respiration, swallowing, coughing and sneezing
Pons	Relays impulses from one side of the cerebellum to another
Midbrain	Relays motor impulses from the cerebral cortex to the pons, and sensory impulses from the spinal cord to the thalamus

assume the names of the cranial bones with which they are in contact, namely:

- frontal lobe
- parietal lobe
- temporal lobe
- occipital lobe.

DEVELOPMENT OF THE BRAIN

The neural tube cranial to the fourth and sixth somites will develop into the brain. Prior to closure of the neural tube, the site of the three primary vesicles is identifiable as large elevated cephalic folds. The three primary brain vesicles develop and form component parts of the brain (Fig. 4.2A), namely the forebrain (*prosencephalon*), midbrain (*mesencephalon*) and hindbrain (*rhombencephalon*).

During week 5 of embryological development, two of the three primary vesicles subdivide further to form five major regions within the developing brain. The forebrain (prosencephalon) divides into two areas: the *telencephalon* from which the cerebral vesicles develop, and the caudal *diencephalon*. The midbrain (mesencephalon) does not divide, but the hindbrain (rhombencephalon) divides into two areas: the *metencephalon*, which gives rise to the pons and the cerebellum, and the *myelencephalon*, which gives rise to the medulla oblongata and the emerging spinal cord (Fig. 4.2B).

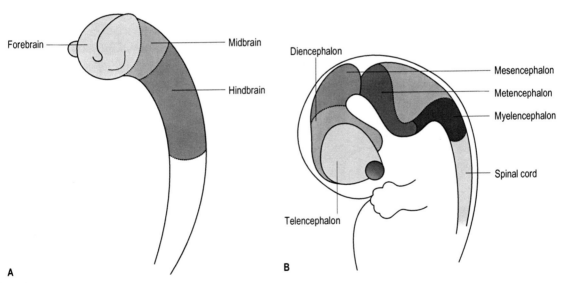

A

Fig. 4.2
A Development of the forebrain, midbrain and hindbrain.
B Major developmental areas within the brain and emerging spinal cord.

FLEXURES OF THE BRAIN

During week 4 of gestation, the brain grows rapidly and bends ventrally with the head fold (Moore & Persaud 1998). During early morphogenesis the primordial brain has the same basic structure as the developing spinal cord. However, the flexures produce variations in the position of the emerging grey and white matter. The three flexures of the brain include:

- midbrain flexure
- cervical flexure
- pontine flexure.

The cervical flexure demarcates the hindbrain from the spinal cord.

FOLDING OF THE BRAIN AND THE FORMATION OF THE CEREBRAL VENTRICLES

During early embryogenesis the lumen of the neural tube is approximately the same shape and size throughout its length, but with the formation of the cerebral flexures and the cerebral hemispheres the shape of the neural tube lumen is altered. Concurrent to these biological activities, the walls of the neural tube begin to thicken and the interconnected spaces that result from these changes develop into the cerebral ventricular system. Thus, the ventricles (little cavities) of the brain are determined by the formation of the cerebral flexures.

The two lateral ventricles (Fig. 4.3A) develop in the cerebral hemispheres; each ventricle is continuous with the developing third ventricle, connected via a narrow interventricular foramen. The third ventricle is wide rostrally and narrow caudally to form the aqueduct of Sylvius and, as a direct result of this formation, the developing thalamus bulges into this area. The aqueduct of Sylvius is continuous

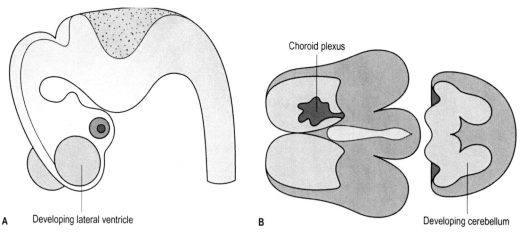

A   Developing lateral ventricle   B   Choroid plexus   Developing cerebellum

Fig. 4.3
A Developing lateral ventricle.
B Development of the choroid plexus.

with the fourth ventricle, which develops as a diamond shape due to splaying of the walls of the hindbrain, caused by the pontine flexure. This ventricle is continuous with the lumen of the spinal cord.

The choroid (membrane-like) plexus is a network of capillaries that develop in the ventricular walls (Fig. 4.3B) and eventually produce cerebrospinal fluid (CSF). The CSF passes through the ventricular system and escapes via three openings to bathe the outer surface of the brain and the spinal cord. These three openings are located in:

- the roof of the hindbrain and the median foramen of Magendie
- the two lateral foramen of Luschka.

The formation of the foramina is attributed to programmed cell degeneration and not to the pressure exerted by the production of CSF rupturing the roof of the hindbrain. The ventricles occupy a large proportion of brain volume in the fetus and early embryo (Jeffrey 2002).

CLINICAL NOTES   **HYDROCEPHALUS**

Each section of the brain plays a critical role in the regulation and control of body functions. Each hemisphere is artificially divided into lobes, so that any damage or pressure to the lobes produces observable signs and/or symptoms directly related to the area of pathology (Wong 1999). The brain is tightly enclosed and protected in the bony cranium, but is highly vulnerable to changes in pressure. The total volume (80% brain tissue, 10% CSF, 10% blood) must remain constant at all times. Any deviation in the proportional volume of one of these elements will be accompanied by a compensatory change in another. Infants and children with open fontanelles compensate for changes in pressure by skull expansion and widened sutures.

Hydrocephalus is a condition in which there is increased pressure in the ventricular system usually secondary to obstruction of CSF flow in the ventricular system (non-communicating) or failure of reabsorption of CSF (communicating).

NON-COMMUNICATING HYDROCEPHALUS

Potential causes of obstruction in the ventricular system include:

- congenital malformation
- aqueduct stenosis
- atresia of the outflow foramina of the ventricle (Dandy–Walker malformation)
- postnatal infection
- vascular malformation
- neoplasm.

COMMUNICATING HYDROCEPHALUS

Potential causes of failure to reabsorb CSF include:

- subarachnoid haemorrhage
- tuberculous meningitis
- Arnold–Chiari malformation
- haemorrhage in preterm infants.

In both types of hydrocephalus the head circumference is disproportionately large, or the rate of growth is excessive; the sutures become separated and the scalp veins congested. The increased pressure in the anterior fontanelle causes bulging and, if untreated, causes the eyes to deviate downwards so that the sclera may be visible above the pupil (setting-sun sign). The infant develops clinical signs and symptoms associated with raised intracranial pressure. Antenatal ultrasonography or routine intracranial scanning in preterm infants may confirm the diagnosis.

The aim of treatment is to minimize the risk of neurological damage and symptomatic relief of raised intracranial pressure. Treatment may involve the insertion of a ventricular shunt.

THE DIENCEPHALON

The walls of the diencephalon thicken and three large swellings develop in each lateral wall that develop into:

- the *epithalamus*
- the *thalamus* (inner chamber)
- the *hypothalamus*.

All three swellings bulge into the third ventricle; the epithalami are initially large but eventually reduce in size. The thalamus develops rapidly on each side, and sometimes the thalami fuse in the midline to form the interthalamic adhesion (Matsumura & England 1992). The hypothalamus develops through the proliferation of neuroblasts in the intermediate zone of the diencephalon. Mamillary bodies and nuclei develop in the hypothalamus and are later involved in physiological functions related to homeostasis and endocrine function. The pineal body (epiphysis cerebri) forms as a cone-shaped gland located in the third ventricle that secretes melatonin (Fig. 4.4). The pituitary gland (hypophysis cerebri) is also a derivative of the diencephalon.

THE METENCEPHALON

The walls of the metencephalon contribute to the formation of the pons and the cerebellum, whereas the medulla oblongata is derived from the myelencephalon. The roof of the hindbrain becomes thin over the lumen of the fourth ventricle and, as the walls splay, the alar plates (sensory afferent) of the pons and medulla oblongata lie lateral to the basal plates (motor efferent).

Fig. 4.4
Development of the pineal gland.

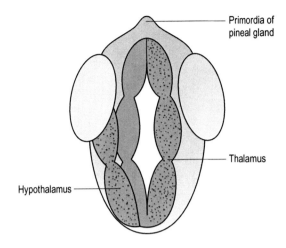

Neuroblasts in each basal plate develop motor nuclei and begin to organize into three columns:

- general visceral efferent
- special visceral efferent
- general somatic efferent.

The sensory alar plates give rise to:

- special somatic afferent
- general somatic afferent
- special visceral afferent
- general visceral afferent.

The *cerebellum* originates from the dorsum of the alar plates, which thicken and project into the fourth ventricle and on to the surface of the metencephalon. Some of the neuroblasts in the intermediate zone of the alar plates migrate and differentiate into neurones at the cerebral cortex. The two cerebellar projections meet and fuse in the midline, forming a 'dumb-bell' shape (Matsumura & England 1992); they enlarge and overgrow the rostral half of the fourth ventricle. The lateral elements of the cerebellum enlarge and form lobes, and fissures develop in the lobes during the fourth month of fetal development.

THE MIDBRAIN (MESENCEPHALON)

This part of the brain undergoes less change than any other part of the developing brain, with the exception of the caudal part of the hindbrain (Moore & Persaud 1998).

THE FOREBRAIN

Two lateral outgrowths—optic vesicles—appear when the rostral neuropores close. These vesicles are the primordia of the retina and

Fig. 4.5
Development of the cerebral
hemispheres.

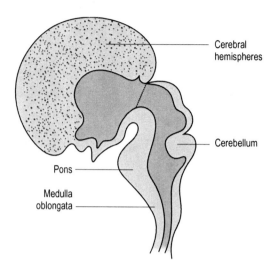

Cerebral
hemispheres

Cerebellum

Pons

Medulla
oblongata

the optic nerves. Furthermore, a second pair of diverticula appears
dorsally and rostrally; these are the primordia of the cerebral hemispheres (Fig. 4.5).

CEREBRAL VESICLES AND DEVELOPMENT OF THE MENINGES

The cerebrum (cerebral hemispheres) is the largest portion of the
brain and comes to occupy the anterior and middle cranial fossa.
Furthermore, the cortex of the brain is identifiable at 8 weeks gestation. The cerebral vesicles grow rapidly and expand to cover the
diencephalon, midbrain and hindbrain. The cortical surfaces of the
hemispheres grow more rapidly than the floor, expanding to form
a 'C' shape. The caudal end of the hemispheres turns ventrally and
laterally to form the temporal lobe and, as the lobe develops in a
forward position, together with the frontal and the developing parietal lobes, these structures grow and immerse the 'insula' of the cerebral cortex. As the temporal lobe continues to grow over the insula, it
carries with it the temporal horn of the ventricle into its definitive
position, forming the lateral sulcus.

Initially the surface of the cerebral hemispheres is smooth, but by
week 18 of gestation sulci (grooves or furrows) and gyri (convolutions
or elevations) develop on the surface. This is an important development that increases the surface area of the brain considerably without
having to increase the size of the cranium.

The meninges

The meninges form from mesenchyme surrounding the spinal cord. The
primitive meninx forms from two layers: an outer layer that forms
the *dura mater* (tough mother), and an inner layer that forms the lep-
tomeninges, which include the *arachnoid* (*arachn* = spider; *oid* = similar
to) mater and the *pia* (*pia* = delicate) mater. The dura mater is the

most superficial layer, composed of dense irregular connective tissue; it forms a close association with the skull. The dura mater is a double layer, the inner of which dips down between the cerebrum and cerebellum and between the cerebral hemispheres to form the intercranial membranes. The *subarachnoid space* is a thin subdural space that contains interstitial fluid (Tortora & Grabowski 2003).

CLINICAL NOTES	**MENINGITIS**

Meningitis is a serious illness in childhood that is commonest in the neonatal period. During the first 10 years of life the incidence is 1 in 200 children.

Meningitis is an acute inflammation of the meninges caused by a variety of bacterial (bacterial meningitis) and viral (viral meningitis) agents. The organisms can enter the cerebrospinal fluid (CSF) via the bloodstream, invading the membranes that overlie the brain and spinal cord. Bacterial infections usually remain confined to the meninges, but viral infections may invade the underlying brain causing meningoencephalitis. Inflammation, exudation and tissue damage to the brain may ensue, causing pyrexia and raised intracranial pressure. Septic shock and rashes may occur in severe infections.

During week 6 of embryological development a swelling appears, known as the *corpus striatum*, on the striatal part of the floor of each cerebral hemisphere. A bundle of fibres (internal capsule) develop and pass to and from the hemispheres, passing through the corpus striatum. These divide the corpus striatum into two parts, known as the medial caudate nucleus and the lentiform nucleus.

LATERALIZATION

The *corpus callosum* is the structure in the brain through which left and right sides of the cerebral cortex grow and mature during the early years of childhood, more so than any other period of life. The growth of this structure within the brain accompanies the functional specialization of the right and left cerebral cortex; a process referred to as lateralization (Bee & Boyd 2004). Furthermore, this relates to right- and left-sided brain dominance, but most individuals have mixed dominance.

CLINICAL NOTES	**CRANIUM BIFIDUM**

Defects in the formation of the cranium are often associated with congenital anomalies of the brain and/or meninges. Defects in the cranium usually occur in the median plane of the calvaria. The defect may be seen in the squamous part of the occipital bone, which may also include the foramen magnum.

Table 4.2 Cranial nerves and origins

Cranial nerve	Origin
Olfactory (I)	Sensory nerve
Optic nerve (II)	Sensory nerve
Oculomotor nerve (III)	Somatic efferent nerve
Trochlear (IV)	Somatic efferent nerve
Trigeminal (V)	Nerves of the pharyngeal arches
Abducens (VI)	Somatic efferent nerve
Facial nerve (VII)	Nerves of the pharyngeal arches
Vestibulocochlear (auditory) nerve (VIII)	Sensory nerve
Glossopharyngeal nerve (IX)	Nerves of the pharyngeal arches
Vagus nerve (X)	Nerves of the pharyngeal arches
Accessory nerve (XI)	Nerves of the pharyngeal arches
Hypoglossal nerve (XII)	Somatic efferent nerve

CRANIAL NERVES

During weeks 5 to 6, 12 pairs of cranial nerves develop (Table 4.2); each is designated by a Roman numeral and a name. The cranial nerves arise as three major groups according to their embryological origins:

- special sensory nerve
- somatic efferent nerve
- branchial arch nerves.

NERVOUS TISSUE

Nervous tissue consists of two basic cell types: neurones and neuroglia. The neurones (Fig. 4.6) provide the most unique functions of the nervous system, whereas the neuroglia support, nourish and protect the neurones and maintain homeostasis in the interstitial fluid that bathes them (Tortora & Grabowski 2003).

NEURONES

Most neurones have three parts:

1. A cell body
2. Dendrites
3. Axon.

The cell body contains the cell nucleus surrounded by cytoplasm that includes organelles (lysosomes, mitochondria and Golgi bodies). Two structures emerge from the cell body of the neurone:

- multiple dendrites
- single axon.

Fig. 4.6
The structure of a neurone.

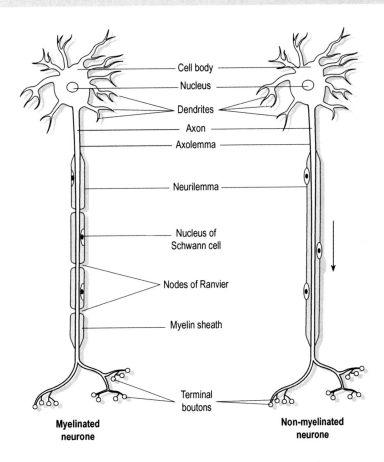

Cell body
Nucleus
Dendrites
Axon
Axolemma
Neurilemma
Nucleus of
Schwann cell
Nodes of Ranvier
Myelin sheath
Terminal
boutons

**Myelinated
neurone**

**Non-myelinated
neurone**

Dendrites (little trees) are the receiving, or input, element of the neurone. They are usually highly branched, forming a 'tree-like' array of structures, short and tapering. The single axon (= axis) propagates impulses towards another neurone, gland cell or muscle fibre. *Axons* are long, thin, cylindrical structures that often join the cell body at a cone-shaped structure known as the axon hillock.

Structurally, neurones are classified according to the number of processes emerging from the cell body:

- multipolar neurones
- bipolar neurones
- unipolar neurones.

In the fetus, neurones are formed in the deeper layers of the neural tube, near to the lumen; they develop as a nucleus surrounded by minimal cytoplasm, and the axon and dendrites are added later. Therefore, neurones form as a cell body that has been developed in one part of the nervous system, that migrates from that location to a point closer to the surface. This process creates three main cell layers within the cerebral cortex, and the anatomical position of each neurone is critical and irreversible (Blows 2003).

All the neurones that the individual will ever have are generated at an extremely rapid rate, between weeks 10 and 26. At the peak of this activity 250 000 cells are produced per minute (Bee & Boyd 2004, Blows 2003, Slater & Lewis 2002, Wong 1999). In the first instance there is a massive overproduction of cells as part of the normal development of the brain, but some neurones are lost naturally through cell death. In the early weeks neurones are simple structures, but in the last 8 weeks of fetal life and the first year of life, axons lengthen and there is major growth of the dendrite arbor. Although mainly occurring at birth, it is estimated that 50–70% of neurones are 'pruned'. This is seen as a key process in the developmental process whereby neurones that have not made connections, or have made inappropriate connections, are removed (Slater & Lewis 2002).

NEUROGLIA

Neuroglia (*glia* = glue), or glia, constitute approximately half the volume of the central nervous system. Historically their name emerged from the work of early histologists, who believed that the glial cells acted like glue holding nervous tissue together (Tortora & Grabowski 2003). Glial cells tend to be smaller than neurones and are more numerous; they do not generate or propagate nervous activity, but are capable of multiplying and dividing in the mature nervous system. Glial cells begin to develop between weeks 13 and 15 of fetal development, and continue to be added to until the age of 2 years (Bee 1997, Bee & Boyd 2004).

DEVELOPMENT OF THE SPINAL CORD

The spinal cord is located within the vertebral column (Fig. 4.7A). The spinal cord is roughly cylindrical and slightly flattened in its anterior–posterior dimension. During early childhood, both the spinal cord and the vertebral column grow longer as part of overall body length. At approximately 4–5 years of age, elongation of the cord ceases but the bony case of the vertebral column continues to elongate. The spinal cord has two principal functions in maintaining homeostasis:

1. Nerve impulse propagation and integrating the information
2. Facilitating the integration of some reflexes.

ORIGINS OF THE SPINAL CORD

The spinal cord develops caudal to the fourth pair of somites. By 9–10 weeks gestation the lateral walls of the neural tube have thickened, a

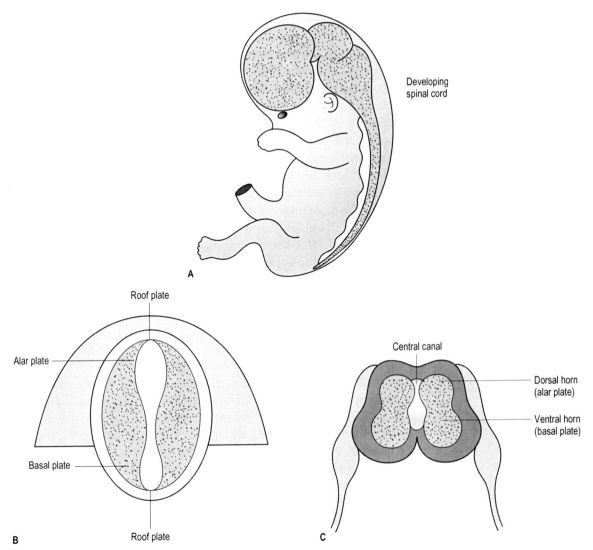

A Developing spinal cord

Roof plate

Alar plate

Basal plate

Roof plate

B

Central canal

Dorsal horn (alar plate)

Ventral horn (basal plate)

C

Fig. 4.7
A Development of the spinal cord.
B Development of alar and basal plates.
C Dorsal and ventral horns.

process that reduces the fetal central canal to a minute canal. The early primitive tube is composed of pseudostratified neuroepithelium, which forms the ventricular (ependymal) zone of the spinal cord and the microglia. Further to these early developments, a second zone composed of neuroepithelial cells develops along the border of the external limiting membrane. This zone eventually forms the white matter of the spinal cord.

As the neuroepithelial cells continue to divide and produce primitive neurones (neuroblasts), a third zone develops. Towards the end of neuroblast formation, the ventricular zone produces glioblasts, or primitive *macroglial cells*. These are the supporting cells of the spinal cord; they eventually form *astrocytes* and *oligodendrocytes*. Macroglial cells are scattered throughout the grey and white matter, and are derived from mesenchymal cells. The microglial cells invade the central nervous system late in fetal life. When the production of neuroblasts and glioblasts is complete, the neuroepithelial cells differentiate into the ependymal lining of the central canal (Matsumura & England 1992).

The proliferation and differentiation of neuroepithelial cells in the developing spinal cord contributes to the thickening of the walls of the spinal cord, but the roof plates remain thin. As the lumen of the spinal canal is reduced in size by these developments, a groove (sulcus limitans) separates the dorsal wall or the alar plate (lamina) from the ventral wall or the basal plate (lamina) (Fig. 4.7B). Both of these plates produce longitudinal bulges extending through most of the length of the developing spinal cord. The cell bodies in the alar plate (afferent) stack into columns of grey matter. Cell bodies in the basal plate (efferent) form the ventral and lateral grey columns. In transverse sections of the spinal cord, these columns are the ventral (grey) horns and lateral (grey) horns (Fig. 4.7C). The axons of the ventral horn cells grow out of the spinal cord and form the ventral roots of the spinal nerves (Moore & Persaud 1998).

ASCENT OF THE SPINAL CORD

Initially the spinal cord and the meninges occupy the entire length of the vertebral canal. In addition, the spinal nerves emerge from the spinal cord through the vertebral foramina of the vertebrae adjacent to them. The vertebral column and the dura mater grow more rapidly than the spinal cord. At birth the spinal cord terminates at the level of the lumbar segment, L2–L3. As a result of the cord ascending, the spinal nerves emerge from the cord. The nerves from the lumbar and sacral regions eventually form the cauda equina (horse's tail). This is appropriately named because arising from the conus medularis is the *filum terminale*, a non-nervous fibrous tissue of the spinal cord that extends inferiorly to attach to the coccyx. The filum terminale consists predominantly of pia mater, and this structure marks the line of the regressing spinal cord. The nerves that leave the spinal column angle inferiorly, like wisps of coarse hair flowing from the end of the cord (cauda equina). Distally, the filum is attached to the periosteum of the first coccygeal vertebra.

CLINICAL NOTES | **SPINA BIFIDA**

Neural tube defects result from the failure of normal fusion of the neural plate to form the neural tube during the first 28 days of development. However, another hypothesis has been proposed: that the defect(s) are due to the 'splitting' of the already closed neural tube, as a result of an abnormal increase in cerebrospinal fluid pressure during the first 12 weeks of gestation.

The term spina bifida denotes non-fusion of the primordial halves of the vertebral arches, which is common in all types of spina bifida. Spina bifida is classified into two types: spina bifida occulta and spina bifida cystica.

Spina bifida occulta is due to failure of fusion of the vertebral arches. There may be associated overlying skin lesions, a tuft of hair, a birthmark or a small dermal sinus in the lumbar region. There may be tethering of the underlying cord, or no obvious external anomaly, with the lesion detected incidentally later in life.

Spina bifida cystica refers to a visible defect with an external sac-like protrusion. The two major forms of spina bifida cystica are *meningocele*, in which the meninges and cerebrospinal fluid are encased and is the rarer form of the condition, and *myelomeningocele*—'myelo' refers to the spinal cord and/or the nerve roots contained within the sac.

Meningocele and myelomeningocele are malformations that tend to be quite severe and account for approximately 90% of spinal cord lesions, which may be located at any point along the length of the spinal column. Usually the 'sac' or the lesion is encased within a fine membrane that may leak cerebrospinal fluid. Equally the sac or lesion may be covered by dura, meninges or skin. Most myelomeningocele lesions are located in the lumbar or lumbosacral area, and the magnitude of the lesion dictates the extent of the impairment.

REFLEXES

A reflex is a fast, involuntary, unplanned sequence of physiological actions and responses that occur in response to a stimulus. Some reflexes are innate or inborn, whereas others are acquired or learned responses.

When integration takes place in the spinal cord grey matter, the reflex is referred to as a spinal reflex. However, if the integration occurs in the brainstem, the reflex is a cranial reflex. Somatic reflexes involve the contraction of skeletal muscles, and autonomic visceral reflexes involve responses of smooth muscles and glands.

Some reflexes persist into adulthood, for example the blink reflex; other reflexes are referred to as adaptive reflexes as they are critical for the infant's survival (Bee & Boyd 2004). These gradually disappear over the first year of life; examples are the Moro, sucking and rooting reflexes. However, newborn infants have a large collection of primitive reflexes that are controlled by the medulla and the midbrain, both of which are close to being fully developed at birth (Bee & Boyd 2004).

DEVELOPMENT OF THE SPINAL GANGLIA

The unipolar neurones in the spinal ganglia (swelling or knot), otherwise referred to as the dorsal root ganglia, are derived from neural crest cells. Initially, the axons of cells in the ganglia are bipolar, soon merging to form a 'T' shape. The *peripheral processes* of the spinal ganglia are dendrites that conduct towards the cell body; they pass in the spinal nerves to sensory endings in visceral or somatic structures. The *central processes* of the spinal ganglia enter the spinal cord and form the dorsal roots of the spinal nerves.

MYELINATION OF NERVE FIBRES

During the latter part of fetal development, myelin sheaths in the spinal cord begin to form and continue to develop for the first year of life. Furthermore, the myelination of fibres is associated with the time that the fibres become functional as the child is developing.

Spinal sheaths surround the axon of the nerve fibres. By approximately 28 weeks gestation, nerve fibres have taken on a whitish appearance resulting from the deposition of myelin. Myelin is a multilayered, white, phospholipid, segmented covering; the function of myelin is to increase the speed of nerve impulses. Axons with this covering are myelinated, and those without the myelin are referred to as unmyelinated.

Myelin is responsible for the colour of the white matter in the brain, nerves and spinal cord. The myelin sheath of axons in the peripheral nervous system is produced by neurolemmocytes or Schwann cells, which are located along the axon of the nerve fibre. The neurolemma found in the peripheral nervous system assists in the regeneration of injured axons and dendrites.

Nerve growth factor is a protein hormone that is found in many tissues and is critical for the survival and development of sensory and peripheral sympathetic neurones. The sensory neurones are stimulated by nerve growth factor for only a short period during fetal development.

DEVELOPMENT OF THE PERIPHERAL NERVOUS SYSTEM

The peripheral nervous system develops from various sources, but mostly from neural crest cells. It can be divided into an afferent and efferent system. The afferent (*ad* = toward; *fero* = to carry) system consists of nerve cells that convey information from receptors in the periphery of the body to the central nervous system. The efferent (*effero* = to bring out) system consists of nerve cells that convey information from the central nervous system to muscles and glands. The efferent nervous system is subdivided into somatic (*soma* = body) and the autonomic (*auto* = self; *nomos* = law) nervous systems.

DEVELOPMENT OF THE AUTONOMIC NERVOUS SYSTEM

The section of the nervous system that is responsible for the regulation of smooth muscle, cardiac muscle and some glands is the autonomic nervous system, which is regulated by higher centres in the brain, particularly the cerebral cortex, hypothalamus and medulla oblongata. Therefore, the autonomic nervous system is neither structurally nor functionally independent from the central nervous system. The autonomic nervous system is divided into two parts:

- the sympathetic nervous system
- the parasympathetic nervous system.

During week 5 of embryological development, neural crest cells in the thoracic region migrate along either side of the spinal cord forming cellular masses (ganglia). These are sympathetic ganglia that are arranged as segments connected by a chain of nerve fibres. These sympathetic trunks forms axons located in the intermediolateral cell column (lateral horn). Sympathetic trunks are composed of ascending and descending fibres because of the routes that the fibres travel.

The preganglionic parasympathetic fibres arise from neurones in nuclei located in the brainstem and sacral region of the spinal cord. Postganglionic neurones are located in peripheral plexuses near, or within, the structure to be innervated. The majority of organs of the body are supplied by both sympathetic and parasympathetic nerves, which oppose each other in a finely balanced way to ensure optimal functioning of organs (Waugh & Grant 2001).

FUNCTIONS OF THE NERVOUS SYSTEM

The complex activities of the nervous system can be organized into three fundamental functions:

- sensory functions
- integrative functions
- motor functions.

Sensory functions	Sensory receptors detect internal stimuli. Neurones convey information from the cranial and spinal nerves to the brain and spinal cord, or from lower to higher levels of the spinal cord or brain.
Integrative functions	The nervous system processes sensory information; the neurones involved in this are called interneurones and they comprise the vast majority of neurones in the body.
Motor functions	Motor functions involve responding to the integrative functions, and both afferent and efferent neurones are involved. Motor neurones convey information from the brain towards the spinal cord, or out of the brain and spinal cord into the cranial or spinal nerves.

GROWTH AND MATURATION OF THE BRAIN AND NERVOUS SYSTEM

Although the human brain is formed before birth, with most of the structure formed but not fully developed or matured, it continues to develop for at least 20 years. There are four recognized developmental stages:

- prenatal
- birth to 5 years
- 5–10 years
- 10–20 years.

Specific developmental skills are attained and developed at each stage (Blows 2003).

The stage from birth to 5 years marks a rapid physical development occurring within the substance of the brain. The maturity of the brain is most advanced in the brainstem and least advanced in the cerebral cortex, which is thin and histologically more primitive at birth. Brainstem maturity is critical so that the newborn infant can sustain life with vital functions (Bee & Boyd 2004, Blows 2003).

The brain is composed of 100 billion cells, and the brain of a newborn infant weighs approximately 350 g, accounting for approximately 20% of bodyweight, compared with a 9 week fetus where the brain comprises 25% of bodyweight and 2% in the adult (Sinclair & Dangerfield 1998). The relative proportion of the brain in comparison to bodyweight decreases as development ensues, and males have slightly heavier brains than females. The brain doubles its weight in the first year of life, and 90% of its adult size is achieved by the age of 5 years, after which time brain growth slows down and progressively achieves adult size by the age of 10 years.

The velocity curve for the weight of the whole brain parallels that of head volume and reaches a peak at 32 weeks gestation. The early development of the brain, compared with that of most other organs, means that from early fetal life the brain weight is closer to the adult value than that of any other organ, with the exception of the eye.

Development within the brain reflects the fact that brain growth is in 'spurts'; each of these spurts is closely associated with particular aspects of development. There are short growth spurts at 1-month intervals until the infant is aged 5 months. As the infant continues to develop, periods of brain growth become longer with spurts occurring at 8, 12 and 20 months. Between the ages of 2 and 4 years, growth is slow, with a major brain growth spurt at 4 years (Bee & Boyd 2004). Neurophysiologists have associated these spurts in brain activity with the achievement of cognitive milestones.

Two major growth spurts occur within the brain during *middle childhood*, usually between the ages of 6 and 8 years, and are closely associated with improvements in fine motor skills and eye–hand coordination. The second spurt occurs at approximately 10–12 years of age when the frontal lobes of the cerebral cortex undergo further development. This manifests in the cognitive processes of logic and the ability to plan—cognitive skills that improve dramatically with the associated development of the cortex.

During the *teenage years* there are two brain growth spurts. The first occurs between the ages of 13 and 15 (Spreen et al 1995). It is during this time that more energy is produced and consumed, and, for the most part, this occurs in the parts of the brain that control perception and motor function (Bee 1997, Bee & Boyd 2004). The second brain growth spurt declares itself at approximately 17 years and continues into adulthood; the primary focus of this spurt is in the frontal lobes of the cerebral cortex.

Synaptogenesis is another feature of brain growth, and is the process whereby connections or synapses (a junction between two neurones) are created as a result of the growth of axons and dendrites. Synaptogenesis occurs rapidly in the cerebral cortex during the first 2 years of life, and results in the brain tripling its birthweight. This initial burst of synaptogenesis is followed by the process of 'pruning', which makes the nervous system more efficient. Synaptogenesis and pruning are heavily dependent upon the child's individual experiences, which stimulate neural pathways. The stimulation leaves behind a chemical signal or marker that is strengthened every time the pathway is stimulated. There appears to be a physiological 'ceiling' or threshold whereby neural connections that reach this critical point can no longer be pruned, and become a permanent part of the brain's architecture (Bee 1997, Bee & Boyd 2004).

Myelination is another crucial process in neural development and maturation. This process follows a cephalocaudal and proximodistal patterning, whereby the nerves supplying the muscles in the upper extremities are myelinated earlier than those supplying the limbs in the lower extremities. Myelination is most rapid during the first 2 years of life, and continues more slowly throughout childhood and adolescence. The neurones of 'association' (motor, sensory and cognitive functions) are largely myelinated by the time the child starts school, and nerve cells in these areas are completely myelinated between 6 and 12 years of age. Progression of myelination contributes to the increased speed of information processing, and may also link into memory (Bee & Boyd 2004). Furthermore, this may also be closely associated with maturation of the hippocampus, which is myelinated in childhood (Rolls 2000, Tanner 1990).

At birth, the *spinal cord* is approximately 15–18 cm long, whereas the adult spinal cord achieves a length in the order of 45 cm. In the infant, the cord extends opposite either the second or the third lumbar vertebra, which is approximately one vertebra lower than in the adult (Sinclair & Dangerfield 1998).

DEVELOPMENT OF THE ENDOCRINE SYSTEM

The endocrine system consists of glands that are widely separated from one another with no direct anatomical links. The glands consist of secretory cells surrounded by a network of capillaries that facilitate the diffusion of hormones (Waugh & Grant 2001). A hormone (*hormon* = excite, or get moving) is a mediator molecule that is released in one part of the body but regulates activity in another part. The influence of the endocrine system is diverse and widespread, as it helps to regulate virtually all types of tissue cells in the body (Tortora & Grabowski 2003).

Two types of gland exist within the system: *endocrine* and *exocrine* glands. Exocrine (*exo* = outside) glands secrete into ducts that carry the secretions into the body cavities, for example sudoriferous (sweat) glands, digestive glands, mucous and sebaceous (oil) glands. In contrast, the endocrine glands secrete their products into the interstitial fluid.

The endocrine system is composed of:

- pituitary gland
- thyroid gland
- parathyroid glands (4)

- adrenal glands (suprarenal) (2)
- pancreatic islets
- pineal gland
- ovaries (female gonads) (2)
- testes (male gonads) (2)
- placenta.

DEVELOPMENT OF THE PITUITARY GLAND

The pituitary gland (hypophysis cerebri), or 'master gland', is ectodermal in origin and originates from two sources: an upgrowth from the ectodermal roof of the stomoderm (the hypophyseal pouch) and a downgrowth from the neuroectoderm of the diencephalon (the neurohypophyseal bud). The double embryonic origin of the pituitary gland accounts for the reason why the gland is composed of two different tissue types. The glandular element, known as the adenohypophysis, arises from ectoderm, and the nervous element arises from the neuroectoderm.

During week 4 of gestation, at approximately 24 days, the hypophyseal or Rathke pouch (a diverticulum from the primitive mouth) projects from the stomadeum and lies adjacent to the diencephalon (Fig. 4.8). By week 5 the pouch has elongated and become constricted at its attachment to the oral epithelium, giving it a 'nipple-like' appearance (Moore & Persaud 1998). The stalk of Rathke's pouch, which connects the developing structures, degenerates and disappears during

Fig. 4.8
Hypophyseal pouch (Rathke pouch).

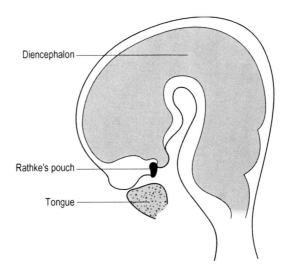

Diencephalon

Rathke's pouch

Tongue

week 6 of gestation. The parts of the gland that form Rathke's pouch are the glandular portions collectively referred to as the anterior lobe or adenohypophysis:

- pars anterior
- pars intermedia
- pars tuberalis.

The pars nervosa infundibulum (stem), a median eminence, gives rise to the posterior lobe or neurohypophysis.

DEVELOPMENT OF THE THYROID GLAND

The thyroid gland is the first endocrine gland to develop, developing from a median endodermal thickening in the floor of the primordial pharynx. This thickening forms a pouch known as the thyroid diverticulum. As the embryo and the embryonic tongue develop, the thyroid gland descends into the neck, and for a short time the tongue and the developing thyroid are connected by the thyroglossal duct (Fig. 4.9).

The primitive thyroid is hollow and, as it solidifies, it divides into lobes that are connected by a structure referred to as the isthmus. By 7 weeks gestation the embryonic thyroid gland has assumed a definitive shape and usually has reached the terminal site within the neck. During week 11 of gestation, colloid begins to appear in the thyroid gland follicles, and subsequently iodine is concentrated and the synthesis of hormones can be facilitated.

Fig. 4.9
Tract of thyroglossal duct.

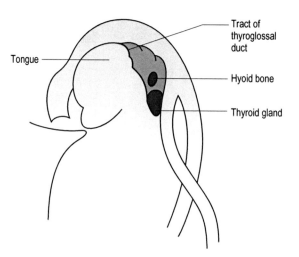

HYPOTHYROIDISM

There is minimal thyroxine transfer from mother to fetus, and the fetal thyroid predominantly produces 'reverse T3', a derivative of T3 that is largely inactive.

After birth, there is a surge in the level of thyroid stimulating hormone, which is accompanied by a marked rise in T4 and T3 levels. Preterm infants may have low levels of T3 and T4 for the first few weeks of life until their thyroid stimulating hormone is within the normal range (Lissauer & Clayden 2001).

Hypothyroidism can be congenital or acquired, and occurs in 1 : 4000 births (Lissauer & Clayden 2001, Smart & Nolan 2000). Causes may include:

- athyrosis
- maldescent of the thyroid
- dishormonogenesis
- iodine deficiency
- thyroid stimulating hormone deficiency.

DEVELOPMENT OF THE PARATHYROID GLANDS

The endodermal epithelial lining of the pharyngeal pouches gives rise to the parathyroid (*para* = beside) glands in the neck.

The third and fourth pharyngeal pouches expand and develop solid bulbar formations with associated elongated ventral structures. A hollow duct forms within the connection between the pharyngeal pouch and the pharynx, but degenerates shortly after development. By 6 weeks gestation the embryological inferior parathyroid glands have developed. The superior parathyroid glands develop from the fourth pharyngeal pouch, and development generally reflects the same pattern as for the inferior parathyroid glands.

Mature parathyroid glands contain two types of epithelial cell. The chief (principal) cells are the most abundant and produce parathyroid hormone; the second cells, oxyphils, are less plentiful and their specific functions are unknown.

DEVELOPMENT OF THE THYMUS GLAND

The thymus gland is located behind the sternum, between the lungs (Fig. 4.10), and has a central role in relation to immunity (see Ch. 10).

Fig. 4.10
Location of the thymus gland.

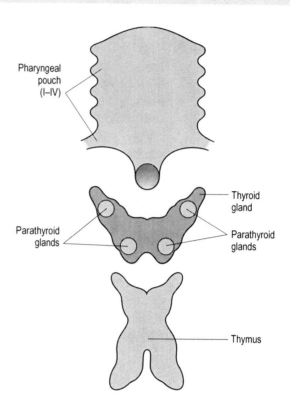

The primordia of the thymus gland originates from behind the third pharyngeal pouch when the bilateral primordia of the thymus fuse in the midline and form the bilobed thymus gland. This is a lymphatic organ, and during week 9 of gestation lymphocytes appear in the tissue. This organ is incomplete at birth; it is quite large and the shape is variable. The gland may have no lobulations, or may be bilobar or trilobar at birth. The functions of the gland are important for the development of the white pulp of the spleen and the immunological development of the infant. During puberty, the thymus reduces in size and is barely recognizable in adulthood.

DEVELOPMENT OF THE PINEAL GLAND (EPIPHYSIS CEREBRI)

The pineal gland, so called because it is shaped like a pine cone, develops as a median diverticulum in the roof of the diencephalon. The gland is covered by a capsule of pia mater and consists of masses of neuroglial cells and parenchymal secretory cells known as pinealocytes. Calcium deposited in the gland is referred to as 'brain sand' – or 'pineal sand'. The pineal gland secretes melatonin, which appears to inhibit reproductive activity by inhibiting gonadotrophic hormones.

Melatonin is released on a 24-hour cycle of activity and inactivity, determined by internal mechanisms. There is some evidence to suggest that the pineal gland produces a second hormone, adrenoglomerulotrophin, which may stimulate the adrenal cortex; however, the physiology of the gland is still unclear.

DEVELOPMENT OF THE ADRENAL GLANDS

The paired adrenal glands have a flattened, pyramid shape; each gland is situated superior to the kidney (see Ch. 8). The cortex and the medulla of the adrenal (suprarenal) glands have different embryological origins. The adrenal cortex is derived from the mesothelial lining of the posterior abdominal wall, and the adrenal medulla is derived from adjacent sympathetic ganglion. The fetal adrenal glands are 10 to 20 times larger relative to weight than the adult glands, and the large adrenal cortex accounts for this. The adrenal cortex produces steroid hormones that are essential for life, and the medulla produces catecholamines.

DEVELOPMENT OF THE PANCREATIC ISLETS

The pancreas (*pan* = all; *creas* = flesh) is described as both an endocrine and an exocrine gland associated with digestion (see Ch. 7). Anatomically, the mature pancreas is located in the curve of the duodenum. It is a flat organ consisting of three parts: head, body and tail.

Embryologically, the majority of the pancreas is derived from the dorsal pancreatic duct and appears before the ventral pancreatic bud. Insulin production begins at week 10 of gestation.

DEVELOPMENT OF THE GONADS: OVARIES AND TESTES

Gonads are the organs of reproduction that produce gametes: oocytes in the female and sperm in the male. The gonads are also affiliated with the respective reproductive systems (see Ch. 9). Embryos with a Y chromosome develop testes, and embryos without the Y chromosome bear genes for the development of ovaries. The gonads normally develop more slowly in female embryos than in male embryos, and the ovary is not usually identifiable until week 10 of gestation.

Chromosomal and genetic sex of an embryo is determined at fertilization; however, the morphological sex characteristics do not develop until week 7 of embryological development. Initially both the male and female systems are similar in development and this initial period is referred to as the 'indifferent stage of sexual development'.

Characteristically the ovaries produce several steroid hormones, including oestrogen and oestradiol; the male gonads produce male sex hormones including testosterone and androgen.

THE ROLE OF THE PLACENTA IN FETAL ENDOCRINE FUNCTION

The syncytiotrophoblast of the placenta synthesizes proteins and steroid hormones using precusors from the fetus and/or the mother. Not only does the placenta play a major role in the production of progesterone and oestrogen, but several hormones are synthesized by the placenta including:

- human chorionic gonadotrophin
- human chorionic somatomammotrophin
- human placental lactogen
- human chorionic thyrotrophin
- human chorionic corticotrophin.

MATURATION AND DEVELOPMENT OF THE ENDOCRINE SYSTEM

At birth the *pituitary gland* is quite large and weighs in the order of 100 mg. It grows at a steady pace, but there are subtle differences in the growth rate and development between the sexes. The anterior lobe of the female pituitary gland is larger than that of the male gland. The *parathyroid glands* are simple structures with one type of secretory cell dominant until the age of 5 or 6 years when a second cell type emerges—oxyphils, whose functions are unclear. The rate of growth of children is governed largely by thyroid hormones and pituitary growth hormone. Thyroid hormone is secreted in greater quantities during the first 2 years of life, after which time the level decreases to a lower level, which remains fairly constant until the time of puberty (Tanner 1989, 1990).

The *thymus gland* has a dual role of endocrine and lymphoid activities, and is the largest gland in the body of the newborn infant, relative to bodyweight and size (Sinclair & Dangerfield 1998). After puberty the thymus diminishes in endocrine activity, but during adulthood it produces thymic hormones.

The *pineal gland* is most active during early childhood. It is responsible for the synthesis of melatonin, which is produced mostly at night. From middle adulthood, calcium is deposited in the cells of the pineal gland, and referred to as 'brain sand' – or 'pineal sand'.

The growth of the *adrenal glands* is comparative to the growth curve of the uterus, but for different reasons. At birth the adrenal glands undergo changes as the adrenal cortex grows rapidly and, in doing so, this changes the structure of the gland. The glands lose approximately one-third of their weight in the first month of life; however, at 3 months the thick cortex begins to regress and a thinner permanent cortex is established. The glands do not begin to develop in size until 2 years of age, and do not regain their birthweight until puberty.

SELF ASSESSMENT

Answer the following questions in relation to your area of professional practice:

- List the major structures in the central (CNS), peripheral (PNS) and autonomic (ANS) nervous systems.
- Compare and contrast the functions of these systems.
- Define the terms endocrine and exocrine.
- List the major structures in the endocrine system.
- Describe the physiological relationship between the nervous system and the endocrine system in maintaining homeostasis.
- Reflect upon this chapter and consider how your new knowledge may be applied to your area of professional practice in caring for children and their families.

References

Bee H 1997 The developing child, 8th edn. HarperCollins, New York

Bee H, Boyd D 2004 The developing child, 10th edn. Allyn Bacon, Boston

Blows W T 2003 Child brain development. Nursing Times 99:28–30

Jeffrey N 2002 Differential regional brain growth and rotation of the prenatal human tentorium cerebelli. Journal of Anatomy 200:135–144

Lissauer T, Clayden G 2001 Illustrated textbook of paediatrics, 2nd edn. Mosby, London

Matsumura G, England M A 1992 Embryology colouring book. Wolfe, London

Moore K L, Persaud T V N 1998 Before we are born: essentials of embryology and birth defects. W B Saunders, London

Rolls E 2000 Memory systems in the brain. Annual Review of Psychology 51:599–630

Sinclair D, Dangerfield P 1998 Human growth after birth, 6th edn. Oxford University Press, Oxford

Slater A, Lewis M 2002 Introduction to infant development. Oxford University Press, Oxford

Smart J, Nolan T 2000 Paediatric handbook, 6th edn. Blackwell Science, London

Spreen O, Risser A, Edgell D 1995 Developmental neuropsychology. Oxford University Press, Oxford

Tanner J M 1989 Foetus into man: physical growth from conception to maturity, 2nd edn. Castlemead Publications, Hertford

Tanner J M 1990 Foetus into man: physical growth from conception to maturity, 2nd edn. Harvard University Press, Cambridge, MA

Tortora G J, Grabowski S R 2003 Principles of anatomy and physiology, 10th edn. John Wiley, New York

Waugh A, Grant A 2001 Ross and Wilson anatomy and physiology in health and illness, 9th edn. Churchill Livingstone, London

Wong D L 1999 Whaley and Wong's nursing care of children, 6th edn. Mosby, London

Bibliography

Bee H, Boyd D 2003 The developing child, 10th edn. Allyn and Bacon, Boston

Campbell S, Glasper A (eds) 1995 Whaley and Wong's children's nursing. Mosby, London

Candy D, Davies G, Ross E 2001 Clinical paediatrics and child health. W B Saunders, London

Crawford D, Hickinson W 2002 An introduction to neonatal nursing, 2nd edn. Nelson Thornes, Cheltenham

Meadow R, Newell S 2002 Lecture notes on paediatrics. Blackwell Science, London

Sweet B 1999 Maye's midwifery, 12th edn. Baillière Tindall, London

Watson R 2002 Anatomy and physiology for nurses, 11th edn. Baillière Tindall, London

Chapter 5

Development of the cardiovascular system

Pauline Carson

CHAPTER OUTCOMES

This chapter will enable the reader to:

- Identify the various stages of development in the heart, veins and arteries
- Outline the circulation in the primitive heart
- Outline the circulation in the fetal heart prior to birth
- Identify the changes that take place in the circulation immediately after birth
- Describe the normal development of the conduction system
- Describe what happens during the cardiac cycle
- Define cardiac output and identify the factors that affect it
- Identify the cardiac abnormalities associated with the various stages of cardiac and vasculature development.

CHAPTER OVERVIEW

The aim of this chapter is to describe the normal embryonic and fetal development of the cardiovascular system. The chapter discusses normal embryological anatomy and physiology, and outlines the changes that take place in the circulation after birth. Clinical Notes address issues of clinical relevance and interest to the reader, and Self Assessment exercises assist in reflecting upon the chapter and guiding the relationship between theory and professional practice.

INTRODUCTION

The cardiovascular system is extremely important in early development and, with blood beginning to circulate by the end of the third week, it is one of the first systems to function in the embryo. As the embryo grows during the third week it reaches a size whereby diffusion, which provides the necessary nutrients and removal of waste products, is no longer adequate. Early development of the heart and circulatory system is therefore imperative to provide an efficient method for the rapidly growing embryo to acquire oxygen and nutrients and to dispose of carbon dioxide and waste products. As such, the heart and circulatory system must grow and develop while at the same time remain fully functional, so that it keeps pace with the growing embryo to meet the needs and demands of the embryo's cells (Carlson 1999).

Functionally the embryonic fetal heart only needs to act as a pump to ensure that blood flows through the embryo, to allow for the exchange of nutrients and oxygen from placenta to fetus and of waste products from fetus to placenta. However, of equal importance is the need to cope with the underdeveloped fetal lungs in utero while anticipating the changes that will occur in the circulation at birth and the complex requirements of the cardiovascular and circulatory system postnatally.

THE EARLIEST DEVELOPMENT OF THE CIRCULATORY SYSTEM

The early development of the cardiovascular system corresponds to the rapid growth of the embryo and the lack of yolk in the yolk sac in the third week. The migration of heart-forming mesoderm through the primitive streak to form bilateral areas of precardiac splanchnic mesoderm signals the earliest aspect of heart and circulatory development (Carlson 1999). The cells that pass through the cranial part will eventually contribute to the development of the outflow tract of the heart, whereas those passing through the posterior part will contribute to the inflow tract (Carlson 1999). It is from these bilateral areas of embryonic mesoderm that the heart and great vessels will develop. The blood and blood vessels have a different origin initially developing in the extra-embryonic mesoderm in the lining of the yolk sac and then in the embryonic mesoderm. It is important to note that, at the same time as the heart is beginning to form in the embryo, many of the major blood vessels are also developing simultaneously.

THE HEART During week 3 of gestation, two tubes begin to develop in a horseshoe-shaped area of embryonic mesoderm known as the *cardiogenic area*.

These two endocardial tubes are initially situated on either side of the foregut, and are brought into the thoracic region when the lateral and cephalic folding of the embryo occurs late in the third week. The tubes then fuse together to form a single heart tube (Larsen 2001).

THE VASCULAR SYSTEM

Initially the embryo obtains nutrition from maternal blood via diffusion across the extraembryonic coelom and the yolk sac. However, this is soon rendered inadequate by the rapid development of the embryo and the increased need for nourishment and oxygen from the maternal circulation. The first evidence of blood vessel formation (*vasculogenesis* and *angiogenesis*) occurs at the beginning of the third week in the extraembryonic mesoderm of the yolk sac, connecting stalk and chorion, with embryonic blood vessel formation beginning at the end of the third week. The yolk sac supplies the first blood cells to the embryonic circulation (Moore & Persaud 2003).

By the end of the third week, this early vascular system and the heart tube have linked up. At the same time the heart begins to beat and blood starts to circulate, resulting in a functioning primitive cardiovascular system—the first system to reach this state (Moore & Persaud 2003).

BLOOD FORMATION

Extraembryonic blood cell production begins on day 17 in the splanchnopleuric mesoderm of the yolk sac where mesenchyme cells developing next to the endoderm, aggregate and cluster together to form blood islands (Fig. 5.1) and then segregate into a core of cells

Fig. 5.1
The early stages of blood cell production and blood vessel development. Blood cell production and blood vessel formation occurs on day 17 in the yolk sac with the formation of blood islands
A blood islands;
B blood cell formation;
C blood cells develop from the endothelial cells of the primitive vessels.
(Adapted from Moore & Persaud 2003.)

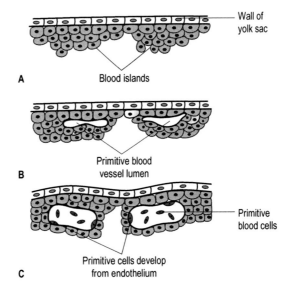

called haemoblasts. These haemoblasts, which are surrounded by flat endothelial cells form the first embryo blood cells while the outer flat endothelial cells develop into blood vessel endothelium (see Blood vessel formation). Blood cells and a primitive form of plasma develop from the endothelial cells of the vessels situated in the walls of the yolk sac and **allantois** and up until week 4 the only blood cells produced are red cells.

Blood cell production in the embryo begins in week 5 in the embryonic yolk sac and then in the liver in week 6. As the embryo grows blood begins to form in the spleen at two and a half months, and at the same time the liver also begins to produce coagulation factors. Blood also begins to form in the bone marrow between two and three months. The source of the haematopoietic stem cells that populate these organs however still remains an enigma (Larsen 1998). By the time of birth all blood formation in the liver and spleen has stopped and **haemopoiesis** takes place in the red marrow of all the bones of the skeleton (Carlson 1999).

The main function of the red blood cells is to transport haemoglobin, which in turn carries oxygen to the cells of the developing fetus. In fetal circulation the red cells contain a particular type of haemoglobin, *fetal haemoglobin*. This haemoglobin has a much greater affinity for oxygen than the normal haemoglobin found in red blood cells after birth, and is therefore suited to the fetal environment (Hockenberry 2003) where oxygen is transferred via the placenta from the maternal circulation. Oxygen saturation in maternal blood in the placenta is at a much lower concentration than in the atmosphere, and thus, if it were not for the greater affinity of fetal haemoglobin for oxygen, the fetus might suffer hypoxia. During the latter part of fetal development, the fetus also begins developing adult haemoglobin.

FURTHER DEVELOPMENT OF THE CARDIOVASCULAR SYSTEM

BLOOD VESSEL FORMATION

Extraembryonic blood vessel formation, like blood, occurs on day 17 in the splanchnopleuric mesoderm of the yolk sac, developing from the same blood islands as the blood (Fig. 5.1). These islands segregate into a core of cells called *haemoblasts*, surrounded by flat endothelial cells (see Blood formation), and it these outer flat endothelial cells that develop into blood vessel endothelium. These early primitive vessels then fuse together forming a network of channels that grow and interconnect, like a river delta, thereby creating an initial vascular network wherein, by the end of the third week, the yolk sac, the connecting stalk

Fig. 5.2
Development of the aortic arches.
A In all 6 arches develop, the first regress as later arches are formed.
B The primitive pattern of aortic arches is transformed into an adult formation during weeks 6–8.
(Adapted from Moore & Persaud 2003.)

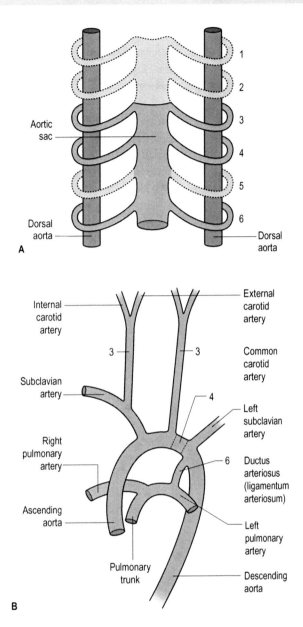

and the chorionic villi are completely vascularized (Larsen 2001). The vessels developing on the yolk sac are known as *vitelline vessels*; they include both arteries and veins, and will eventually supply and drain the gut. Those vessels developing in the connecting stalk and chorion are called *umbilical and chorionic vessels* respectively. The umbilical vessels include the umbilical arteries that will carry deoxygenated blood from the embryo to the placenta, and the umbilical vein that will carry oxygenated blood from the placenta to the embryo.

Embryonic blood vessel formation includes development of both the arterial system and the venous system, with the latter beginning development on day 18 in the splanchopleuric mesoderm of the embryonic disc. Cells within the mesoderm (*angioblasts*) that develop into flattened endothelial cells join together and form *angiocysts*, which in turn form a network of vessels throughout the embryonic disc called angioblastic *cords*. This network of angioblastic cords, or the *angioplastic plexus*, forms the embryo's initial circulatory system, growing and spreading throughout the embryo in the following ways:

- angiocysts continuing to form and fuse
- new vessels budding and sprouting from existing angioblastic cords (*angiogenesis*)
- insertion of angioblasts into existing vessel walls (Larsen 2001).

DEVELOPMENT OF THE ARTERIAL SYSTEM

THE DORSAL AORTA

The two dorsal aortae develop through the process of vasculogenesis in the dorsal mesenchyme of the embryonic disc and will eventually form the outflow tract of the heart. During the early stages of arterial development when the dorsal aortae are still paired, three sets of arterial branches sprout from them: the ventral segmental branches, the

Table 5.1 Major arterial branches of the aorta (Carlson 1999)

Embryonic vessels	Adult derivatives
Dorsal intersegmental branches (paired)	
Cervical intersegmental (1–6)	Lateral branches joining to become vertebral arteries
Seventh intersegmentals	Subclavian arteries
Thoracic intersegmentals	Intercostal arteries
Lumbar intersegmentals	Iliac arteries
Lateral segmental branches	
Up to 20 pairs of vessels supplying the mesonephros	Adrenal arteries, renal arteries, gonadial (ovarian or spermatic) arteries
Ventral segmental branches[a]	
Vitelline vessels	Coeliac artery, superior and inferior mesenteric arteries
Allantoic vessels	Umbilical arteries

[a]Originally paired in areas where the embryonic aorta itself consists of paired components.

dorsal intersegmental branches and the lateral segmental branches (Carlson 1999).

The ventral segmental branches initially fuse with arteries of the vitelline system and the vascular plexus of the future gut as the embryo folds and the yolk sac begins to shrink. Eventually these vessels become disconnected from the yolk sac, forming the arteries that will supply blood to the gastrointestinal tract from the dorsal aorta. The arteries supplying blood to the limbs and vertebrae arise from the dorsal intersegmental branches, whereas those supplying the adrenals, kidneys and gonads arise from the lateral segmental branches (Larsen 2001). All of these branches will undergo further modifications before reaching what is considered to be their adult state. Table 5.1 shows a summary of the embryonic vessels and their adult derivatives.

During week 4, the two dorsal aortae fuse together to form one dorsal aorta, except for the area around the aortic arches where they remain separate. The fused dorsal aortae form the descending thoracic and abdominal parts of the aorta (Fitzgerald & Fitzgerald 1994).

THE AORTIC ARCHES

Prior to embryonic folding, the dorsal aortae connect with the endocardial tubes and then, between days 22 and 24 as the embryo folds, they are pulled until they form a loop called the *dorsoventral loop*, which results in the first pair of aortic arches lying in the thickened mesenchyme of the first pair of pharyngeal arches (Larsen 1998). Four other aortic arches will also develop between days 26 and 29 in their respective pharangeal arches, and in turn will develop into an adult arterial formation. During the fourth week of life, the *pharyngeal arches* develop and receive blood vessels from the heart. These blood vessels that arise from the aortic sac develop via vasculogenesis and angiogenesis within their respective pharyngeal arches (Larsen 2001) and terminate in the dorsal aorta of the corresponding side. These are known as aortic arches.

In all, six aortic arches develop but not all at the same time, as the first two will regress as the later arches form. During weeks 6 to 8, this primitive pattern of aortic arches changes, with some arches disappearing while others transform into an adult arterial formation (Fig. 5.2).

The first and second pairs of aortic arches are the two that disappear, while the proximal part of the third forms the right and left *common carotid arteries*, and the distal part joins with the dorsal aortas to form the proximal part of the right and left *internal carotid arteries*. The distal part of the internal carotid arteries derives from the cranial extensions of the dorsal aortas. The right and left *external carotid arteries* sprout from the common carotid arteries.

Unlike the third aortic arches, the fourth and sixth pairs of aortic arches are remodelled asymmetrically to form different vessels on each side. The fourth arch on the left forms part of the *aortic arch of the aorta*, while the right forms the proximal part of the *right subclavian artery*. The distal part of the right subclavian derives from the right dorsal aorta, while the *left subclavian artery* arises from the left *seventh intersegmental artery*, which itself has sprouted directly from the left dorsal aorta. Likewise, the sixth arch also forms different vessels on each side, with the proximal part of the right forming the proximal part of the *right pulmonary artery*, the distal part degenerating while the proximal part of the left forms the *left pulmonary artery* and the distal part forms the *ductus arteriosus*. This vessel, which connects the pulmonary trunk and the aorta, allows blood to be shunted from the pulmonary artery to the aorta, thus bypassing the lungs, throughout fetal life and closing at birth. The fifth aortic arch and artery, which is often rudimentary and may even be absent, has no derivatives (Moore & Persaud 2003).

CLINICAL NOTES   **ANOMALIES ARISING DURING PHARYNGEAL ARCH DEVELOPMENT**

The pharangeal aortic arch undergoes extensive remodelling as it becomes transformed into the adult arterial pattern. As a result of the many changes that take place during this period of remodelling, a variety of defects can occur. These are usually due to the persistence of parts of the arches that should normally disappear or to the disappearance of parts that should normally remain (Moore & Persaud 2003). These include:

- interrupted aortic arch
- aortic atresia
- vascular ring
- double aortic arch
- anomalous right subclavian artery
- patent ductus arteriosus
- coarctation of the aorta
- right arch aorta.

THE UMBILICAL ARTERIES

The umbilical arteries are among the first arteries to develop. They arise from the connecting stalk during week 4, and initially connect to the ventral segmental branches. In week 5 they then connect to a pair of lumbar intersegmental branches called the *internal iliac arteries*, and the initial ventral segmental connection disappears leaving the intersegmental branches as their primary branch off the aorta

(Larsen 2001). These arteries will carry deoxygenated blood from the embryo to the placenta where carbon dioxide and waste products will be removed.

THE HEAD ARTERIES AND THE CIRCLE OF WILLIS

The arteries that supply the face arise from external carotid arteries, whereas those supplying the brain arise from the internal carotid arteries and the vertebral arteries. As the vertebral arteries grow towards the brain they eventually join together, forming the basilar artery. Pairs of arteries arising from this artery supply the brainstem as it runs along it, and eventually branches from both the basilar artery and the internal carotid artery meet and fuse, thus joining both circulations together. At the same time, two other branches of the internal carotid arteries also fuse, leading to the development of a vascular ring at the base of the brain called the *cerebral arterial circle* or the *circle of Willis* (Carlson 1999). The arteries arising from this circular arrangement supply most of the brain.

CLINICAL NOTES | **FUNCTION OF THE CIRCLE OF WILLIS**

The circle of Willis equalizes blood pressure to the brain and also ensures that there is a continuous blood supply to the brain by providing alternative routes for blood flow should some of the arteries supplying the brain become occluded or damaged (Tortora & Grabowski 2003).

DEVELOPMENT OF THE VENOUS SYSTEM

In the 4-week-old embryo, three sets of veins are draining the heart tube: the umbilical veins, the vitelline veins and the common cardinal veins. Oxygenated blood from the chorion enters the heart via the umbilical veins, while the vitelline veins bring poorly oxygenated blood back from the yolk sac. The intraembryonic cardinal veins return blood from the head and body of the embryo, and are the vessels that will form the basis of the venous circulation in the embryo, the other vessels being primarily extraembryonic (see Blood vessel formation).

CARDINAL VEINS

The cardinal veins are the embryo's main venous drainage system developing initially as a pair of anterior and posterior cardinal veins, draining the head and body parts of the embryo respectively, and joining the common cardinal veins entering the sinus venosus (Moore & Persaud 2003). Remodelling and anastomosis of the anterior cardinal veins leads to the development of the left and right brachiocephalic veins, internal jugular veins and superior vena cava, with the definitive superior vena cava draining blood from both sides of the head, both upper limbs and the thoracic body wall by the end of the eighth week (Larsen 2001).

The posterior cardinal veins are, for the most part, replaced by a pair of subcardinal and supracardinal veins, the remaining remnant of the posterior cardinal veins which are not replaced are remodelled to develop the common iliac veins and the sacral portion of the inferior vena cava with the common iliac veins and the root of the azygos vein, the only adult derivatives of the posterior cardinal veins (Moore & Persaud 2003). The subcardinal veins are the first to appear and will be further developed through an extensive process of anastomosis and remodelling to form the left renal vein, suprarenal veins and gonadal veins, draining the kidneys and gonads respectively and a segment of the inferior vena cava. As the subcardinal veins are being remodelled the supracardinal veins begin to develop. These veins become disrupted in the kidney region (Moore & Persaud 2003) thereby giving rise to separate thoracic and abdominal venous components (Larsen 2001). Remodelling and anastomosis of the supracardinal veins in the thoracic region leads to the development of the azygos and hemiazygos veins while remodelling of the supracardinal veins in the abdominal region results in the formation of the inferior segment of the inferior vena cava.

THE VITELLINE VEINS

The two vitelline veins that arise in the yolk sac drain into the sinus venosus, the venous end of the developing heart. As they pass through the mesenchyme of the septum transversum, they develop channels that connect and anastomose both inside and outside the developing liver. The network of blood vessels developing within the liver forms the hepatic veins, while those outside form the portal vein, which drains the intestines, via the anastomosis of a network of vitelline veins around the duodenum (Moore & Persaud 2003). The part of the right vitelline vein that is closest to the liver disappears, while the superior portion becomes the terminal portion of the IVC. By the end of the third month the left vitelline vein has disappeared completely in the region of the sinus venosus (Larsen 2001).

THE INFERIOR VENA CAVA

The IVC is made up of four segments, all derived from remnants of earlier vitelline and cardinal vein systems. As outlined above, the right vitelline vein becomes the terminal or hepatic segment while the right subcardinal forms the prerenal segment, the part between the liver and the kidneys. The right supracardinal vein gives rise to the renal or abdominal segment, with the sacral or postrenal segment arising from the posterior cardinal veins (Moore & Persaud 2003).

THE UMBILICAL VEINS

As with the vitelline veins, the two umbilical veins also pass through the septum transversum from the placenta to the sinus venosus. During the second month, the right umbilical vein disappears and the left remains. At the same time as the right umbilical vein disappears, the left also loses its connection with the sinus venosus and instead joins to the *ductus venosus* (Larsen 2001). This new channel between the umbilical vein and the IVC allows purified, oxygenated blood from the placenta to be shunted directly through the liver from the umbilical vein into the IVC. In so doing the liver capilliary network is bypassed, thus allowing organs in most need of well oxygenated blood, such as the heart and brain, to receive it.

THE PULMONARY VEINS

Unlike the development of the rest of the venous system, the pulmonary veins do not develop or arise from part of an earlier, more primitive, venous system. Instead they form independently at the beginning of the fourth week when a pulmonary vein sprouts from the left atrium and immediately branches into a right and left pulmonary vein and then bifurcates again forming a total of four vessels. These vessels then grow towards the lungs, where they connect and *anastomose* with veins that are developing in the mesoderm investing the bronchial buds (Larsen 1993). As the left atrium grows and develops during week 5, the common pulmonary vein trunk becomes incorporated into the atrium wall, and eventually the first two branches and then the second two branches are also absorbed into the growing atrium (Carlson 1999). This absorption results in first two and eventually four separate openings of the definitive pulmonary veins into the left atrium.

THE CORONARY VESSELS

The coronary vessels start to develop in week 5 as blood islands in the epicardium of the developing heart. The developing capilliary network then joins with coronary arteries sprouting from special branches of the aorta emerging just above the cusps of the semilunar valves, and with coronary veins that sprout from the coronary sinus (Larsen 1998).

CLINICAL NOTES

ANOMALIES ARISING DURING DEVELOPMENT OF THE ARTERIAL AND VENOUS SYSTEMS

Owing to the many changes that take place during the development and subsequent remodelling of the arterial and venous systems, in order to reach their adult state, variations and anomalies can occur.

Arterial system

- Coractation of the aorta—narrowing of the aorta, which usually occurs just after the junction of the ductus arteriosus (postductal) but can also be proximal to this juncture (preductal). If the coarctation is postductal, the embryo develops other collateral circulation routes during development to allow blood to get to the trunk and lower extremities. This anomaly is more common in males than females; although the cause is unclear, genetic and environmental factors appear to play a role (Moore & Persaud 1998)
- Absence or stenosis of one of the coronary arteries
- Vascular ring and double aortic arch—the right aorta does not regress and surrounds the oesophagus and trachea
- Anomalous right subclavian artery.

Venous system

- Double inferior vena cava—caudal part of the left supracardinal system persists and does not regress, resulting in an abnormal left inferior vena cava (Larsen 1998)
- Double superior vena cava—persistence of left anterior cardinal system
- Anomalous pulmonary venous drainage—the embryonic pulmonary vascular plexus connects with one or more of the great veins and drains blood into the right atrium instead of the left.

DEVELOPMENT OF THE HEART

THE PRIMITIVE HEART

As outlined earlier, the heart begins to develop towards the end of the third week (Fig. 5.3) in a horseshoe-shaped area of splanchnopleuric mesoderm known as the cardiogenic area (Larsen 2001) with the appearance of a pair of endothelial strands called *angioblastic cords* (Moore & Persaud 2003). These two cords or strands of cells, which have formed through the process of vasculogenesis, soon canalize and form two thin-walled endocardial heart tubes (Moore & Persaud

2003) on either side of the foregut. At the same time the two dorsal aortae, which form the outflow tract of the heart, are also developing and will connect with the two heart tubes prior to embryonic folding, which takes place towards the end of the third week. When lateral and cephalic folding of the embryo takes place, the tubes are brought

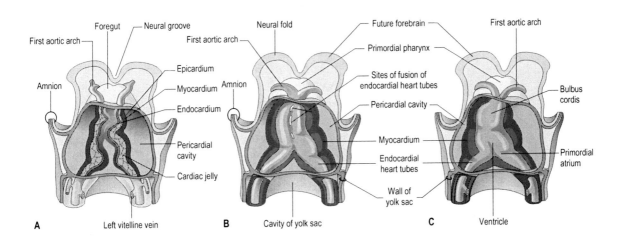

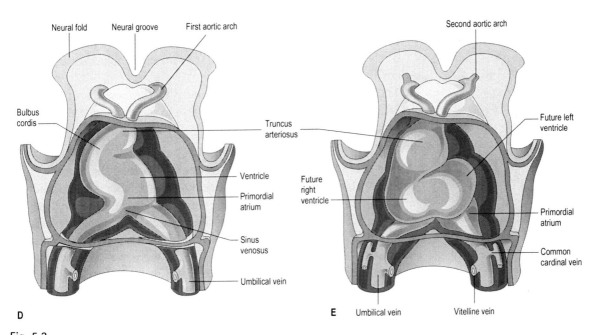

Fig. 5.3
A–C The developing heart and pericardial region days 22–35.
D–E As the heart elongates it forms regional segments and bends upon itself to form an S shape. (From Moore & Persaud 2003, with permission.)

into the thoracic region where they fuse together to form a single tubular heart (Larsen 2001).

Between day 22 and 28 the heart tube expands and elongates, developing areas that dilate and constrict alternately to form distinct regions that will be further developed as the heart is formed. Beginning at the inflow end and working towards the outflow end, these regions of dilatations and constrictions are:

- *Sinus venosus*—a dilatation that opens out into the primitive atrium and consists of left and right sinus horns which receive blood from each side of the body from the cardinal veins, umbilical veins and vitelline veins via the common cardinal veins
- *Primitive atrium*—a dilatation that will eventually give rise to parts of both atria
- *Atrioventricular sulcus*—a constriction separating the primitive atria from the primitive ventricle
- *Primitive ventricle*—a dilatation that will eventually give rise to most of the left ventricle
- *Bulboventricular sulcus* or *interventricular sulcus*—a constriction separating the next dilatation, the bulbus cordis, from the primitive ventricle
- *Bulbus cordis*—a dilatation that will eventually give rise to part of the right ventricle. At its superior end this dilatation, which is called the conotruncus, is the region that will eventually form the distal outflow tract of the right and left ventricles including the conus cordis and the truncus arteriosus
- *Truncus arteriosus*—attached cranially to the aortic sac; its aortic arches will eventually split to give rise to the pulmonary trunk and ascending aorta.

At the same time as the heart tube begins to elongate, constrict and dilate, it also starts to loop and, because it is attached both caudally and cranially, it bends on itself to form a U-shaped loop called the *bulboventricular loop*. As it does so, the bulbus cordis gets displaced to the right, the ventricle to the left and the atrium is carried towards the back of the ventricle (Larsen 2001). Thus, what was once a straight symmetrical structure now becomes the first asymmetrical structure to appear in the embryo (Carlson 1999). By day 26 the truncus arteriosus is visible and the major chambers can be identified with a common atria and common ventricle present. Looping is completed by day 28; the heart has already started to beat and blood is flowing through the primitive heart. Further remodelling, including septation of the atria and ventricles and division of the truncus arteriosus, now takes place.

DEXTROCARDIA

During this period of looping, malpositioning of the heart can occur. One of the most frequent positional abnormalities of the heart is dextrocardia. If the heart tube bends towards the left instead of the right, the heart is displaced to the right and results in transposition, whereby the heart and its vessels are reversed left to right as in a mirror image (Moore & Persaud 2003). When dextrocardia occurs alongside transposition of other organs, such as the liver, it is known as *dextrocardia with situs inversus.* When the abnormal position is not accompanied by displacement of other organs, it is known as *isolated dextrocardia.*

The incidence of accompanying cardiac defects in dextrocardia with situs inversus is low and, as long as there are no other associated vascular abnormalities, these hearts usually function normally. Isolated dextrocardia is usually complicated by severe cardiac anomalies (Moore & Persaud 2003).

THE LAYERS OF THE HEART

The heart tubes are initially made up of endothelium, but as they fuse they are surrounded by a thick mass of splanchnopleuric mesoderm. This differentiates into two layers: an outer layer of *myocardium* or heart muscle, and an inner layer of gelatinous connective tissue called *cardiac jelly.* This gelatinous layer, which is secreted by the outer layer of developing myocardium, separates the myocardium from the endothelial layer of the heart tube, which itself becomes the endothelial layer of the heart called the *endocardium.* The *epicardium* or *visceral pericardium* develops from other splanchnopleuric mesoderm, arising from the area of the sinus venosus and then migrating across the surface of the myocardium (Larsen 2001, Moore & Persaud 2003) (Fig. 5.4).

The myocardium is composed of specialized muscle tissue called cardiac muscle that is found only in the heart. These muscle fibres are in very close contact with one another and are connected by irregular thickenings called *intercalated discs* (Fig. 5.4) containing *desmosomes,* which hold fibres together, and gap junctions, which allow the electrical impulses that stimulate contraction of the heart muscle to conduct from one fibre to the next (Tortora & Grabowski 2003). Thus, when an action potential or electrical impulse is initiated in the sinoatrial node, the pacemaker region of the heart, this arrangement allows it to spread rapidly from cell to cell.

FORMATION OF THE FOUR CHAMBERS OF THE HEART

By the time that looping is completed, around day 28, the primitive heart with its identifiable regions and common atria and ventricle continue to undergo further development and remodelling with the

Fig. 5.4
A The layers of the heart, the inner endocardium layer, a middle muscle layer of myocardium and an outer epicardium layer.
B The myocardium layer is composed of specialist cardiac muscle tissue where the fibres are connected by intercalated discs.

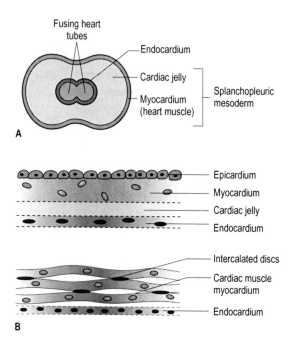

development of endocardial cushions and a septum to form a four-chambered heart, development of the valves and partitioning of the truncus arteriosus. These different processes take place simultaneously, beginning around week 4.

The primitive atrium and ventricle begin to enlarge and expand, and remodelling and development of the sinus venosus occur. The right horn of the sinus venosus, which itself enlarges to keep up with the rapidly growing heart, eventually becomes incorporated into the right atrium forming the smooth portion of the right atrial wall. As it does so it displaces the original right half of the primitive atrial wall, which remains as a rough-walled appendage of the right atrium called the *right auricle*. At the same time the common cardinal veins are undergoing development, so that systemic venous blood enters the right sinus horn via the developing inferior and superior vena cava. As a result of this diminished blood flow, the left horn of the sinus venosus stops growing and becomes the *coronary sinus* (Larsen 2001).

While the right atrium undergoes development during the fourth and fifth week, the left is also developing simultaneously and sprouting a pulmonary vein. As the primitive left atrium enlarges, eventually the trunk and first branches of this pulmonary vein system become incorporated and absorbed into the wall of the left side through a process of intussusception (see The Pulmonary Veins); they then form the smooth-walled part of the left atrium. The primitive atrium is displaced to the left as a result, and remains as the left auricle (Larsen 2001).

While the atria are undergoing further development, the ventricles are also being remodelled and developed. This process involves remodelling of both the primitive ventricle and the bulbus cordis, and is described further under septation of the ventricles and partitioning of the bulbus cordis.

At the same time as the above processes are being carried out, the primitive heart is also being divided into the four chambers of the heart through the formation of endocardial cushions and the simultaneous division of the atria and ventricles.

ENDOCARDIAL CUSHION DEVELOPMENT

The endocardial cushions begin to develop from a proliferation of mesenchymal cells situated on the dorsal and ventral walls in the atrioventricular canal area. As the cushions grow into the canal towards one another they meet and fuse, thereby separating the atrioventricular canal into right and left atrioventricular canals. The lateral cushions that are formed act as primitive atrioventricular valves, which help to propel blood through the heart; however, later in development definitive valves will develop in the region of these endocardial cushions (see Valve formation) (Carlson 1999).

CLINICAL NOTES

ANOMALIES ARISING DURING ENDOCARDIAL CUSHION DEVELOPMENT

Defects that may occur during endocardial cushion development include:

- ostium primum atrial septal defects
- ventricular septal defects
- anomalies of the tricuspid and mitral valves
- complete atrioventricular septal defects.

ATRIAL AND VENTRICULAR PARTITIONING

While the endocardial cushions are taking shape, partially separating the atrium from the ventricles, other structural formations and changes are also taking place to divide and partition the primitive atrium and the ventricle into two separate atria and ventricles.

THE ATRIA

Partitioning of the primitive atrium (Fig. 5.5) begins in week 5 when a crescent-shaped membrane called the *septum primum* grows from the dorsal wall towards the atrioventricular canal. As it grows, the gap formed between its free end and the endocardial cushions is known as the *ostium primum* or *foramen primum*. This gap acts as a shunt, allowing blood to pass from the right to left side of the heart, but it reduces and disappears as the septum primum grows towards and eventually fuses with the endocardial cushions. Just before the ostium primum closes, however, small perforations appear on the septum primum, as

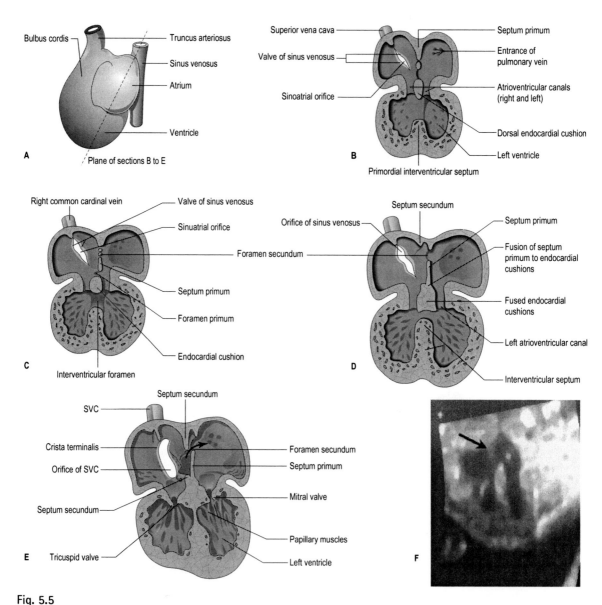

Fig. 5.5
Partitioning of the heart.
A Plane of sections B-E.
B-D Partitioning of the atrioventricular canal, primordial atrium and ventricle from about days 28–35.
E About 8 weeks showing the heart after it is partitioned into 4 chambers.
F Sonogram of 2nd trimester fetus showing the 4 chambers of the heart. (From Moore & Persaud 2003, with permission of W B Saunders.)

a result of genetically programmed cell death, and join together to form a new opening called the *ostium secundum* or *foramen secundum*, thereby creating a new opening for blood to pass from the right to the left side (Moore & Persaud 2003).

At the same time as the septum primum is growing, another crescent-shaped membrane grows from the ventrocranial wall (the ceiling) of the atrium on the right side of the septum primum. This is a thicker and more muscular membrane than the septum primum, and it grows into the atrium gradually overlapping the foramen secundum before stopping and leaving a gap between its free end and the dorsal wall (floor) of the right atrium, the *foramen ovale*. The remains of the septum primum then form the flap-like valve of the foramen ovale (Moore & Persaud 2003).

Throughout the remainder of fetal development and up until birth, the foramen ovale allows most of the blood entering the right atrium to pass from the right atrium to the left atrium through two staggered openings: the foramen ovale itself at the bottom of the right atrium and the foramen secundum near the roof of the left atrium (Larsen 2001). After birth, the foramen ovale closes and the interatrial septum becomes completely closed (see discussion on changes in circulation).

CLINICAL NOTES | **ATRIAL SEPTAL DEFECTS**

An atrial septal defect (ASD) can occur during partitioning of the atrium as a result of abnormal development of the interatrial septum. An ASD is a common congenital heart anomaly that occurs more commonly in females than in males.

Defects include (Moore & Persaud 2003):

- *Ostium secundum* ASDs—these occur in the area of the oval fossa. They are relatively common and include defects of the septum primum and septum secundum. Septum secundum ASDs are one of the most common types of congenital heart defect.
- *Endocardial cushion defects with ostium primum* ASDs—a less common form of ASD occurring when the septum primum does not fuse with the endocardial cushions.
- *Sinus venosus* ASDs—rarest type of ASD, located in the superior part of the interatrial septum near the entry of the superior vena cava.

Atrial septal defects are characteristic of several partial and complete trisomies, including trisomy 21, and are associated with almost all documented autosomal and sex chromosome aberrations (Larsen 1998).

The ventricles

The partitioning of the primitive ventricle (Fig. 5.5) is first indicated at the end of week 4 when a muscular ridge forms in the floor of the ventricle as a result of the bulboventricular sulcus protruding into the cardiac lumen (Larsen 2001). This muscular ridge forms the muscular part of the interventricular septum and grows from the apex of the ventricle towards the fused endocardial cushions, stopping before it reaches them and leaving a gap between the free end of the septum and the endocardial cushions. This gap, called the *ventricular foramen*, allows communication between the right and left ventricle, and prevents the left ventricle from being shut off from the ventricular outflow tract while it also develops. By the seventh week the ventricular foramen closes as a result of fusion between the interventricular septum, membranous extensions of the endocardial cushions and the aorticopulmonary septum that divides the outflow tract of the heart. This membranous area of fusion is known as the *interventricular septum* (Moore & Persaud 2003).

The wall of the early ventricle is composed of the three layers detailed above: an inner layer of endothelial tissue, a middle layer of cardiac jelly and an outside layer of myocardium. Ingrowths from this outer layer spread into the cardiac jelly, while at the same time epithelial tissue grows outward eventually clothing the ingrowths in epithelium. The cardiac jelly disappears, leaving the epithelium-covered myocardial ingrowths to form the trabeculae carneae, chordae tendineae and papillary muscles (Matsumura & England 1992).

CLINICAL NOTES   VENTRICULAR SEPTAL DEFECTS AND HYPOPLASTIC LEFT HEART SYNDROME

Ventricular septal defects

Ventricular septal defects (VSDs) are the most common congenital heart defects. They occur more frequently in males than in females, accounting for approximately 25% of all cardiac defects, and may occur in any part of the interventricular septum. During the first year of life many small VSDs close spontaneously (30–50%). Children with a large VSD will have a left to right shunt of blood (Moore & Persaud 2003).

Ventricular septal defects can occur during the partitioning of the ventricles as a result of abnormal development of the interventricular septum due to muscular and membranous ventricular septa failing to fuse:

- *Membranous VSD*—most common type of VSD, occurring as a result of the membranous part of the interventricular septum failing to develop. A large VSD with excessive pulmonary blood flow and pulmonary hypertension will result in dyspnoea and cardiac failure in early infancy.
- *Muscular VSDs*—less common, they can appear anywhere in the muscular part of the interventricular septum. If multiple small defects occur, they produce what is known as a *Swiss Cheese VSD*.

Ventricular septal defects can occur as isolated defects or in conjunction with other more complex cardiac defects, such as Tetralogy of Fallot and Transposition of The Great Vessels.

Single ventricle or *common ventricle* is a rare congenital cardiac defect that occurs when there is an absence of the interventricular septum. Failure of the interventricular septum to form results in a three-chambered heart wherein both atria empty into the single ventricle through either a common valve or two separate atrioventricular valves, and the pulmonary artery and aorta also arise from the single ventricle (Moore & Persaud 2003).

Hypoplastic left heart syndrome (HLHS)

Underdevelopment of the left side of the heart results in a hypoplastic left ventricle and aortic atresia. Once the patent ductus arteriosus closes, the infant will progressively deteriorate with cyanosis and decreased cardiac output leading to cardiovascular collapse. Without intervention, infants with HLHS will die in the first months of life. Surgical intervention involves a staged approach with a *Norwood procedure* done initially, followed by a *bidirectional Glen shunt* at 6–9 months of age; the final stage is a *modified Fontan procedure* (Hockenberry 2003).

FORMATION OF THE OUTFLOW TRACT OF THE HEART: TRUNCUS ARTERIOSUS AND BULBUS CORDIS PARTITIONING

In the primitive heart the outflow tract is the bulbus cordis and the truncus arteriosus. As the heart develops, the interventricular foramen and the expanded base of the conus cordis allow the two ventricles to communicate within one another. However, as septation continues and nears completion, the outflow tract develops (Fig. 5.6) in a tightly coordinated way to ensure that proper heart function is maintained. In week 5, ridges known as *bulbar ridges* are formed in the walls of the bulbus cordis. Similar ridges called *truncal ridges*, which are continuous with the bulbar ridges, also form in the walls of the truncus arteriosus. These spiral ridges—it is suggested that their spiral nature is a result of the streaming of blood from the ventricles—grow towards one another, meeting in the middle and fusing together to form a spiral *aorticopulmonary septum*, and dividing both the bulbus cordis and the truncus arteriosus into two separate ventricular outflow channels, the pulmonary trunk and the ascending aorta (Moore & Persaud 2003). The separation of these two channels into the aortic and pulmonary outflow tracts takes place when the aorticopulmonary septum fuses with the endocardial cushion and muscular interventricular septum as part of the final process of ventricular partitioning (Larsen 2001) (see The Ventricles above). As a result of the spiralling nature of the bulbar and truncal ridges, and the resulting spiralling aorticopulmonary septum, the aorta and pulmonary trunk twist

Fig. 5.6
A Development of the aortic and pulmonary trunk begins in the 5th week with the formation of ridges in the bulbar cordis and truncus arteriosus.
B which fuse to form the aorticopulmonary septum.
C and then spiral to form the aorta and pulmonary trunk.
(Adapted from Moore & Persaud 2003.)

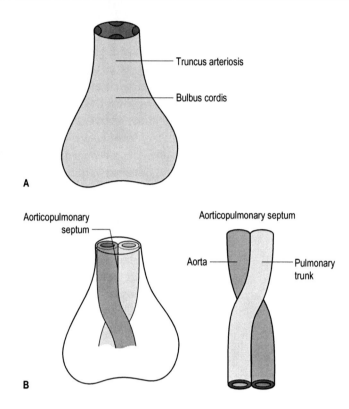

around one another, accounting for the partial spiralling of the aorta and pulmonary artery seen in the adult heart (Carlson 1999).

As the outflow tract is being remodelled and divided, the ventricles are simultaneously being partitioned and the bulbus cordis is incorporated into the right ventricle.

CLINICAL NOTES | **ANOMALIES ARISING DURING PARTITIONING OF THE OUTFLOW TRACT**

A variety of cardiac defects can occur as a result of abnormal partitioning of the outflow tract of the heart, some of which are very complex and may or may not occur in conjunction with a ventricular septal defect or other cardiac abnormality. They include:

- *Truncus arteriosus*—the failure of normal septation and division of the bulbar trunk into the aorta and pulmonary artery results in a single vessel that overrides both ventricles. The blood from both ventricles mixes in the common great artery and causes hypoxaemia and desaturation. Surgical treatment is required with early repair in the first few months of life. Future operations will also be required to replace the conduits (Hockenberry 2003).

- *Tetralogy of Fallot*—a group of four defects that include overriding aorta, ventricular septal defect, pulmonary stenosis and right ventricular hypertrophy. Surgical correction is required, with an elective repair usually performed within the first year of life. A palliative procedure to increase pulmonary blood flow and increase oxygen saturation may be performed on infants who cannot undergo a primary repair; however, in general shunts are avoided because they may result in pulmonary artery distortion (Hockenberry 2003).
- *Transposition of The Great Arteries (TGA)*—the pulmonary trunk arises from the morphological left ventricle and the aorta arises from the morphological right ventricle. TGA is the most common cause of cyanotic heart disease in newborn infants and is often associated with other cardiac defects such as ASD and VSD (Moore & Persaud 2003). Surgical correction is required, with the procedure of choice being the arterial switch procedure, which is performed in the first weeks of life (Hockenberry 2003).
- *Aortic Valve Stenosis*—stricture or narrowing of the aortic valve. Valvular stenosis, caused by a malformation or fusion of the cusps is the most common type, or subvalvular stenosis, a fibrous ring below a normal valve, produces a stricture. Supravalvular stenosis occurs infrequently. This is a serious defect because obstruction tends to be progressive, and sudden episodes of low cardiac output or myocardial ischaemia can result in sudden death (Hockenberry 2003).
- *Aortic Valve Atresia*—complete obstruction of the aortic valve.
- *Pulmonary Valve Stenosis*—the entrance to the pulmonary artery is narrowed.
- *Pulmonary Valve Atresia*—an extreme form of pulmonary stenosis and therefore no blood flow to the lungs. Occurs when division of the truncus is so unequal that the pulmonary trunk has no lumen, or there is no orifice at the level of the pulmonary valve. It may or may not be associated with a VSD (Moore & Persaud 2003).

VALVE FORMATION

The atrioventricular valves

The atrioventricular valves are designed to allow blood to enter the ventricles and prevent it from flowing back when the ventricles contract. Between weeks 5 and 8 these valves begin to form as tissue swellings on either side of the left and right atrioventricular canals, eventually hollowing out and developing into leaflets or cusps. Both valves initially develop with an anterior and posterior cusp, with the right atrioventricular valve developing a third septal cusp in the third month. The valves have been named with reference to the number of cusps in each valve. The two-cusped left atrioventricular valve is known as the *bicuspid valve* or *mitral valve,* and the three-cusped right atrioventricular valve is known as the *tricuspid valve* (Larsen 2001).

To allow the cusps to close and thus prevent blood from flowing back into the ventricles, the free edge of each cusp is attached to the anterior and posterior walls of their respective ventricles by thin tendon-like chords called *chordae tendineae*, which themselves are imbedded into small raised areas of myocardium called *papillary muscles*. The chordae tendineae and papillary muscles develop from ingrowths of the myocardium (Larsen 2001).

The aortic and pulmonary valves

The aortic and pulmonary valves begin to develop (Fig. 5.7) in the middle of week 5, around the same time as partitioning of the bulbus cordis and truncus arteriosus is taking place; their development is completed by week 9. Small bulges or tubercles develop on the end of each truncal swelling in the right and left lateral walls at the inferior end of the truncus arteriosus (Larsen 2001). As the truncal swellings fuse together as part of aorticopulmonary septum development, the small bulges divide into two with half of each in each of the two outflow tracts (Larsen 2001). At the same time, two more bulges develop at the same level on the anterior and posterior walls of the truncus arteriosus with the result that, after septation, the one on the anterior wall will lie in the newly developing pulmonary trunk and the one on the posterior wall will lie in the newly developing ascending aorta (Larsen 2001). Consequently, each newly developing outflow tract contains three bulges in a triangle formation, which will then give rise to the three-cusped semilunar valves of the aorta and pulmonary trunk that will prevent blood from flowing back into the ventricles (Larsen 2001).

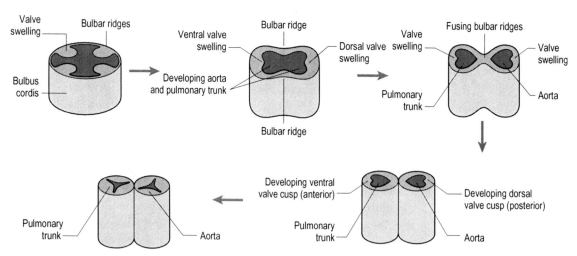

Fig. 5.7
Semi-lunar valve formation. The aortic and pulmonary valves begin to develop in the middle of week 5 as the truncus arteriosus and bulbus cordis are partitioning and are completed by week 9.
(Adapted from Moore & Persaud 2003.)

DEVELOPMENT OF THE CONDUCTING SYSTEM

The heart is one of the first organs to function in the embryo, starting to beat and propel blood throughout the embryo and placenta by day 22 (Larsen 2001). In order for it to maintain regular effective pumping, the heart needs to beat regularly and rhythmically. As such, the heart has a specialized conduction system whereby electrical impulses, or *action potentials*, generated within the heart are conducted throughout the atria and ventricles, in turn leading to contraction of the heart muscle and the circulation of blood. These electrical impulses are *myogenic*, that is, they arise spontaneously in the cardiac muscle itself and spread from cell to cell (Larsen 1998). All cardiac cells are capable of developing action potentials, but only certain specialized cardiac muscle cells, known as autorhythmic cells, that make up the heart's normal conduction system do so spontaneously. These include the sinoatrial node, the atrioventricular node, the bundle of His and the Purkinje fibres. The electrical impulses are initiated in an area known as the pacemaker region, where a network of specialized cardiac muscle fibres repeatedly generate action potentials, which in turn trigger heart contraction. The heart itself is innervated by sympathetic and parasympathetic nerves; however, these do not initiate beats and serve only to speed up or slow down the heart rate (Larsen 2003).

During embryonic development approximately 1% of cardiac muscle fibres become autorhythmic fibres, acting as a pacemaker to set the rhythm of electrical excitation, and a conduction system consisting of a network of specialized cardiac muscle fibres that provides a route for each cycle of cardiac excitation to progress through the heart (Tortora & Grabowski 2003).

In early heart development the pacemaker region is initially located in the primitive atrium but is quickly taken over by the sinus venosus where, during the fifth week, a cluster of pacemaking cells forms a distinct oval-shaped structure called the *sinoatrial node*. As the heart develops the sinoatrial node becomes incorporated into the wall of the right atrium with the sinus venosus, close to the entrance of the superior vena cava (Moore & Persaud 2003). Soon after the sinoatrial node develops, a second pacemaker region begins to develop in the interatrial septal region, just above the endocardial cushion region. This second pacemaker area is called the *atrioventricular node* and is connected to the sinoatrial node by strands of specialized cardiac muscle cells that are able to conduct the stimulus from the sinoatrial node to the atrioventricular node.

At the same time as the atrioventricular node is forming, a bundle of specialized conducting cells called the *atrioventricular (AV) bundle*, or *bundle of His*, also appears, and extends from the atrioventricular node in the base of the atrium to the ventricles along both sides of the interventricular septum. This specialized bundle of tissue forming the AV bundle will form the only pathway between the atria and ventricles as connective tissue grows in from the epicardium during development of the four chambers, separates the muscles of the atria and the ventricles, and forms what is known as the *fibrous skeleton of the heart* (Moore & Persaud 2003). On entering the ventricle the AV bundle splits into two bundles, extending down the interventricular septum towards the apex of the heart, one branch going into the left ventricle (the left bundle branch) and one going into the right ventricle (the right bundle branch). These right and left branches then distribute conducting tissue known as *Purkinje fibres* throughout the ventricular myocardium.

SEQUENCE OF CONDUCTION

Once the conduction system has completed development, the sequence of conduction is as follows (Fig. 5.8):

1. An electrical impulse, or action potential, is initiated in the sinoatrial node.
2. The impulse is conducted throughout the atrial muscle from cell to cell via the gap junctions in the intercalated discs, and the atria contract. This process also accounts for the spread from the right atrium to the left atrium as the atria contact each other at their shared interatrial wall; the spread is so rapid that both atria contract at the same time (Vander et al 1990).
3. As the action potential spreads down the atrial muscle fibres, it reaches the atrioventricular node situated at the base of the right atrium, where it then enters the AV bundle, or bundle of His.
4. Once the AV bundle is stimulated, the action potential spreads down both the right and left bundle branches towards the apex of the heart and the Purkinje fibres. The Purkinje fibres then rapidly conduct the impulse back up from the apex and distribute it throughout the rest of the ventricular myocardium. This rapid conduction along

Fig. 5.8
Conduction.

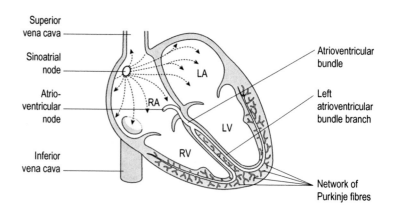

the Purkinje fibres ensures a single coordinated contraction of both ventricles, although the contraction does begin very slightly earlier in the bottom of the ventricles.

ACTION POTENTIALS AND CARDIAC CONTRACTION

The action potential that is initiated in the sinoatrial node depolarizes or excites the atrial and ventricular contractile muscle fibres and triggers their contraction. The development of cardiac action potentials is beyond the remit of this text, and thus the reader is advised to consult a detailed physiology text.

CLINICAL NOTES   AUTORHYTHMIC FIBRES

Autorhythmic fibres repeatedly generate action potentials and thus continue to stimulate a heart to beat even after it is removed from the body and all its nerves have been cut, for example for the purposes of transplantation (Tortora & Grabowski 2003).

CLINICAL NOTES   ARRYTHMIAS FOLLOWING SURGERY

There is risk of damage to the conduction system resulting in arrythmias during surgical repair of defects occuring in areas close to the conduction pathways for example following repair of Fallots Tetralogy (Archer & Burch 1998)

THE CARDIAC CYCLE

The cardiac cycle is the orderly sequence of events associated with the contraction and relaxation of the atria and ventricles, *systole* and *diastole*, and as such is the period of time from the beginning of one heart beat to the start of the next one. During a cardiac cycle the atria and ventricles alternately contract and relax, with each cycle consisting of three phases:

- *Atrial systole*—the atria contract and blood is ejected into the relaxed ventricles.
- *Ventricular systole*—as the atria relax, the ventricles contract ejecting blood into the aorta and pulmonary artery. During this phase the atrioventricular valves are closed, thus preventing blood from flowing back into the atria.
- *Complete cardiac diastole*—during this phase both the atria and the ventricles are relaxed and blood flows into the atria from the superior and inferior vena cava and pulmonary veins.

CARDIAC OUTPUT AND STROKE VOLUME

In order for the cardiovascular system to meet the metabolic oxygen needs of the body effectively, an adequate *cardiac output* is required. The cardiac output is the amount of blood ejected from the left ventricle (or right ventricle) in 1 minute, and is calculated by multiplying the heart rate by the stroke volume—the amount of blood ejected by the ventricle during a contraction (Tortora & Grabowski 2004). Stroke volume is influenced by three factors:

- *Preload*—put simply, this is the volume of blood that returns to the heart (Wong 1999) and thus the amount of *pressure* put on the heart muscle before it contracts. If the amount of blood increases, the stretch on the muscle fibres will be greater, which in turn will increase the force of contraction and so increase the amount of blood being pumped out. Thus, the more the heart fills with blood during diastole, the greater the force of contraction will be during systole. This principle is known as the *Frank Starling Law of the Heart* (Tortora & Grabowski 2004).
- *Contractility*—the efficiency of the myocardial fibre; in other words, the ability of the cardiac muscle to contract at any given fibre length (i.e. the strength of contraction at preload).
- *Afterload*—the resistance against which the ventricles have to pump when ejecting blood. Any condition that makes it more difficult to pump blood into the circulation, such as hypertension, increases the afterload (Wong 1999); any increase in afterload decreases stroke volume, which in turn means that more blood remains in the ventricles after systole (Tortora & Grabowski 2003).

Cardiac output (CO) is determined by multiplying the heart rate (HR) by the stroke volume (SV) and is reported in millilitres or litres per minute:

$$CO = HR \times SV$$

As children of different sizes have different normal ranges of cardiac output (Table 5.2), the term *cardiac index* is used. Cardiac index (CI) is

Table 5.2 Normal paediatric cardiac output and stroke volume in children at different ages (Hazinski 1992)

Age	Heart rate (beats/min)	Cardiac output (L/min)	Stroke volume (mL)
Newborn	145	0.8–1.0	5
6 months	120	1.0–1.3	10
1 year	115	1.3–1.5	13
2 years	115	1.5–2.0	18
4 years	105	2.3–2.75	27
5 years	95	2.5–3.0	31
8 years	83	3.4–3.6	42
10 years	75	3.8–4.0	50
15 years	70	6.0	85

equal to the child's cardiac output divided by the child's body surface area in metres squared (Hazinski 1992):

$$CI = CO \div \text{body surface area } (m^2)$$

Normal cardiac index in the child is approximately 3.5–4.5 L per min per m^2 of body surface. (Hazinski 1992).

BLOOD PRESSURE

Blood pressure is the pressure exerted by blood on the walls of the blood vessels and is generated by contraction of the ventricles. It is highest in the aorta and large arteries, and gradually decreases as the blood flows through the systemic circulation and the distance from the left ventricle increases (Tortora & Grabowski 2003). When the left ventricle contracts and blood is forced out into the aorta, the pressure that results is the highest arterial pressure that will be attained during systole, and is therefore called the *systolic pressure*. The lowest arterial pressure occurs when the heart is at rest during diastole and is therefore called the *diastolic pressure*. Several factors are involved in the control of blood pressure; these include cardiovascular factors such as cardiac output, blood volume, peripheral vascular resistance, artery wall elasticity, venous return and other factors including hormones and the nervous system.

A more detailed discussion of the above cardiac physiology is beyond the remit of this text and the reader is advised to consult a detailed physiology text for further reading.

NB: *The cardiac cycle described above is that of the postnatal circulation.* Anatomical differences in the fetal circulation and postnatal circulation mean that blood flow through the fetal heart is different (see Fetal circulation below).

FETAL CIRCULATION

THE PRIMITIVE CIRCULATION

By the end of week 3 a primitive cardiovascular system has developed into a functional state, with the primitive heart tube linking up with the primitive blood vessels in the embryo, the yolk sac, the connecting stalk and the chorion, and blood beginning to circulate. On day 21–22 contractions begin as peristaltic waves initiating in the region of the sinus venosus. These waves propel the blood through the heart; at first it ebbs and flows, but by the end of week 4, when coordinated contractions begin, the blood flows in only one direction entering the heart at the sinus venosus (Moore & Persaud 1998). Blood from the vitelline veins, formed in the wall of the yolk sac, enters the heart via the sinus venosus, as does blood from the chorionic and umbilical veins. As the yolk sac is no longer able to provide nourishment to the growing embryo, blood that has derived oxygen and nutrition from the maternal blood through the primitive placenta travels via the chorionic and umbilical veins and drains into the sinus venosus.

Once the blood enters the heart, it flows through the primitive atrium and then through the atrioventricular canal into the primitive ventricle, where it is pumped through the bulbus cordis and truncus arteriosus into the aortic arches. From there it is distributed to the rest of the embryo's body via the dorsal aorta and its branches, as well as to the yolk sac and placenta via the chorion, vitelline and umbilical arteries (Moore & Persaud 1998).

FETAL CIRCULATION

The fetal circulation (Fig. 5.9) is designed to ensure that the vital organs and tissues in the developing fetus receive the best oxygenated blood while also bypassing the uninflated lungs and preparing for the modifications that are needed at birth to establish postnatal circulation, when the lungs will take over oxygenation from the placenta. Carlson (1999) suggests that the embryonic circulation is perhaps a more complex system than is necessary for the growth and development of the fetus, but points out that the fetal plan of circulation is essential as the embryo must prepare for the moment at birth when it suddenly shifts to a completely different pattern of oxygenation of blood via the lungs rather than through the placenta.

Prenatally the lungs are essentially non-functioning and the pulmonary vessels are vasoconstricted (Moore & Persaud 2003). The liver is also only partially functioning and thus requires less blood than other organs such as the brain, which requires the highest oxygenation concentration (Wong 1999). The fetal circulation is therefore designed in such a way that the blood carrying oxygen and nutrients from the placenta is diverted to such organs. As such, the fetal circulation has three important structures or fetal shunts to facilitate this process: the *ductus venosus*, the *ductus arteriosus* and the *foramen ovale*. Their purpose and function are discussed below.

Blood, which has been well oxygenated and is nutrient rich, travels from the placenta via the *umbilical vein* and enters the fetal system through the umbilicus. From here the blood travels to the liver, where it is divided. Half of the blood will enter the hepatic and portal systems, through the liver sinusoids, before eventually returning to the IVC via the hepatic veins, while the other half bypasses the liver completely and drains directly into the IVC via the *ductus venosus*, a fetal vessel that joins to the IVC (Moore & Persaud 2003).

Once in the vena cava, this blood now has immediate access to the heart, although it has now also received poorly oxygenated blood

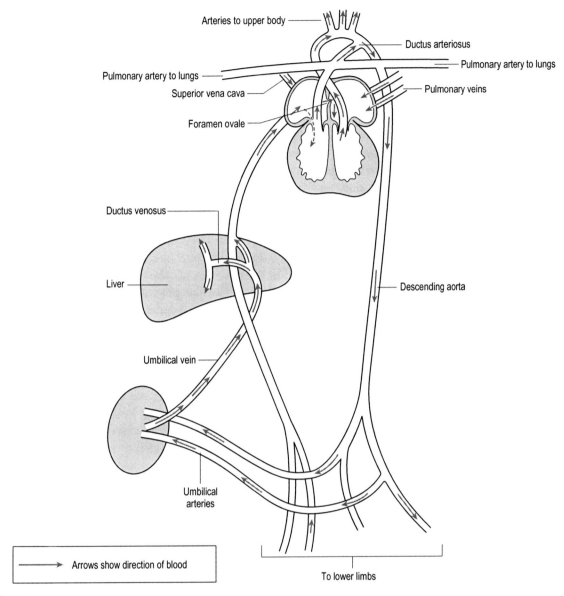

Arteries to upper body

Ductus arteriosus

Pulmonary artery to lungs

Pulmonary artery to lungs

Superior vena cava

Pulmonary veins

Foramen ovale

Ductus venosus

Liver

Descending aorta

Umbilical vein

Umbilical arteries

Arrows show direction of blood

To lower limbs

Fig. 5.9
The fetal circulation.
(Adapted from Moore & Persaud 2003.)

returning from the abdomen, pelvis and lower limbs, which means it is less well oxygenated than in the umbilical vein but does nevertheless still have a high oxygen content (Moore & Persaud 2003). As the blood reaches the right atrium, the majority is directed through the *foramen ovale* and *foramen secundum* into the left atrium. Thus, better oxygenated blood enters the left atrium and then the left ventricle to be pumped through the aorta to the heart, head and upper limbs. Some of the first vessels going off the aorta supply the heart and brain, and therefore these organs will receive blood with the high concentration of oxygen necessary for their development.

Although the majority of blood passes through the foramen ovale, a small amount remains in the right atrium, possibly because the opening of the foramen ovale is smaller than that of the IVC, this blood mixes with poorly oxygenated blood returning from the head and upper limbs via the superior vena cava and from the heart via the coronary sinus, and is directed through the tricuspid valve into the right ventricle (Carlson 1999). This blood is then pumped via the pulmonary artery towards the lungs; however, because the lungs are not yet functioning and thus require only a very small amount of blood for their growth and development, the majority of the blood in the pulmonary artery is shunted back across the ductus arteriosus into the aorta. The ductus arteriosus enables the right atrium to exercise in preparation for working at full capacity at birth, while at the same time protecting the lungs from circulatory overload (Carlson 1999). The blood in the descending aorta perfuses the caudal part of the fetus and is also returned to the placenta via the two umbilical arteries.

In the fetal circulation, unlike the postnatal and adult circulation, pressure on the right side of the heart is greater than that on the left. The reason for this is twofold; first, the uninflated fetal lungs create a high pulmonary vascular resistance in the right side of the heart and pulmonary artery, and, second, the presence of the ductus arteriosus and the free-flowing placental circulation creates a low systemic vascular resistance in the remainder of the fetal vascular system. At birth, when the umbilical cord is clamped and the lungs inflate, this immediately changes and the haemodynamics of the fetal vascular system undergo a vast abrupt change. This process of change is described below.

CHANGES OCCURRING AT BIRTH FROM FETAL TO NEONATAL CIRCULATION

Important changes and adjustments take place at birth to convert from a fetal circulation to that of a functioning neonatal circulation, two of the most important being the initiation of respiration and expansion of the lungs, and the cessation of blood flow through the placenta (Moore & Persaud 2003). This transition from fetal to neonatal circulation involves the closure of the three fetal shunts, which up to this point have allowed blood to bypass the liver and lungs but are no longer required once the baby is born.

This process begins as soon as the baby takes its first breath, the lungs inflate and the umbilical cord is clamped. Once the lungs have inflated, the inspired oxygen dilates the pulmonary vessels, which in turn decreases pulmonary vascular resistance and thus increases pulmonary blood flow. As a result of the increased blood flow through the pulmonary vessels in the lungs, the pressure in the right atrium and pulmonary artery decreases. This coincides with an increase in systemic vascular resistance and thus increased pressure on the left side as a result of constriction of the umbilical arteries (which also prevents loss of the infant's blood) and clamping of the umbilical cord.

The cord, however, is not clamped for a minute or so to allow blood flow to continue through the umbilical vein and thus transfer fetal blood from the placenta to the infant (Moore & Persaud 1998). The fetal shunts that allowed blood to bypass the liver and lungs are no longer required after birth and will close either immediately or over the first few hours or days after birth.

Closure of the foramen ovale

The increased pressure in the left atrium and decreased pressure in the right atrium effect the closure of the foramen ovale. The pressure in the left atrium, which is greater than that in the right, presses the valve or flap of the foramen ovale against the septum secundum and functionally closes the foramen ovale at or soon after birth (Moore & Persaud 2003). A proliferation of endothelial and fibrous tissue later causes an anatomical closure of the foramen ovale.

Constriction of the ductus arteriosus

The ductus arteriosus constricts at birth, with the most important factor in this process being the increased oxygen concentration of the blood. A substance called bradykinin, which has potent contractile effects on smooth muscle, is released from the lungs during initial aeration and appears to act on the wall of the ductus arteriosus when there is a high oxygen content in the aortic blood; however, the mechanisms by which oxygen causes the ductus to restrict is not yet well understood (Moore & Persaud 2003). Other factors, including the fall in prostaglandin levels after birth, are also involved. The ductus arteriosus is closed functionally within 24 hours of birth, although anatomical closure takes longer and has usually occurred by the 12th week as a result of fibrin deposits forming a fibrous ligament called the *ligamentum arteriosum* (Moore & Persaud 2003).

The ductus venosus

The sphincter of the ductus venosus constricts, thus allowing all blood entering the liver to pass through the hepatic sinusoids (Moore & Persaud 2003). The ductus venosus itself also constricts and is eventually converted into a fibrous ligament called the *ligamentum venosum*, which passes through the liver from the left branch of the portal vein to the IVC (Moore & Persaud 2003).

The umbilical vessels

The majority of the intra-abdominal parts of the umbilical arteries form the *medial umbilical ligaments*, while the proximal parts persist as the superior vesical arteries supplying the superior part of the urinary bladder (Moore & Persaud 2003). The intra-abdominal parts of the umbilical vein become the *ligamentum teres*, passing from the umbilicus to the left branch of the portal vein (Moore & Persaud 2003).

The transition from fetal to adult circulation is not a sudden occurrence and, although major changes do occur when the infant takes its first breath, some are merely functional and more permanent changes take place over a longer period (Moore & Persaud 2003).

CLINICAL NOTES   PROBLEMS ASSOCIATED WITH THE CLOSURE OF
THE FETAL SHUNTS

Cardiac defects can arise as a result of ineffective closure of some of the fetal shunts, including patent ductus arteriosus (PDA) and patent foramen ovale. Patency of the ductus arteriosus after birth results in blood flowing from the higher pressure aorta to the lower pressure pulmonary artery, causing a left to right shunt with increased blood flow to the lungs. Closure of the duct is done either surgically, by dividing or ligating the patent vessel via a left thoracotomy, or non-surgically, by occluding the duct with a coil inserted via cardiac catheterization (Hockenberry 2003).

As a result of reversible flow of blood through the ducts in the early neonatal period, functional murmurs are occasionally heard and the increased pressure associated with crying and straining can shunt unoxygenated blood from the right side of the heart across the ductal opening, causing transient cyanosis (Wong 1999).

Complex cardiac anomalies such as transposition of the great arteries or truncus arteriosus rely on a patent ductus arteriosus to sustain life. In infants with these conditions, closure of the duct signals the onset of cyanosis and a rapid deterioration in the infant's condition. In these infants the administration of intravenous prostaglandins is usually started (Wong 1999) to ensure that patency of the duct is maintained until a balloon atrial septostomy (Rashkind procedure) can be performed via cardiac catheterization or surgery can be carried out during the first few hours or days of life.

POSTNATAL CIRCULATION (ADULT CIRCULATION)

After birth the cardiovascular and circulatory system assumes that of an adult circulation (Fig. 5.10) whereby blood is oxygenated by the lungs and distributed around the systemic circulation. Blood returns to the heart via the superior vena cava and inferior vena cava, and drains into the right atrium. As the atria contract, blood is forced through the tricuspid valve into the right ventricle. As the ventricles contract, the blood is pumped through the pulmonary valve into the pulmonary artery to the lungs, where it becomes oxygenated. The oxygenated blood then returns to the heart via the pulmonary veins from where it drains into the left atrium. As the atria contract, the blood is forced through the mitral valve into the left ventricle and finally, as the ventricle contracts, it is pumped through the aortic valve into the aorta and around the heart and systemic circulation. The thick-walled arteries carry oxygenated blood away from the heart to the capilliary bed where the tissues are supplied with oxygen and nutrients. Carbon dioxide and deoxygenated blood are then transported from the tissues back to the heart via the thin-walled veins.

Fig. 5.10
A Interior of the heart.
B Direction of the flow of
blood through the heart.

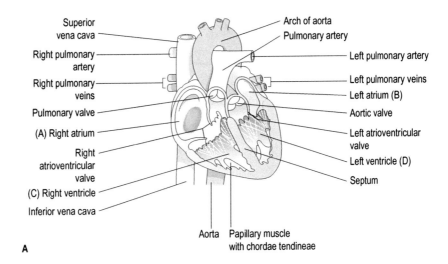

A

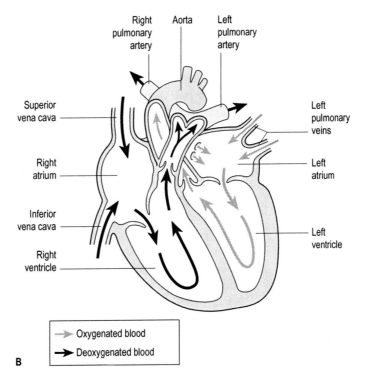

B

POSTNATAL CARDIAC DEVELOPMENT

THE HEART AND VASCULATURE

In the infant the size of the heart, in relation to its body size, is larger; in the newborn infant the heart weighs approximately 0.75% of the bodyweight. It also lies transversely, but as the lungs expand the

Table 5.3 Normal ranges of
heart rates for children
(Wong 1999)

Age	Heart rate (beats/min)	
	Resting awake	Resting asleep
Birth	100–180	80–160
1 week to 3 months	100–220	80–180
3 months to 2 years	80–150	70–120
2 to 10 years	70–110	60–100
10 years to adult	55–90	50–90

heart gets pushed downwards until it lies more obliquely and lower in relation to the rib cage, as in the adult (Sinclair & Dangerfield 1998). At birth the walls of the ventricles are largely the same thickness; however, with the increased systemic vascular resistance that occurs after birth, the walls of the left ventricle become thicker than those of the right ventricle. The right ventricle pumps blood to the lungs, and there is a much lower pressure in the pulmonary bed than that which is exerted by the systemic vascular resistance on the left (Wong 1999). Consequently the walls of the right ventricle grow less, and so they are only half as thick as those of the left ventricle in the adult.

After birth the systolic blood pressure is low and is a reflection of the neonate's weak left ventricle. This changes, however, as the left side of the heart increases in strength and power, with a sharp rise in systolic pressure occurring during the infant's first 6 weeks. This rise in systolic pressure continues as the child grows, although at a much slower rate until just before puberty when it again rises rapidly, this time to adult levels (Wong 1999).

As a child grows, changes also take place in the arteries and veins. The walls of the vessels thicken to cope with the increased pressure, while the vessels themselves also grow and elongate in order to keep up with the child's increasing height and weight. However, at present there is still very little known about how blood vessels grow in order to keep up with the changes in body dimensions (Sinclair & Dangerfield 1998).

Changes also take place in heart rate and blood pressure. Younger children have smaller hearts and higher heart rates, and as their hearts grow the heart rate slows (Table 5.3). Children's maximal heart rates are higher than those of adults, to a rate of approximately 200 beats per minute (MacGregor 2000). As the heart strengthens and grows, resting blood pressure rises (Table 5.4), nearing the adult range by the time the young person reaches the age of 15 years.

During adolescence, the growth spurt associated with this period of development is accompanied by a related spurt in the heart muscle, an increase in blood pressure and a decrease in heart rate. While there is little or no increase in the number of cardiac muscle fibres during growth, the size of the fibres themselves increases about sevenfold.

Table 5.4   Changes in blood pressure throughout childhood (MacGregor 2000)

Age	Blood pressure (mmHg)	
	Male	Female
Newborn	70/55	65/55
5 years	95/56	94/56
10 years	100/62	102/62
15 years	115/65	111/67
Adult	121/70	112/60

This then brings about a related increase in the number of cardiac blood vessels supplying the fibres, and an associated reduction in the number of fibres supplied by each vessel, from six in the newborn to about one in the adult. The number of vessels per unit volume of tissue remains unchanged, however, as the whole system is increasing in size (Sinclair & Dangerfield 1998).

BLOOD AND BLOOD CELL FORMATION

The blood volume of the full-term infant is approximately 80–85 ml per kg bodyweight. In the newborn immediately after birth, the total blood volume averages 300 mL; however, this amount depends on the amount of placental transfer of blood that takes place after birth, which itself depends on how long the infant remains attached to the placenta before it is clamped. As much as 100 mL can be added to the blood volume (Wong 1999).

As with the structural and circulatory aspects of the cardiovascular system, significant changes also take place in relation to *haemopoiesis* during the first year after birth. During the first 5 months, fetal haemoglobin (HbF) remains present as the level of adult haemoglobin increases steadily throughout this period. At 2–3 months of age, physiological anaemia is common as a result of the propensity for fetal haemoglobin to shorten the life of red blood cells, which in turn results in a decreased number of red blood cells. High levels of HbF are thought to depress the production of erythropoietin, the hormone released by the kidney that stimulates red blood cell production (Wong 1999). Another factor that accounts for lower haemoglobin levels is the decreasing amount of maternal iron stores. These stores, which are present for the first 5–6 months, gradually diminish by the end of the first 6 months (Wong 1999).

By the time of birth, all blood cell production takes place in the red marrow of all the bones in the skeleton and continues throughout infancy and childhood. As bone growth ceases near the end of adolescence, however, red bone marrow has been replaced in many of the bones by yellow bone marrow containing fat; red blood cell production ceases to takes place in most bones, and remains only in the upper shaft of the femur, ribs, vertebrae, sternum and arm bones in adults.

SELF ASSESSMENT

- Draw and label a diagram of the primitive heart and describe the flow of blood through it.
- Describe the process involved in separating the heart into four chambers.
- Draw and label a diagram of the fetal circulation.
- Identify the changes that take place during the transition from fetal circulation to neonatal circulation.
- Explain what happens during the cardiac cycle, including the sequence of conduction, in the postnatal (adult) heart.
- Cardiac physiology:
  (a) Define cardiac output and the factors that affect it.
  (b) What three factors regulate stroke volume?
- Name at least two defects associated with the following stages of cardiovascular development:
  (a) Development of the arteries
  (b) Development of the veins
  (c) Looping of the primitive heart
  (d) Endocardial cushion development
  (e) Atrial and ventricular septation
  (f) Partitioning of the outflow tract
  (g) Transition from fetal to neonatal circulation.

References

Archer N, Burch M 1998 Paediatric cardiology: an introduction. London, Chapman and Hall Medical.

Carlson B M 1999 Human embryology and developmental biology, 2nd edn. Mosby, St Louis

Fitzgerald M J T, Fitzgerald M 1994 Human embryology. Baillière Tindall, London

Hazinski M F 1992 Nursing care of the critically ill child, 2nd edn. Mosby, St Louis

Hockenberry M J 2003 Wong's nursing care of infants and children, 7th edn. Mosby, St Louis

Larsen WJ 2001 Human embryology, 3rd edn. Churchill Livingstone, Philadelphia

Larsen W J 1998 Essentials of human embryology. Churchill Livingstone, Edinburgh

MacGregor J 2000 Introduction to the anatomy and physiology of children. Routledge, London

Matsumura G, England M A 1992 Embryology colouring book. Mosby, London

Moore K L, Persaud T V N 1998 Before we are born: essentials of embryology and birth defects, 5th edn. W B Saunders, Philadelphia

Moore K L, Persaud T V N 2003 The developing human: clinically orientated embryology, 7th edn. W B Saunders, Philadelphia

Sinclair D, Dangerfield P 1998 Human growth after birth, 6th edn. Oxford University Press, Oxford

Tortora G J, Grabowski S R 2003 Principles of anatomy and physiology. John Wiley, New York

Tortora G J, Grabowski S R 2004 Introduction to the human body: essentials of anatomy and physiology, 6th edn. Wiley, New Jersey

Vander A J, Sherman J H, Luciano D S 1990 Human physiology, international edition, 5th edn. McGraw–Hill, New York

Wong D L 1999 Whaley and Wong's nursing care of infants and children. Mosby, St Louis

Chapter 6

Development of the respiratory system and respiration

Duncan Randall

CHAPTER OUTCOMES

This chapter will enable the reader to:

- Identify the elements that make up the respiratory system
- Describe the development of the respiratory system in the fetus and child
- Explore the factors that affect lung development in the fetus and child
- Identify changes to the fetal respiratory system at birth
- Examine the interaction of respiratory system development and childhood respiratory conditions.

CHAPTER OVERVIEW

The aim of this chapter is to describe the development of the respiratory system in children in terms of embryonic, fetal and childhood development. This chapter looks at the development of the upper airways of the nasal cavity and trachea, and the lower airways of the bronchus and bronchial tree. The development of the supporting structures for the airway, such as the diaphragm and rib cage, is examined, as well as the physiology that enables development of the lungs, such as surfactant production and action. Clinical Notes will draw out the relationship between the developmental anatomy and clinical issues of respiratory distress syndrome, chronic lung disease, Robin sequence, sudden infant death syndrome and respiratory difficulties following elective caesarean section. Self Assessment exercises are given to assist in reflection on the material in the chapter and its relevance to the reader's own area of professional practice.

INTRODUCTION

For all of us respiration is vital. Without a constant supply of oxygen, cells within the body would be unable to oxidize glucose to produce energy or store energy in the phosphate bond of adenosine triphosphate (ATP). This is just one of the *oxidation* reactions for which oxygen is required in the human body.

The Earth's mass allows for the escape of lighter atoms such as hydrogen and helium while retaining heavier gases such as nitrogen (78.08% of the atmosphere), oxygen (20.95% of the atmosphere) and carbon dioxide (0.0036% of the atmosphere). When the Earth first formed, high levels of carbon dioxide provided a greenhouse effect, which maximized the weak solar radiation before the sun began hydrogen fusion. The subsequent trapping of carbonates in silica and in photosynthesis reduced the level of carbon dioxide, and its warming effect as the sun's radiation grew. This has allowed the Earth to have surface water for the past 400 million years—water in which life has evolved. This life adapted to an oxygen-rich environment by the incorporation of mitochondria to utilize the benefits of aerobic metabolism and avoid the toxic effects of oxygen and its free radicals.

In humans, respiration, or gaseous exchange of oxygen and carbon dioxide across the cell membrane, is facilitated by the respiratory tract and cardiovascular systems. Here we are concerned with the development of the respiratory tract, as the cardiovascular system was considered in Chapter 5.

The respiratory tract consists of the upper airway structures (Fig. 6.1): external nares (nostrils), vestible and internal nares (conchae) that lead to the *oropharynx*, the structures of the mouth and oral cavity that join in the oropharynx to form the *laryngopharynx*, which extends from the hyoid bone into the *oesophagus*, posteriorly and anteriorly past the *epiglottis* into the trachea. The epiglottis divides the oesophagus and the *trachea*, separating the gastric and respiratory functions of the oropharynx. The epiglottis also divides upper and lower respiratory tracts.

The thyroid cartilage, thyroid gland and tracheal cartilage encase and support the trachea, which houses the vocal folds (cords) that help to generate speech. The trachea terminates at the carina, where it separates into the right and left bronchus, which divide repeatedly to form secondary and tertiary bronchi, terminal bronchioles, respiratory bronchioles and finally alveolar ducts, leading to a single cell layer of alveoli. The continual dividing of the lumen gives a branching appearance to the structure, commonly referred to as the bronchial tree.

Fig. 6.1
Adult respiratory organs.

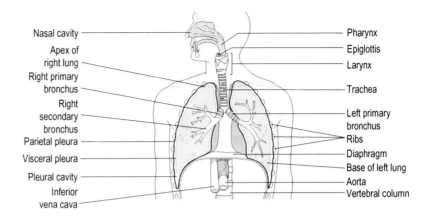

The respiratory tract is supported by gross anatomy in the structures of the lungs, diaphragm and thorax.

The bronchial tree is organized into alveolar sacs, which in turn are contained within the lobes of the lung, two on the left and three on the right. A dense network of capillaries, lymphatic vessels and neural pathways serves the lungs. The lung is enclosed in the pleural membrane, which consists of an outer layer attached to the thoracic cavity, the *parietal pleura*, and an inner layer that encapsulates the lung lobes, the *visceral pleura*; between these is the fluid-filled pleural cavity. The pleural cavity allows the lungs to expand within the thorax with minimal friction.

Below is the diaphragm, a thin flat layer of muscle and connective tissue that divides the thorax from the abdomen. The diaphragm is especially important in the breathing of the fetus, neonate and child, as the movement of the diaphragm creates most of the pressure difference in the thorax, combined with the upward and outwards motion of the ribcage.

Respiratory disease in childhood is common and appears to be increasing in the UK (Austin et al 1999). It is respiratory symptoms that most concern parents when they consult their general practitioner about their child's health (Kai 1996). Children's lungs do not reach adult volume until early adulthood (18–24 years), making them more susceptible to respiratory collapse, especially in early childhood (Allen & Gripp 2002, Rosenthal et al 1993). Because of their relative size and the increased rate of breathing, children are exposed to larger volumes of air than adults, increasing their risk of environmental hazard exposure (Bunn & Grigg 2000).

It is clear, then, that an understanding of the developmental anatomy and physiology of the respiratory system is essential for all healthcare professionals dealing with children.

EMBRYOLOGY

UPPER AIRWAYS: EXTERNAL NARES AND MOUTH TO EPIGLOTTIS

In the fourth to fifth week of embryonic development, folds or clefts appear in the ventral surface of the hindbrain of the embryo that delineate into ridges of tissue called the pharyngeal pouches, producing a gill-like appearance (brachia) characteristic of the embryo at this stage. The clefts of the pharyngeal pouches deepen but do not connect to internal structures, forming the pharyngeal arches each with its own musculature, nerves and skeletal features. In the human embryo there are six pairs of pharyngeal arches, although the fifth and sixth arches are rudimentary and only four arches appear on the surface. The pharyngeal arches, together with the stomodeum, form the structures of the face and neck (Figs 6.2 & 6.3).

At this time, a slit appears in the cranial (head) end of the laryngo-tracheal tube, forming the laryngeal aditus or inlet. Splanchnic mesenchyme cells from the sixth pharyngeal arches proliferate to form bilateral arytenoid swellings, and above an epiglottal swelling occurs in the midline of the hypobranchial eminence (or copula; an area in the midline of the third pharyngeal arch). These swellings pull the laryngeal aditus into a T shape.

Above the T, the epiglottis forms from the epiglottal swelling from the midline of the fourth pharyngeal arch; the root of the tongue and the palatine tonsils develop from the second and third pharyngeal arches; and the anterior section of the tongue develops from the first pharyngeal arch.

These swellings and the proliferation of epithelial cells occlude the canulae until week 10, when recanalization occurs. Incomplete recanalization results in *laryngeal webbing*, giving the infant a *stridor*.

The nerve supply to the structures of the tongue and laryngopharynx can be determined from the pharyngeal arch from which they developed; thus, the epiglottis and vocal fold (cords) are innervated by the superior laryngeal nerve, reflecting their fourth arch derivation. Tissue developing from the third arch, such as the tongue root, is supplied by the *glossopharyngeal nerve*, and the taste sensation in the anterior two-thirds of the tongue is from the first arch, from the corda tympani branch of the facial nerve VII.

Each pharyngeal arch also gives rise to cells that ossify into the cartilage and bones that form the upper airway (Fig. 6.3). The first arch provides the cells that ossify into Meckel's cartilage, which forms the lower jaw and the incus and malleus bones of the inner ear. The second arch provides the stapes bone in the ear and the styloid process and ligaments, as well as the lesser horn of the hyoid bone. The body and greater horn, which make up the lower parts of the hyoid bone,

Fig. 6.2
Development of pharyngeal arches and nerve structures at 4–5 weeks.

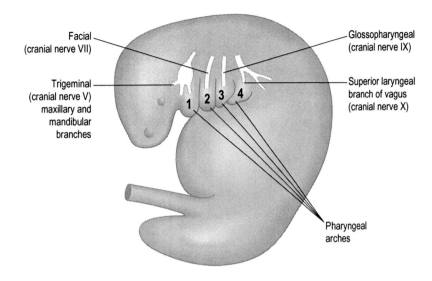

Facial (cranial nerve VII)

Trigeminal (cranial nerve V) maxillary and mandibular branches

Glossopharyngeal (cranial nerve IX)

Superior laryngeal branch of vagus (cranial nerve X)

Pharyngeal arches

Fig. 6.3
Pharyngeal arches and development of structures of the upper airway.

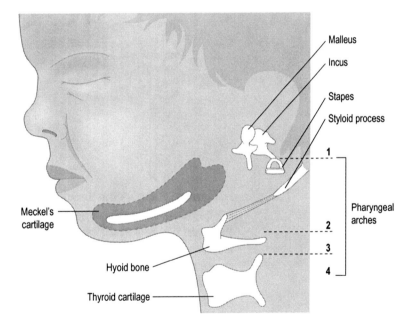

Malleus

Incus

Stapes

Styloid process

Meckel's cartilage

Pharyngeal arches

Hyoid bone

Thyroid cartilage

come from the third arch, and the thyroid cartilage and cricoid cartilage derive from the fourth and sixth arches respectively.

In weeks 5 to 6 of gestation, the second pharyngeal arch extends toward the epicardial ridge of the chest, effectively overlapping pharyngeal arches 3–6. This can result in cervical cysts that persist in childhood, found under the mandible anywhere below the ear and above the cricoid cartilage.

CLINICAL NOTES | **ROBIN SEQUENCE**

This range of congenital malformations can be linked to development of the first pharyngeal arch. It may occur as part of other syndromes or separately, and affects 1 in 8500 births. Infants have three features: *micrognathia*, cleft palate and *glossoptosis*. In classical Robin's sequence, children have small lower jaws and chin, reflecting the skeletal development of the first pharyngeal arch.

Fig. 6.4
Embryonic development of the nasal cavity and nose at 4–5 weeks.

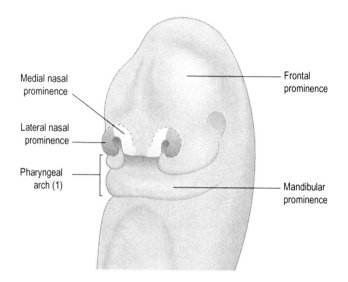

Medial nasal prominence

Lateral nasal prominence

Pharyngeal arch (1)

Frontal prominence

Mandibular prominence

Figure 6.4 shows the development of the face. The structures of the nose and nasal cavity develop alongside the structures of the larynx. Between weeks 4 and 5 of gestation, cells for the forebrain delineate to form nasal placodes, which form nasal pits in the fifth week. This produces ridges of tissue that form in semicircles—the lateral prominences and the medial nasal prominences. The nasal pit deepens until it is separated from the oral cavity only by the thin oronasal membrane, which in turn breaks down, joining the nasal and oral cavity until fusion of the secondary palate occurs. Externally the lateral prominences form the *alae* of the nose, while the medial prominences fuse in the midline to form the *philtrum* of the upper lip, the crest and tip of the nose in the midline. This fusion of tissues occurs with the fusion of the palatine shelves derived from maxillary prominences in the first pharyngeal arch. Fusion in the midline occurs between 7 and 10 weeks gestation; failure of this fusion gives rise to cleft lip and palate (Fig. 6.5).

During this time conchae appear above the secondary palate in the nasal cavity as diverticula (folds) in the lateral nasal cavity wall.

Fig. 6.5
Fusion of the palatine shelves
(7–10 weeks).

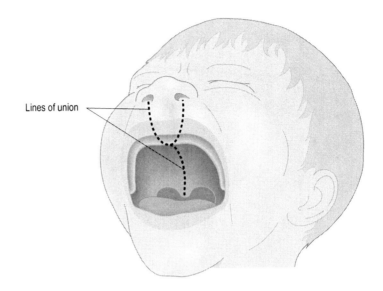

Lines of union

LOWER AIRWAYS: LUNGS, EPIGLOTTIS TO ALVEOLI

In the fourth week of gestation a small diverticulum appears in the ventral aspect (front) of the foregut. This soon forms two lung buds and separates from the gut. Thus the lung is derived from endodermal tissue, whereas the supporting musculature and cartilage of the lung are from the splanchnic mesoderm.

Failure of the trachea to separate from the oesophagus gives rise to tracheo-oesophageal fistulas (see Fig. 6.8). The separation of these canulae and the branching of the bronchial tree has been shown in animal studies to be mediated by transcriptive morphoregulatory molecules (Minoo et al 1999).

In the fifth week the lung buds divide into the right and left bronchi. The right main bronchi forms three secondary bronchi, predictive of the three lobes of the right lung; the left forms two secondary bronchi and therefore two left lobes. Throughout the embryonic and fetal periods the lungs continue to branch and grow into the *pericardioperitoneal* canals on each side of the gut (Figs 6.6–6.7).

The mesoderm covering the developing lung lobes forms the visceral pleura, while the somatic mesoderm that lines the pericardioperitoneal cavity develops into the parietal pleura; the space between these forms the pleural cavity.

Between 6 and 16 weeks of gestation the lung structure is described as being in the pseudoglandular period (Fig. 6.9A). In this period of lung development the conductive branchial tree, together with epithelial cell structures such as ciliated cells, develops centrally and extends peripherally. Some have suggested that at the end of this stage the precursors of gas-exchanging cells appear at the peripheral edges of the tree structure (Burri & Moschopulos 1992).

Fig. 6.6
Branching of lung buds from
the foregut.

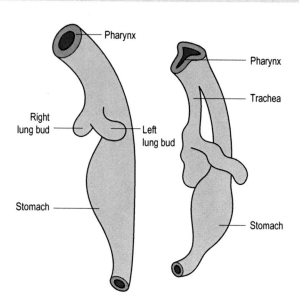

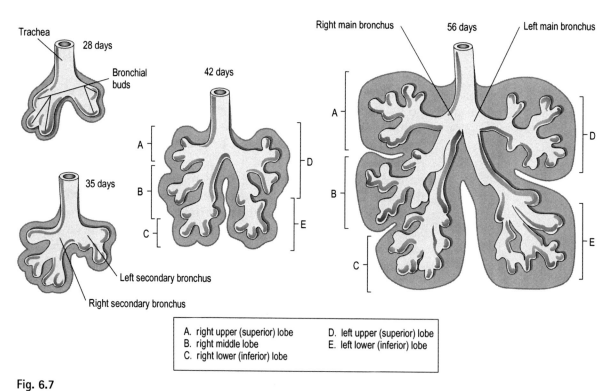

A. right upper (superior) lobe   D. left upper (superior) lobe
B. right middle lobe   E. left lower (inferior) lobe
C. right lower (inferior) lobe

Fig. 6.7
Development of the branching structure of the lungs into lobes. (From Moore & Persaud 2003, with permission of
W B Saunders.)

Fig. 6.8
Tracheo-oesophageal
malformations.

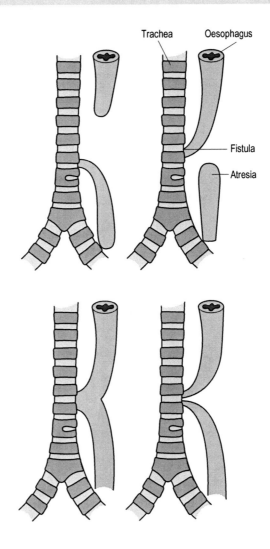

DEVELOPMENT OF
THE DIAPHRAGM

During the fourth week of gestation as the head and body become delineated, the septum transversum forms from mesenchyme cells. This lateral plate of tissue does not completely separate thorax and abdomen, but leaves large spaces into which the budding lungs grow and through which the oesophagus and gut pass (Fig. 6.10). The pleuroperitoneal membranes, which surround the developing lungs, grow from the dorsal aspect of the fetus towards the septum transversum. In week 6 the structures of the septum transversum, pleuroperitoneal membranes and the peripheral tissue of the oesophagus fuse to separate the thorax and abdomen. Failure of fusion results in a herniation of the diaphragm where the gut is pushed into lung space, affecting lung development. Once the diaphragm has fused, myoblasts from the body wall invade the rim of the diaphragm giving it its muscular and domed nature. Although the main nerve supply to the diaphragm

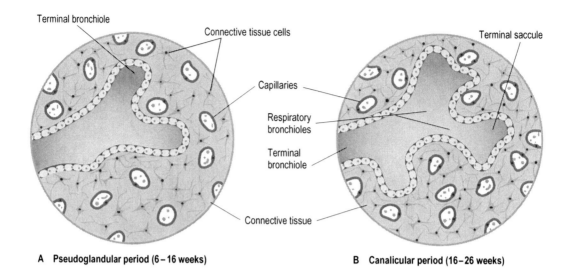

A   Pseudoglandular period (6–16 weeks)   B   Canalicular period (16–26 weeks)

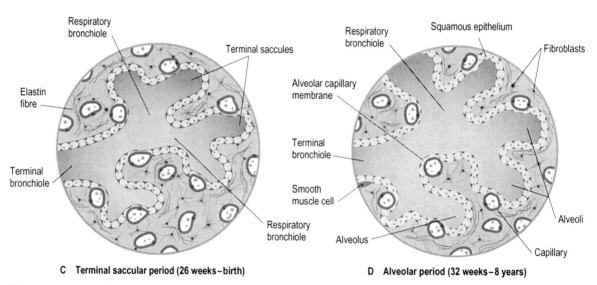

C   Terminal saccular period (26 weeks–birth)   D   Alveolar period (32 weeks–8 years)

Fig. 6.9
A–D Structural development of the lungs. (From Moore & Persaud 2003, with permission of W B Saunders.)

comes from the phrenic nerve originating in the pleurocardial folds, some nerves serving the lower thorax also invade with the myoblasts.

FETAL DEVELOPMENT

Although the conchae in the nasal cavity continue to divide and develop during the fetal and childhood periods, the structures of the upper airway are on the whole formed in the embryo, continuing to delineate and grow during weeks 8–40 of gestation. However, the

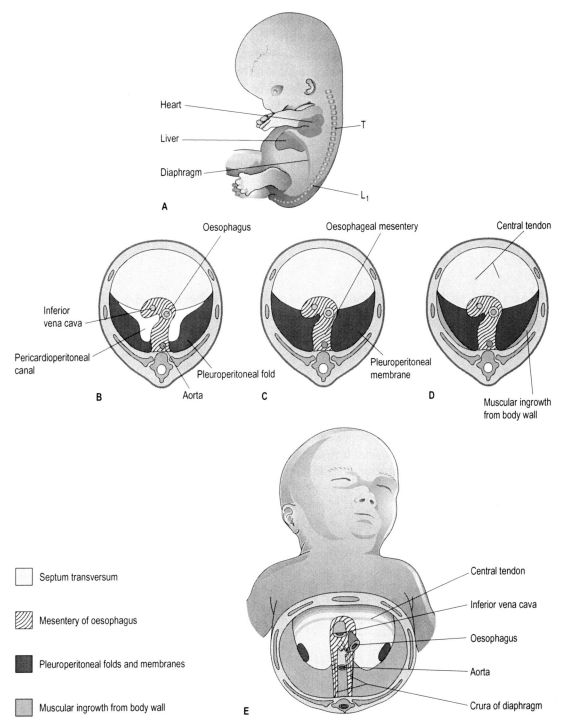

Fig. 6.10
A–E Development of the diaphragm. (From Moore & Persaud 2003, with permission of W B Saunders.)

transformation of the lung during this period is remarkable. The lung volume increases and the structure of the lungs alter as they become ready to take on gaseous exchange.

This development is influenced by intrinsic factors such as the production and regulation of morphoregulatory molecules, which can be grouped into three classifications:

- transcription factors, which act to differentiate cells into new structures
- signalling factors, which initiate the differentiation of cells into new structures
- extracellular matrix and receptors, which form networks such as collagen.

Lung development is also influenced by extrinsic factors, such as fetal lung liquid.

FETAL LUNG LIQUID

Fetal lung liquid is produced by epithelial lung cells creating osmotic gradients via the active transport of chloride ions into the lumen of the lung by means of the sodium–potassium adenosine triphosphatase pump (Fig. 6.11), thereby drawing fluid into the lung lumen. Studies in sheep have demonstrated relatively high chloride levels in fetal lung liquid (140–150 mmol/L) in comparison to amniotic fluid (90–100 mmol/L), as well as a steady increase in the secretion of fetal lung liquid over the fetal period. Various studies have shown that during apnoea and fetal breath movement the pressure gradient between the fetal lungs and the amniotic sac is maintained at 1–2 mmHg. Thus, during fetal development the lung is constantly stretched by the

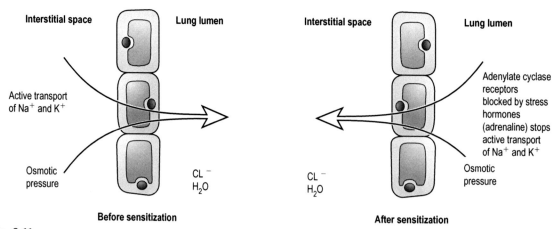

Fig. 6.11
Sensitization of pulmonary epithelium by adrenaline.

hydrostatic pressure of fetal lung liquid and fetal breath movements. Experiments in animals to increase or decrease the pressure within the fetal lung have shown a direct relationship to fetal lung development. Such an effect can also be observed where the fetal lung has been compressed, such as when gastric contents have herniated through the diaphragm. Conversely, congenital malformations of the upper airways can lead to overexpansion, affecting lung growth.

This stretching of the developing lung causes the mesenchymal cells to differentiate into smooth muscle; cells that are not elongated do not develop into smooth muscle. The development of type II pneumocytes, important in the production of surfactant, is also influenced by fetal lung liquid pressure. Compression of the alveolar surface also appears to enhance surfactant functioning, as discussed below.

LUNG STRUCTURE

In the fetal stage, lung structure progresses from the pseudoglandular stage of weeks 6–16 into the canalicular stage, which lasts from week 16 to 26 of gestation, and finally into the saccular stage, from 26 weeks to birth (Fig. 6.9A–C).

In the canalicular stage, the branching structure of the lungs extends into the mesenchyme surrounding the growing structure and acquires a capillary sleeve from the capillary network, which will grow with each bronchiole and connect it to the main cardiovascular network. During the canalicular stage, pulmonary epithelium begins to differentiate as the cuboid cells elongate into type I pneumocytes. The type II pneumocytes remain spherical, but develop laminar bodies crucial to surfactant production (see below). As lung development moves into the saccular stage, the last bronchioles divide. Each saccule divides irregularly to produce a cluster of saccules connected to the bronchiole. Thus the capillary network becomes squeezed between saccules, giving a characteristic structure of a layer of connective tissue with capillary layers on either side, covered by a single cell layer of alveolar epithelium. It is during this stage that elastic tissue begins to appear, facilitated by the constant stretching of the lung (Demayo et al 2002). This elastic tissue forms extracellular matrix, which extends internally to the lung from the axial fibre network, from the hilum to the terminal respiratory unit, and eventually forms a ring of tissue around each alveolus. This network is braced by an external network, which extends from the plural cavity connective tissue into the lung, subdividing lobes and segments and alveolar units. This network of collagen fibres limits the expansion of the lung on inspiration and is thought to help model and remodel the developing lung.

This double layer of capillaries and elastic tissue is the prerequisite for alveolization. During alveolization, each saccule is divided by the elastic tissue, forming a ridge in the saccule lumen. Elastic tissue then forms a ring about the entrance to the newly formed alveoli. Thus, the double layer of capillaries is split and alveoli are formed with a single cell layer of pulmonary epithelium fused to a capillary, creating the, on average, 0.5-μm thick blood–air membrane for effective gaseous exchange. This begins the process of increasing the fetal lung surface area from 1–2 m^2 to the adult surface area of more than 50 m^2.

Although debate continues regarding the exact extent of alveolization before birth and when adult levels are reached, it is proposed that there is a 'bulk alveolar formation' beginning at 36 weeks of gestation and slowing down by 6 months of age postnatally.

FETAL BREATH MOVEMENTS

Fetal breath movements appear in humans at about 10–11 weeks gestation (De Vries et al 1986). These movements of the diaphragm and intercostal muscles act to lower intrathoracic pressure, and arise from the activation of neural pathways of the respiratory region in the brain (phrenic and intercostal nerves), as do postnatal breathing movements. Although fetal breath movements increase over the fetal period, prolonged apnoea can still be observed at term. However, attempts to link fetal breath movements with an increased risk of neonatal respiratory problems have not been reliable (Patrick et al 1980).

As well as rhythmic fetal breath movement, hiccupping and asphyxial gasping have been observed in the human fetus. Although the function of hiccupping is unclear, it has been observed to decrease during the fetal period from 10% of observed time to 2–4% at term (Pillai & James 1990).

Asphyxial gasping is associated with severe hypoxia in the fetus and appears to be an early innate response to low levels of oxygen or high levels of carbon monoxide.

It would appear that the mechanical expansion and contraction of the fetal lung interacts with the biochemical regulation of the developing lung. This can be seen in the production and functioning of surfactant.

SURFACTANT

The pliability of the fetal lung comes in part from a single molecular layer (monolayer) of a complex mixture of lipids and proteins. This monolayer alters the surface tension of peripheral air spaces to allow expansion, but also to prevent the collapse of alveoli. Primarily this is achieved by a high dipalmitoyl phosphatidylcholine (DPPC) content, approximately 45% by weight. However, surfactant also contains surfactant-specific proteins SPA, SPB, SPC and SPD, which play a vital role in the functioning of surfactant and the lungs.

These lipids and surfactant proteins (SPA–D) are synthesized in pneumocyte type II cells. At about 20 weeks' gestation, laminar bodies appear in type II cells. These laminar bodies consist of bilayers of phosphoid lipids, newly synthesized SPB and SPC with some recycled SPA. The laminar bodies are fused with the surface membrane, and unravel to combine with synthesized SPA and calcium forming a complex lattice structure of tubular molecules intersecting with lipids called tubular myelin. At the lung–lumen interface, non-DPPC lipids are removed by the expansion and contraction caused by fetal breath movements; thus the monolayer created from the tubular myelin is enriched with DPPC. This gives the monolayer the ability to reduce surface tension when compressed, so that during fetal expiration movements smaller alveoli are prevented from emptying into larger spaces, thereby preventing collapse.

Most of the lipids removed from the epithelial surface are recycled or destroyed by vesicles within type II cells. Some are absorbed by alveolar macrophages. SPA is thought to influence both of these processes. In vitro experiments on lung tissue have shown that the carbohydrate and collagenous binding properties of SPA, which resemble those of complement factor C1q, promote *chemolysis* and *phagocytosis* by alveolar macrophages and intracellular lysis by oxygen free radicals (Van Iwaarden 1992).

During the second and third trimesters, saturated lipid levels rise, until around week 20 when the saturated lipid level is at 30% of the adult level. Animal studies show a 7-fold increase in saturated lipid levels in the last quarter of the third trimester. This seems to be related to increased production rather than decreased absorption, as the increase relates directly to increased levels of the enzyme fatty acid synthetase, which is likely to be the key factor regulating lipid production. Human amniotic fluid shows a similar increase in saturated lipid levels towards term (40 weeks), and correlates to lung maturity.

Surfactant proteins have different gene (and RNA) profiles during gestation. SPA is hardly detectable in the fetus from 13 to 24 weeks, whereas SPB gene expression rises from its first detection at about 13 weeks to 50% of adult levels at 24 weeks, and SPC reaches 15% in the same time frame (Liley et al 1989). Thus it appears that the SPA gene expression is linked to the appearance of type II alveolar cells, whereas that of SPB and SPC is independent. Levels of surfactant proteins detected by means of immunoassay are increased during the second and third trimester (24 weeks onwards).

Studies in sheep suggest that surfactant production is regulated by endogenous glucocorticoids (e.g. cortisol) and thyroid hormones. Surgical removal of secreting organs results in poor lung maturation and reduced surfactant production, whereas replacement therapy induces lung maturation. Steroid treatment of infants expected to be born prematurely has been shown to increase lung maturity at birth (Halliday et al 2003). However, this Cochrane review of early dexamethasone treatment warns that the advantages for lung development may be outweighed by the disadvantages of steroid treatment.

CLINICAL NOTES   **RESPIRATORY DISTRESS**

Respiratory distress syndrome (RDS)
This is a syndrome of prematurity seen in neonates born before they have sufficient surfactant to enable their lungs to function in air. Typically these neonates have severe respiratory distress and a ground-glass appearance to their lungs on radiography. Often these children need ventilation for some time and treatment with artificial surfactant.

Chronic lung disease
Often a sequela to RDS, chronic lung disease describes an enduring state of lung failure in which oxygen supplements may be required to maintain blood oxygen saturation levels (oxygen dependence). In children it is a disease of prematurity where the following features are common: a history of artificial ventilation for 3 days or more, a 'ground glass' appearance on chest radiography, signs of respiratory distress, hypersensitivity of the lungs, and poor weight gain (Carey & Totton 1996). This group of children included those previously diagnosed as having bronchopulmonary dysplasia.

For children with chronic lung disease, oxygen dependency can be prolonged and the majority will require community care. It has been estimated that at any one time in the UK there are some 730 infants dependent on oxygen (Southall & Samuels 1990). Children with chronic lung disease often present as medically fragile with repeated admissions to hospital.

CHANGES AT BIRTH

At birth, fetal lungs filled with fetal lung fluid and with a high-pressure, low-flow vascular system must empty of fluid; by closure of the ductus arteriosus, the vascular system becomes low pressure and high flow, as the two sides of the heart separate and establish an adult circulation. The structures of the lungs and chest held in place by the fetal lung liquid and amniotic fluid must stiffen to resist atmospheric pressure and gravity. That this transformation must occur within moments of birth surely makes it one of the most remarkable transformations in human anatomy.

The process begins a few days before term when pulmonary epithelium becomes sensitive to stress hormones, mainly adrenaline. This process of sensitization appears to be mediated by triiodothyronine (T3) and cortisol acting together (Barker et al 1991), with levels of T3 being kept low by various conversions of the hormone to T2 or T4, giving a short fetal half-life for T3 until late in pregnancy when levels of both T3 and cortisol rise. Before this sensitization, adrenaline present in the pulmonary epithelium will slow fetal lung fluid production, but after sensitization it blocks the active transport of sodium and chloride ions across the pulmonary epithelium, reversing the osmotic pressure and causing fetal lung liquid to be reabsorbed into the interstitial spaces where it is slowly redistributed by the lymph system (Fig. 6.11).

Thus, as labour begins and stress hormones in the fetus rise, fetal lung liquid begins to be reabsorbed. During delivery, as the head emerges and the baby proceeds along the birth canal, the chest wall is compressed, so increasing intrathoracic pressure. This action drains the lungs of fetal lung fluid.

CLINICAL NOTES METHOD OF DELIVERY AND LUNG FUNCTION AT BIRTH

Babies born by elective caesarean section, who do not experience labour or the effects of uterine contractions and compression by the birth canal, may show signs of retention of fetal lung fluid, including grunting, tachypnoea and respiratory distress. Such babies require careful neonatal nursing and are more frequently admitted to neonatal units for observation with respiration-related disease (Levine et al 2001).

Although these babies have similar levels of stress hormones, as sampled from cord blood at birth, the length of exposure appears to be crucial. As suggested by animal studies, a period of labour rather than the method of delivery is the major factor determining lung function at birth.

POSTNATAL DEVELOPMENT

Lung development continues thoroughout childhood. Although alveolization may be mainly complete by 6 months of age, the structure of the lungs changes over childhood. In the term baby the chest wall is highly compliant with incomplete ossification of the ribs, which are horizontal rather than downward sloping as in the adult (see Ch. 3). Ossification is not complete until 25 years of age, and adult rib positioning at about the age of 10 years (Allen & Gripp 2002). The structure of the diaphragm is also different in the newborn; it is flatter and has a smaller, less convex, curvature into the thorax. The horizontal positioning of the ribs reduces the 'bucket handle' motion, which expands the thoracic cage (Fig. 6.12). These factors, together with the

Fig. 6.12
Rib positions in the adult (A)
and the child (B).

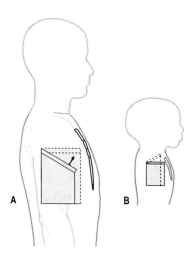

high compliance of the neonatal chest wall, make the neonate's chest a less effective pump. This results in a smaller resting volume, which predisposes the neonate to *atelectasis* and reduced reserves of oxygen.

To compensate for this reduced efficiency, the expiratory time is prolonged by the diaphragm and slight tracheal collapse in the upper airways to maintain an end-expiratory pressure (EEP). In addition, the neonate has a higher haemoglobin concentration (mean level 16.8 (range 13.7–20.1) g/dL) and a higher haematocrit of 55% (adult haemoglobin level is 14–16 g/dL and haematocrit 42–47%), better gaseous exchange and a higher respiratory rate (25–40 breaths per minute).

The neonate's ability to control breathing also develops in the postnatal period. The long periods of apnoea tolerated in the womb cannot be sustained now that the neonate is reliant on gaseous exchange. Although chemoreceptors in the brainstem and carotid begin from birth to drive adult responses to low oxygen and increases in carbon monoxide levels, some patterns of fetal breathing persist such as periodic breathing where rates and tidal volume change slowly with regular apnoea. Infants under 2 months of age may use this type of breathing for 50 minutes per day (Richards et al 1984). This pattern is not associated with reductions in heart rate or hypoxia. Periodic apnoea where the neonate stops breathing, with breaths in between at irregular intervals, may occur more than 200 times per day in infants aged under 2 months, and is associated with bradycardia and temporary hypoxia (Richards et al 1984). These types of breathing pattern increase as gestational age and birthweight decrease. The newborn's response to hypoxia is also subject to developmental change. When exposed to low levels of oxygen (e.g. at high altitude or in an aircraft cabin), a two-phase response occurs: first, an increased expiratory volume, and, second, a progressive decline which affects oxygen saturation and can fall below the 95% norm (Richard et al 1993).

This hypoxic reaction may be heightened in rapid eye movement (REM) sleep, while carbon dioxide response is less during REM sleep.

CLINICAL NOTES	SUDDEN INFANT DEATH SYNDROME

Sudden infant death syndrome (SIDS) affects children, generally under 2 years of age, who appear to have a respiratory arrest while sleeping, with the highest prevalence in 2–4-month-old children. Links have been drawn between SIDS and the preterm infant's breathing pattern. These theories suggest an altered arousal response.

For ethical reasons, testing infants' responses to hypoxia is unacceptable. However, auditory response and arousal is seen as a similar mechanism and has been used to show decreased arousal in infants in the prone position, in infants who do not use a pacifier and in those whose mothers smoked during pregnancy (Chang et al 2003).

Prevention of SIDS—the 'back to sleep' public health campaign—has reduced the incidence of SIDS by concentrating on encouraging parents to place babies on their backs (supine) and to avoid parental smoking (Douglas et al 1998).

As the child grows, although the compliance of the lung as a whole remains stable, the chest wall compliance gradually decreases over the lifespan. The balancing of the compliance of the lung and chest wall as well as the structural changes in the ribcage, diaphragm and abdominal muscles gradually increases the child's respiratory efficiency and resilience. Thus between 1 and 2 years of age, delayed expiration disappears (Allen & Gripp 2002).

During this early period of childhood, hyperreactivity in the lungs also diminishes. Hyperreactivity refers to the natural reaction of the airway to constrict if stimulated by an irritant; under laboratory conditions this is simulated by the inhalation of histamine or methacholine (Hill et al 1992).

Hyperreactivity in young children is also increased by environmental tobacco smoke (parental history of smoking), a family history of asthma and upper airway viral infection (Hill et al 1992). Hyperreactivity in children presents as an expiratory wheeze heard on auscultation of the chest. This developmental predisposition to wheezing may mask the development of asthma in young children.

Over the course of childhood, lung volumes increase and resistance decreases in a linear relationship to age and height until puberty, when there is a large increase in lung volume (McKenzie et al 2002, Rosenthal et al 1993). Boys' lung growth exceeds that of girls'. This extra spurt of growth means that, whereas in girls growth is proportional throughout the airways, in boys the larger airways grow faster than the smaller airways. However, maximal female lung growth is reached at around 18 years, whereas that of the male continues into young adulthood (24–30 years); the periods of growth and lung volume achieved are both decreased by tobacco smoking. These periods of growth, up to 18 years of age in females and 24 years in males, may also constitute a critical period of 'field cancerization', when cells exposed to tobacco smoke may become precursors of lung cancer cells, so that smoking during this period may lead to malignancy in later life (Wiencke & Kelsey 2002).

The development of the respiratory system over the span of childhood and early adulthood shows that children are not born with lungs that are small replicas of adult lungs. This developing system requires understanding in its own right. Many questions remain unanswered in the embryonic and fetal development of human lungs, which could inform this understanding of our children's developing respiratory system.

SELF ASSESSMENT

- Outline why respiration and respiratory disorders are important in childhood.
- Describe the development of either the upper airways or the bronchial tree in the embryo and fetus.
- How is surfactant produced and regulated, and why is it important in lung development?
- Identify the factors that affect lung growth in the fetus.
- Describe the changes to the lungs that occur at birth.
- Outline the changes to children's respiratory system from birth to adult maturation.

References

Allen J, Gripp K W 2002 Development of the thoracic cage. In: Haddad G G, Chernick V, Abman S H (eds) Basic mechanisms of pediatric respiratory disease, 2nd edn. B C Decker, London, p 124–137

Austin J B, Kaur B, Anderson H R et al 1999 Hay fever, eczema, and wheeze: a nationwide UK study (ISAAC, International Study of Asthma and Allergies in Childhood). Archives of Disease in Childhood 81:225–230

Barker P M, Walters D V, Markiewicz M, Strang L B 1991 Development of the lung liquid reabsorption mechanism in fetal sheep: synergism of triiodothyronine and hydrocortisone. Journal of Physiology 433:435–449

Bunn H J, Grigg J 2000 Air pollution and respiratory disease in children: evidence for an association. Asthma Journal 5:168–172

Burri P H, Moschopulos M 1992 Structural anaysis of fetal rat lung development. Anatomical Record 234:399–418

Carey B E, Totton C 1996 Bronchopulmonary dysplasia. Neonatal Network 15(4):73–77

Chang A B, Wilson S J, Masters I B et al 2003 Altered arousal response in infants exposed to cigarette smoke. Archives of Disease in Childhood 88:30–33

Demayo F, Minoo P, Plopper C G, Schuger L, Shannon J, Torday J S 2002 Mesenchymal–epithelial interactions in lung development and repair: are modeling and remodeling the same process? American Journal of Physiology. Lung Cellular and Molecular Physiology 283:L510–L517

De Vries J I P, Visser G H A, Precht H F R 1986 Fetal behaviour in early pregnancy. European Journal of Obstetrics, Gynecology, and Reproductive Biology 21:271–276

Douglas A S, Helms P J, Jolliffe I T 1998 Seasonality of sudden infant death syndrome in mainland Britain and Ireland 1985–95. Archives of Disease in Childhood 79(3):269–270

Halliday H L, Ehrenkranz R A, Doyle L W 2003 Early postnatal (<96 hours) corticosteroids for preventing chronic lung disease in preterm infants (Cochrane Review). In: The Cochrane Library, Issue 1. Update Software, Oxford

Hill M, Szefier S J, Larsen G L 1992 Asthma pathogenesis and the implications for therapy in children. Pediatric Clinics of North America 39(6):1205–1224

Kai J 1996 What worries parents when their preschool children are acutely ill, and why: a qualitative study. British Medical Journal 313:986–993

Levine E M, Ghai V, Barton J J, Strom C M 2001 Mode of delivery and risk of respiratory disease in newborns. Obstetrics and Gynecology 97(3):439–442

Liley H G, White R T, Warr R G, Benson B J, Hawgood S, Ballard P L 1989 Regulation of messenger RNAs for the hydrophobic surfactant proteins in the human lung. Journal of Clinical Investigation 83:1191–1197

McKenzie S A, Chan E, Dundas I et al 2002 Airway resistance measured by the interrupter technique: normative data for 2–10 year olds from three ethnicities. Archives of Disease in Childhood 87:248–251

Minoo P, Su G, Drum H, Bringas P, Kimura S 1999 Defects in tracheoesophageal and lung morphogenesis in Nkx2.1 deficient mouse embryos. Developmental Biology 209:60–71

Moore K L, Persaud R V N 2003 Developing human clinically orientated embryology, 7th edn. W B Saunders, Philadelphia

Patrick J, Campbell K, Carmicheal L, Natale R, Richardson B 1980 Patterns of human fetal breathing during the last 10 weeks of pregnancy. Obstetrics and Gynecology 56:24–30

Pillai M, James D 1990 Hiccups and breathing in human fetuses. Archives of Disease in Childhood 65:1072–1075

Richard D, Poets C F, Neale S, Stebbens V A, Alexander J R, Southall D P 1993 Arterial oxygen saturation in preterm neonates without respiratory failure. Journal of Pediatrics 123:963–968

Richards J M, Alexander J R, Shinebourne E A, de Swiet M, Wilson A J, Southall D P 1984 Sequential 22 hour profiles of breathing patterns and heart rate in 110 full term infants during their first 6 months of life. Pediatrics 74:763–777

Rosenthal M, Bain S H, Cramer D et al 1993 Lung function in white children aged 4 to 19 years: I—Spirometry. Thorax 48:794–802

Southall D P, Samuels M P 1990 Bronchopulmonary dysplasia: a new look at management. Archives of Disease in Childhood 65:1089–1095

Van Iwaarden J F 1992 Surfactant and the pulmonary defence system: In: Robertson B, van Golde L M G, Batenburg J J (eds) Pulmonary surfactant: from molecular biology to clinical practice. Elsevier Science, Amsterdam, p 215–227

Wiencke J K, Kelsey K T 2002 Teen smoking, field cancerization and a critical period hypothesis for lung cancer susceptibility. Environmental Health Perspectives 110(6):555–557

Bibliography

Ballard P L 1989 Hormonal regulation of pulmonary surfactant. Endocrine Reviews 10:165–181

Behrman R E, Kliegman R M (eds) 2002 Nelson essentials of pediatrics, 4th edn. W B Saunders, Philadelphia

Demayo F, Minoo P, Plopper C G, Schuger L, Shannon J, Torday J S 2002 Mesenchymal–epithelial interactions in lung development and repair: are modeling and remodeling the same process? American Journal of Physiology. Lung Cellular and Molecular Physiology 283:L510–L517

Hanson M A, Spencer J A D, Rodeck C H, Walters D (eds) 1994 Fetus and neonate physiology and clinical application. Vol. 2: Breathing. Cambridge University Press, Cambridge

Harding R, Bocking A D (eds) 2001 Fetal growth and development. Cambridge University Press, Cambridge

Moessinger A C, Harding R D, Adamson T M, Singh M, Kiu G T 1990 Role of lung liquid volume in growth and maturation of the fetal sheep lung. Journal of Clinical Investigation 86:1270–1277

Nunn J F 2000 The atmosphere. In: Lumb A B (ed.) Nunn's applied respiratory physiology, 5th edn. Butterworth Heinemann, Oxford

Sadler T W 1995 Langman's medical embryology, 7th edn. Williams & Wilkins, Baltimore

Chapter 7

The gastrointestinal tract

Mary Sandwell

CHAPTER OUTCOMES

This chapter will enable the reader to:

- Describe the embryological and fetal development of the gastrointestinal tract
- Identify the changes that occur within the gastrointestinal tract from birth to maturity
- Identify the organs that make up the gastrointestinal tract and describe the structure and function of each
- Define digestion and explain how the end products of digestion are absorbed.

CHAPTER OVERVIEW

The aim of this chapter is to explore the development of the gastrointestinal tract during the embryo stage (weeks 4 to 8 after conception), the fetal stage (week 9 to birth) and after birth to maturity. It also discusses digestion and absorption after birth. The Clinical Notes address issues of clinical relevance and interest to the reader. The Self Assessment exercises assist in reflecting upon the chapter and guiding the relationship between theory and professional practice.

INTRODUCTION

Food is vital for sustaining life, building and repairing damaged tissues; it is the source of energy that drives the chemical reaction in every cell. When food is first taken into the body, it is not in a suitable state for use as an energy source for the cell; therefore it needs to be broken down into molecules that are small enough to cross the cell membrane. This process is called digestion. The passage of the molecules into the blood and lymph is known as absorption. The organs that perform these functions compose the digestive system.

The digestive organs are divided into two main groups:

1. The gastrointestinal tract or alimentary (*alimentum* = nourishment) canal—a continuous tube that extends from the mouth to the anus and is open at both ends.
2. The accessory structures—the teeth, tongue, salivary glands, liver, gall bladder and pancreas.

The activities of digestion are grouped under six basic processes:

- *ingestion*—taking food into the mouth
- *secretion*—cells within the walls of the gastrointestinal tract and accessory organs secrete water, acid, buffers and enzymes into the lumen of the tract
- *mixing and propulsion*—smooth muscle in the gastrointestinal tract mixes food and secretions, and moves them along the alimentary tract
- *digestion*—mechanical breakdown by chewing (mastication), chemical breakdown by the enzymes present in the secretions
- *absorption*—digested food substances pass through the lining of the gastrointestinal tract by either active or passive diffusion; the material then passes into the lymph and blood and is circulated around the body
- *elimination*—of indigestible substances and bacteria through the anus as faeces.

EMBRYOLOGY AND FETAL DEVELOPMENT

About 14 days after fertilization, the cells of the endoderm form a cavity referred to as the *primitive* gut. The primitive gut has a double-layered wall:

- *endodermal layer*—this gives rise to the epithelial lining and glands of most of the gastrointestinal tract

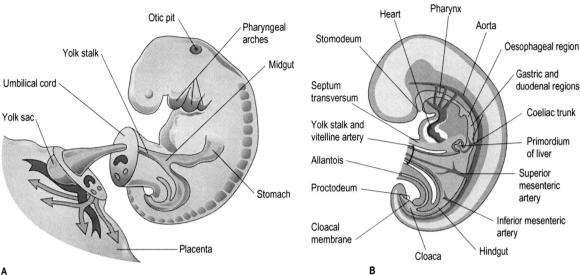

A

Fig. 7.1

A Lateral view of a four week old embryo showing the relationship of primordial gut to the yolk sac.

B Cross section of the embryo showing early digestive system and its blood supply. The blood vessels are derived from the vessels that supplied the yolk sac.

(From Moore & Persaud 2003, with permission of W B Saunders.)

● *mesodermal layer*—this produces the smooth muscle and connective tissue of the gastrointestinal tract.

During the third week the gut grows and there is differentiation, with an anterior *foregut*, an intermediate *midgut* and a posterior *hindgut*.

The headfold of the embryo becomes the foregut, the fold in the tail becomes the hindgut, and the middle, which is still in direct communication with the yolk sac, becomes the midgut (Fig. 7.1). Thus the gastrointestinal tract forms a continuous tube from mouth to anus, which are fixed areas of endoderm and ectoderm; the tube is therefore anchored at both ends. The formation of the gut involves continuous elongation, herniation, and histogenesis and functional maturation.

Figure 7.2 shows the origins of the primitive gut. The *foregut derivatives* are:

● pharynx and its derivatives
● lower respiratory tract
● oesophagus
● stomach
● liver
● pancreas
● gall bladder
● biliary duct system
● duodenum cephalic to the opening of the bile duct.

The blood supply to these parts is the *coeliac artery*.

Fig. 7.2
Origins of the primitive gut.

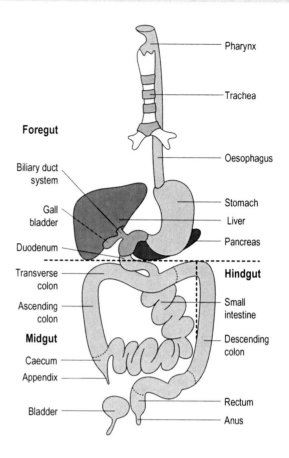

The *midgut derivatives* are:

- small intestine including the duodenum distal to the opening of the bile duct
- caecum
- vermiform appendix
- ascending colon
- proximal two-thirds of transverse colon.

The blood supply to these parts is the *superior mesenteric artery.*
The *hindgut derivatives* are:

- distal one-third of transverse colon
- descending colon
- sigmoid colon
- rectum
- superior part of the anal canal
- epithelium of urinary bladder and most of urethra.

The blood supply to these parts is the *inferior mesenteric artery.*

Between weeks 6 to 8 of development, the proliferation of the epithelial cells lining the gut obliterates the lumen, which is then gradually recanalized. Early growth of the gut is extremely rapid so that it extrudes into the amniotic cavity.

The normal growth of the gastrointestinal tract before birth depends on the fetus swallowing; by the 16th week of development, the fetus will swallow about one-third of the total amniotic fluid every hour. Amniotic fluid provides approximately 10% of fetal protein requirements and is also associated with the effective development of the gastrointestinal mucosa, pancreas and liver, and with the promotion of growth.

DEVELOPMENT OF THE TONGUE

The development of the tongue starts in the fourth week when the first arch forms—*tuberculum impar* (median tongue bud). In a 5-week-old embryo the tongue is represented by a pair of *lateral lingual swellings* (distal tongue buds), which are derivatives of the first arch; these enlarge and fuse in the midline. Their line of fusion is seen in the adult as the *median sulcus and septum*. These swellings continue to grow and form the anterior two-thirds of the tongue.

The posterior one-third of the tongue (root) forms the *copula* (ventromedial ends of the second arch) and the hypobranchial eminence. During growth, the hypobranchial eminence overgrows the copula. The anterior two-thirds and the posterior one-third of the tongue meet in the position of a V shape—the *terminal sulcus* region of the adult tongue.

The taste buds develop in weeks 7 and 8. The buds of the anterior two-thirds are supplied by a special branch of the facial nerve, the *chorda tympani* (cranial nerve VII). A row of taste buds flanking the terminal sulcus is supplied by the *glossopharyngeal nerve.*

All the muscles, with the exception of the palatoglossus, are activated by the *hypoglossal nerve* (cranial nerve XII). The palatoglossus is activated by the *vagus nerve* (cranial nerve X).

After birth   The tip of the tongue in the infant is stubby and rounded; the mobile and more pointed tip of the adult tongue develops gradually with chewing and swallowing.

DEVELOPMENT OF THE SALIVARY GLANDS

There are three pairs of salivary glands: the parotid, the submandibular and the sublingual. The largest glands, the parotids, originate from ectoderm; the other two pairs originate from endoderm. The different origins are based on the position of each in relation to the oropharyngeal membrane in the future mouth.

After birth   The salivary glands triple their birthweight by 6 months of age. By the age of 2 years they are five times as large as at birth, and at this stage they have developed the adult structure and functions.

The salivary glands of the neonate produce only small amounts of saliva containing the enzyme amylase.

DEVELOPMENT OF THE OESOPHAGUS

The area of the foregut just caudal to the lung bud is the oesophagus. At first, the segment of the oesophagus is very short and the stomach seems to reach the pharynx. During the second month, the gut grows and the oesophagus nearly reaches the proportions of the mature infant in relation to the position of the stomach.

In the early stages the lining of the oesophagus is stratified columnar. By week 8 the epithelium has partly closed off the lumen, and large vacuoles appear. During the following weeks these vacuoles merge and the lumen of the oesophagus recanalizes, but with multi-layered ciliated epithelium. At about 4 months this epithelium is replaced with stratified squamous epithelium, which characterizes the mature oesophagus.

By 5 weeks of gestation the primoderm of the inner circular muscle is present, and by 8 weeks the outer longitudinal muscle begins to form. The oesophageal wall contains both smooth and skeletal muscle.

After birth   The pharyngeal–oesophageal swallow is a primitive autonomic reflex for the first 3 months of life. The infant's mouth learns discriminative and motor skills as the stratified muscles in the throat establish cerebral connections.

DEVELOPMENT OF THE STOMACH

From week 4 the stomach is attached to the dorsal body by the dorsal mesentery (*dorsal mesogastrium*) and to the ventral wall by the ventral mesentery (*ventral mesogastrium*). From about 6 weeks' gestation, the stomach is identified as a dilated area similar in shape to the adult stomach.

The J-shaped stomach gradually rotates so that the lesser curvature faces the right side of the body and the greater curvature the left. As

Table 7.1 Stomach capacity by age (Moules & Ramsey 1998)

Age	Capacity (mL)
Newborn	10–20
1 week	30–90
2–3 weeks	75–100
1 month	90–150
3 months	150–200
1 year	210–360
2 years	500
10 years	750–900
16 years	1500
Adult	2000–3000

this rotation occurs, the stomach also tilts 90° clockwise; the dorsal mesogastrium is carried with it, leading to the formation of a pouch-like structure called the *omental bursa*. The dorsal mesogastrium and omental bursa enlarge considerably, and part of the dorsal mesogastrium becomes the *omentum*. The omentum hangs over the transverse colon and a portion of the small intestine as a large double flap of fatty tissue. The cavity of the entire abdomen is referred to as the greater sac of the peritoneum.

The cells of the gastric mucosa begin to secrete hydrochloric acid shortly before birth.

After birth   The position and shape of the stomach is high in the abdomen and is oriented horizontally rather than vertically as in the older child (ages 2–10 years). As feeding begins, the stomach capacity increases rapidly, tripling during the first 2 weeks (Table 7.1).

DEVELOPMENT OF THE LIVER

The liver is the heaviest gland of the body and, after the skin, is the second largest organ. During week 4 a ventral endodermal bud arises from the caudal foregut to form the hepatic diverticulum. This will give rise to the liver, gall bladder and pancreas. As the endodermal bud continues to grow, cords of cells extend into the mesenchymal mass of the septum transversum and the bud soon divides into two. The most cranial of these forms the liver, the caudal forms the gall bladder and pancreas.

The liver initially has two lobes of approximately the same size; as it develops, the right lobe grows faster than the left and the adult shape is formed. As it continues to grow, the liver remains covered by a glistening, translucent layer of mesenteric tissue that now serves as the connective tissue capsule of the liver.

A major function of the embryonic liver is to produce blood cells. The liver functions as a *haemopoietic centre*, beginning in week 6, peaking between the third and sixth month, and stopping by birth.

At about 12 weeks the *hepatocytes* begin to produce bile, largely from the breakdown of haemoglobin. The bile drains down the bile duct and is stored in the gall bladder, and by week 13 it colours the intestinal contents (meconium) dark green.

Blood enters the fetus via the umbilical vein, where it travels to the inferior vena cava by two routes. About half enters the hepatic sinusoids and the remainder goes through the ductus venosus and bypasses the liver. More blood can be made to enter the liver substance when the sphincter of the umbilical vein contracts and forces blood into the portal sinus and to the portal vein and sinusoids.

After birth   At birth the liver is relatively large, occupying 40% of the peritoneal cavity and displacing the bowel; the lower margin is palpable below the costal margin. In the infant the liver is 5% of the total bodyweight, compared with 2.5% in the adult. Its size reflects the importance of the functions it performs during fetal development.

CLINICAL NOTES   PHYSIOLOGICAL JAUNDICE

The most common form of physiological jaundice, or *icterus neonatorum*, is relatively mild and self-limiting. Most newborns have raised bilirubin levels and about 50% demonstrate observable signs of jaundice. Newborns produce twice as much bilirubin as adults because they have a higher concentration of circulating erythrocytes and a shorter life of red blood cells (70–90 days instead of 120 days in older children and adults). Normal changes in the hepatic circulation after birth may contribute to excessive demands on liver function.

Two phases of physiological jaundice have been identified (Wong 1999):

- Bilirubin levels gradually increase to approximately 6 mg/dL on the third day of life, then decrease to a plateau of 2–3 mg/dL by day 5.
- Bilirubin levels maintain a steady plateau with no increase or decrease until approximately 12–14 days of age, at which time the bilirubin concentration decreases to the normal level of less than 1 mg/dL.

CLINICAL NOTES   BILIARY ATRESIA

Biliary atresia, or extrahepatic biliary atresia, is a progressive inflammatory process that causes both intrahepatic and extrahepatic bile duct fibrosis, eventually causing ductal obstruction. The condition arises in approximately

50 babies a year in England and Wales. If untreated, biliary atresia will lead to cirrhosis, liver failure and death within the first 2 years of life.

The cause of biliary atresia is unknown; although viral infections with cytomegalovirus, rubella virus, Epstein–Barr virus, rotavirus or reovirus type 3 have been implicated, no specific agent has been found in every case (McEvoy & Suchy 1996, cited in Hockenberry et al 2003). Biliary atresia is not seen in the fetus or stillborn or newborn infant; this suggests that it is acquired late in gestation or in the perinatal period, and its symptoms are manifested within a few weeks of birth.

Many infants with biliary atresia appear well at birth; if jaundice persists beyond the first 2 weeks of life, biliary atresia should be suspected. The urine becomes dark and the stools become progressively paler (Hockenberry et al 2003).

The primary treatment of biliary atresia is hepatic portoenterostomy (Kasai procedure); this involves using a loop of bowel to form a duct to drain the bile from the liver, which results in bile drainage in approximately 80–90% of infants. However, 80–90% will eventually require a liver transplant.

DEVELOPMENT OF THE GALL BLADDER

During week 4 the gall bladder (*galla* = bile) develops from a solid endodermal outgrowth at the caudal part of the hepatic diverticulum. The stalk of the gall bladder forms the adult cystic duct. The stalk connecting the hepatic and cystic ducts to the duodenum forms the adult bile duct.

By the seventh week, vacuoles and degeneration appear in the solid extrabiliary apparatus, and the apparatus is recanalized. The duodenum rotates during weeks 5 to 7, and the entrance to the bile duct, which was initially on the ventral surface, is carried round to the dorsal aspect of the duodenum. By week 13, bile pigment is secreted.

DEVELOPMENT OF THE PANCREAS

In the fifth week the pancreas (*pan* = all areas; *kreas* = flesh) develops from the dorsal and ventral endodermal buds arising from the caudal foregut; these give rise to the parenchyma of the gland. The septa and connective tissue capsule arise from adjacent splanchnic mesenchyme.

The dorsal pancreatic bud is larger and lies on the dorsal aspect of the foregut. Its origin is cephalic to the smaller ventral pancreatic bud, which lies on the ventral aspect near to the entrance of the bile duct into the duodenum. Each bud has a duct system. The dorsal bud grows into the dorsal mesentery and forms most of the pancreas, the body, tail and most of the head.

When the stomach and midgut rotate, the ventral pancreatic bud and its duct are carried clockwise, where they fuse with the dorsal pancreatic duct and its bud system. The ventral pancreatic bud forms the uncinate process and part of the head of the adult pancreas.

The pancreas is a dual organ with both exocrine and endocrine functions. Some 99% is exocrine. Large numbers of *acini* are connected to a sensory duct system. The acini produce digestive enzymes and fluid called pancreatic juice. One per cent is endocrine, consisting of approximately 1 000 000 richly vascularized *islets of Langerhans*, which are scattered among the acini. These produce the hormones glucagon and insulin, which are present by week 12.

DEVELOPMENT OF THE INTESTINES

The intestines are formed from the posterior part of the foregut, the midgut and the hindgut. It is important to understand two points when considering the enormous transformation that takes place in the gut, changing it from a primitive tube to the complex folded arrangement of the adult intestinal tract:

- The yolk stalk extends from the floor of the midgut to the yolk sac. In the adult, the site of attachment of the yolk sac in the small intestine is between the small and large intestine at the ileocaecal junction.

- On the dorsal side of the primitive gut, an unpaired ventral branch of the aorta, the superior mesenteric artery and its branches provide the blood supply to the midgut. The superior mesenteric artery acts as a pivotal point around which the later rotation of the gut occurs.

By the seventh week, rapid growth of the gut tube causes it to buckle out into a hairpin-like loop (Figure 7.3A). The major change that causes the intestines to assume an adult position is an anticlockwise rotation of the caudal limb of the intestinal loop (with yolk sac and superior mesenteric artery as reference points) around the cephalic limb from its ventral aspect. The main result of this rotation is to bring the future colon across the small intestine so that it can assume its C shape position along the ventral abdominal wall.

Behind the colon the small intestine undergoes great elongation and becomes packed into its usual place in the abdominal cavity.

During weeks 9 to 11, the volume of expanded gut is greater than the abdominal cavity can accommodate; as a result the developing

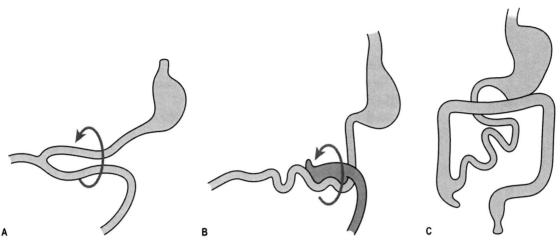

Fig. 7.3
Rotation of the midgut.
A Week 7. B Week 10.
C Week 12.

intestines are herniated into the umbilical cord (Fig. 7.3B). By the tenth week the abdominal cavity has grown sufficiently to accommodate the intestinal tract, and the herniated loops begin to move back into the abdominal cavity. Coils of small intestine return first, and force the distal part of the colon (which was never herniated) to the left side of the peritoneal cavity, thereby establishing the position of the descending colon. After the return of the small intestine, the proximal part of the colon returns with its caecal end swinging to the right and downwards (Fig. 7.3C).

| CLINICAL NOTES | OMPHALOCELE AND GASTROSCHISIS (WONG 1999) |

Omphalocele
This is related to a true failure of embryonic development. It occurs when there is a failure of the caudal or lateral unfolding of the abdominal wall at approximately 3 weeks of gestation. Because of this deficiency in the abdominal wall, the bowel is unable to complete its return to the abdomen between 10 and 12 weeks. A translucent peritoneal sac usually covers the omphalocele; it may contain a small portion of bowel, or most of the bowel and abdominal viscera such as the liver.

Gastroschisis
This occurs when the bowel herniates through a defect in the abdominal wall to the right of the umbilical cord and through the rectus muscle. There is no membrane covering the exposed bowel. It has been suggested that at some point between the bowel being in the umbilical cord and after fixation a tear occurs at the base of the cord allowing the cord to herniate.

During fetal development many functional capabilities are developed, but no major digestive functions occur until feeding starts after birth. Digestive enzymes are present (with the exception of lactase) from about 24–28 weeks of gestation. From about 14 weeks peristalsis of the gut has developed; by 34 weeks there is a coordination of sucking, swallowing and peristalsis.

As the gastrointestinal tract matures it produces mucus, which will lubricate the passage of food and faeces after birth. The mucus, which accumulates in the fetal colon, is *meconium*.

After birth

The digestive system 'descends' with growth, and the length of the small intestine is doubled by puberty. At birth the intestines are thin walled because the musculature is not well developed; the mucosa and submucosa are stronger. Villi continue to form in the small intestine up to puberty.

In infancy the pelvis is small and can accommodate very little of the small intestine. The caecum in the fetus is conical and the appendix is related to the apex of the cone. As the infant grows, the caecum descends relative to the abdominal wall; greater growth of its lateral aspect alters its shape to a rounded cup, and the appendix moves round to its inner side. The ileocaecal recesses are more distinct in children than in adults.

ANOMALIES OCCURRING IN THE GASTROINTESTINAL TRACT DURING FETAL DEVELOPMENT

Mouth

Cleft lip and/or cleft palate is the most common craniofacial congenital abnormality, occurring in about 1 in 800 live births. Cleft lip results from the incomplete fusion of the embryonic structure surrounding the primitive cavity. Cleft palate occurs when the primary and secondary palatine plates do not fuse during embryological development.

Oesophagus

Stenosis and atresia often occur as a result of incomplete recanalization. If the oesophagus and laryngotracheal channels fail to separate completely, tracheo-oesophageal fistula and atresia of the oesophagus may result.

Stomach

The most common condition is pyloric stenosis.

Extrabiliary apparatus

Failure of the extrabiliary apparatus to recanalize in the seventh week can result in atresia; the baby becomes jaundiced because bilirubin can no longer be excreted across the placenta.

Intestines
- omphalocele and gastroschisis (see Clinical Notes box)
- umbilical hernia—the abdominal contents herniate after their return through an imperfectly closed linea alba (the tendinous area of the abdominal wall)
- Meckel's diverticulum—persistent yolk sac
- stenosis and atresia—occurs most commonly in the ileum and duodenum; results from incomplete recanalization
- volvulus—parts of the bowel may twist and obstruct their own blood supply.

Anal canal   Malformations includes several types of imperforate anus with or without a fistula resulting from the anomalous development of the urorectal septum.

DIGESTION AND ABSORPTION

'At birth the full term infant is capable of adapting to extrauterine nutrition. This adaptation is due to:

- Coordination of sucking and swallowing
- Efficient gastric emptying
- Intestinal motility
- Regulation of digestive secretions and enzymes
- Excretion of waste products.'

(Wong 1999).

The two main functions of the gastrointestinal tract are digestion and absorption. *Mechanical digestion* occurs through a series of neuromuscular activities that move and mix food along the digestive tract at a rate suitable for digestion and absorption. *Chemical digestion* involves five types of gastrointestinal secretion:

- enzymes
- hormones
- hydrochloric acid
- mucus
- water and electrolytes.

Absorption occurs after the digestion of food is completed. The simplified nutrients are transported from the gastrointestinal tract to the blood or lymph.

DIGESTION

MOUTH   Once food has been placed in the mouth, chemical and mechanical digestion begin.

Chemical digestion

- Food is broken down into small particles by chewing.
- Food is mixed with saliva. Salivary amylase breaks down the particles into maltose.
- The optimum pH for the action of salivary amylase is 6.8.

Mechanical digestion

- When food has been taken into the mouth it is masticated and moved around the mouth by the tongue and cheek muscles until it forms a bolus.

- The mouth is closed and the voluntary muscles of the tongue and cheeks push the bolus backward into the pharynx, where it is swallowed.

- The muscles of the pharynx are stimulated by a reflex action in the walls of the oropharynx, coordinated by the lower pons and the medulla in the brain. Contraction of these muscles propels the bolus down into the oesophagus.

- The presence of the bolus in the pharynx stimulates a wave of peristalsis, which propels the bolus into the stomach.

- Peristalsis occurs in the oesophagus after swallowing; otherwise the walls are relaxed.

- The cardiac sphincter at the entrance to the stomach relaxes when food presses against it, allowing the bolus to enter the stomach.

- 'The movement of food through the pharynx and the oesophagus is so automatic that a person can swallow, and food will reach the stomach even if he is standing on his head' (Marieb 1999).

Stomach

- When a meal has been eaten, mixing with the gastric juice takes place gradually; it may be some time before food is sufficiently acidified to stop the action of salivary amylase.

- Several minutes after food enters the stomach, gentle rippling peristaltic movements called *mixing waves* pass over the stomach every 15–25 seconds.

- These waves macerate the food, mix it with secretions of the gastric juice, and reduce it to a liquid known as *chyme*.

- As digestion proceeds, more vigorous mixing waves begin at the body of the stomach and intensify as they reach the pylorus.

- As food reaches the pylorus (which is almost, but not completely, closed), each wave forces several millilitres of chyme into the duodenum through the pyloric sphincter.

- Most of the chyme is forced back into the stomach where it is subjected to further mixing.

- The next wave pushes it forward again, and forces a little more into the duodenum.

A newborn's stomach will empty in 2.5–3 hours.
A 5-year-old stomach will empty in 3–6 hours.
In adults, a carbohydrate meal leaves the stomach in 2–3 hours; a protein meal remains longer, and a fatty meal remains the longest.

CLINICAL NOTES	PYLORIC STENOSIS

Pyloric stenosis occurs when the circumferential muscle of the pylorus becomes thickened, causing an obstruction to the outlet of the stomach and resulting in compensatory dilatation, hypertrophy and hyperperistalsis of the stomach.

First-born males are affected four to six times more frequently than any female infants. Pyloric stenosis is more likely to affect full-term babies. It is rarer in infants of African or Asian descent than in white infants.

Clinical signs include projectile vomiting that occurs during or immediately after some feeds; the infant is hungry and irritable; prolonged vomiting leads to dehydration and weight loss. Visible peristalsis is present from the upper left quadrant to the right; it is most prominent immediately after a feed or just before vomiting. Palpation should reveal a hard mobile tumour (the pylorus), which feels like an olive just to the right of the epigastrium.

Treatment is surgical—Ramstedt's operation, which consists of splitting the pyloric muscle. Feeding is introduced within a few hours of surgery and the infant usually makes a full recovery.

GASTRIC JUICE

Gastric juice consists of:

- water and mineral salts secreted by the gastric glands
- mucus secreted by goblet cells in the glands of the stomach surface
- hydrochloric acid and the intrinsic factor secreted by parietal cells in the gastric glands
- inactive enzyme precursors—pepsinogens secreted by chief cells in the glands.

Functions of gastric juice:

- Water further liquefies the food.
- Hydrochloric acid acidifies the food and stops the action of salivary amylase; kills ingested microbes; and provides the acid environment needed for effective digestion by pepsins.

CLINICAL NOTES	HYDROCHLORIC ACID

The concentration of hydrochloric acid, which is present at birth, falls too low to permit much peptic digestion of protein in the stomach. The pH is neutral (pH 7) at birth owing to the swallowing of amniotic fluid. Gastric secretions commence during the first 8 hours of life and reach adult levels at about 10 years of age (MacGregor 2000).

- Pepsinogens are activated to pepsins by hydrochloric acid and by pepsins already present in the stomach. They begin the digestion of proteins, breaking them down into smaller molecules. Pepsins are most effective at a pH of 1.5–3.5.
- Intrinsic factor (a protein) is necessary for the absorption of vitamin B12 from the ileum.
- Mucus prevents damage to the stomach wall by lubricating its contents.

SECRETION OF GASTRIC JUICE

There is always a small quantity of hydrochloric acid in the stomach, even when there is no food present; this is known as the fasting juice. Secretions reach their peak level about 1 hour after eating and return to their fasting level after about 4 hours. There are three phases of gastric juice secretion (Fig. 7.4):

- cephalic phase
- gastric phase
- intestinal phase.

Cephalic phase

This flow of juice occurs before food reaches the stomach. It is stimulated by the sight, smell or taste of food, and is due to a reflex stimulation of the vagus nerve.

Gastric phase

The presence of food stimulates the *enteroendocrine cells* in the pyloric antrum and duodenum to secrete *gastrin*, a hormone that passes directly into the bloodstream. The blood, which contains gastrin and is circulating to the stomach, stimulates the gastric glands to produce more gastric juice, which is continued after the completion of a meal and the cephalic phase.

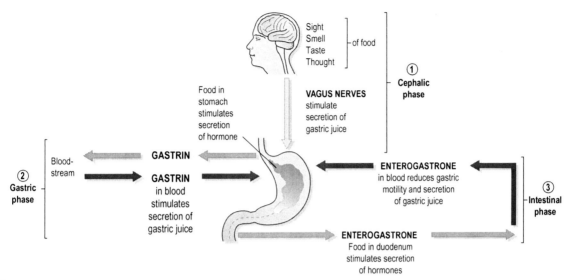

Fig. 7.4
The three phases of secretion
of gastric juice.

Intestinal phase   When the partially digested food reaches the small intestine, the
hormone *enterogastrone* is produced by the endocrine cells in the
intestinal mucosa; this slows down the secretion of gastric juice and
reduces gastric motility.

FUNCTIONS OF THE STOMACH

- Temporary storage, allowing time for the digestive enzymes,
  pepsins to act

- Chemical digestion—pepsins convert proteins to polypeptides

- Mechanical breakdown—the three smooth muscle layers allow the
  stomach to act as a churn; gastric juice is added and the contents
  are liquefied to chyme

- Limited absorption of water, alcohol and some lipid-soluble drugs

- Non-specific defence against microbes provided by hydrochloric
  acid in gastric juice

- Preparation of iron for absorption further along the tract; the acid
  environment of the stomach solubilizes iron salts, which is
  required before iron can be absorbed

- Production of the intrinsic factor that is needed for the absorption
  of vitamin B2 in the terminal ileum

● Regulation of the passage of gastric contents into the duodenum. When the chyme is sufficiently acidified and liquefied, the pyloric antrum forces small jets of gastric content through the pyloric sphincter into the duodenum.

CLINICAL NOTES	INFANT FEEDING

INFANT FEEDING

Milk is the only form of nutrition that an infant requires for the first 4–6 months of life. Breast milk is ideal for human babies and has many advantages over artificial milk formulae, both to the mother and to the infant; for example (Huband & Trigg 2001):

● Infant—gastrointestinal illnesses, middle ear infection, respiratory infections, urinary tract infection, insulin-dependent diabetes, allergies
● Mother—reduced risk of breast cancer and ovarian cancer.

Formula milks are based on cow's milk but are highly developed to meet the basic nutritional needs of infants. Most formula feeds have added carbohydrate, usually in the form of lactose or maltodextrins. The fat content is usually replaced with polyunsaturated vegetable oil or butterfat blend; this alters the fatty acid composition to resemble that of breast milk more closely. The protein base is usually demineralized whey to which the appropriate mixture of minerals, vitamins and trace elements is added. Casein-predominant milks are normally given to babies of 4–6 months who are perceived to be still hungry. This process produces formula milk that is similar to mature breast milk (Rudolf & Levene 1999).

Whey moves through the duodenum within an hour; casein may stay in the stomach and be gradually broken down in the pyloric antrum over 24 hours (MacGregor 2000).

SMALL INTESTINE

The small intestine is continuous with the stomach at the pyloric sphincter, and leads into the large intestine at the ileocaecal valve. It is approximately 250–300 cm long at birth, and grows a little in childhood to approximately 3 m by adulthood. Its length provides a large surface area for digestion and absorption, as circular folds, villi and microvilli further increase the area.

The small intestine consists of three main sections:

● The duodenum is about 25 cm long and circles around the head of the pancreas.
● The jejunum is the middle section, and is about 1 m long.
● The ileum (or terminal section) is about 2 m long and ends at the ileocaecal valve.

The movements of the small intestine are divided into two types:

1. *Segmentation*—this is the major movement of the small intestine; it is a localized contraction in areas containing food. It mixes chyme with digestive juices and brings particles of food into contact with the mucosa for absorption.

2. *Peristalsis*—this movement propels the chyme through the intestinal tract. These movements are very weak in the small intestine, and chyme can remain for 3–5 hours.

Chemical digestion in the small intestine depends on the activities of three accessory structures: the pancreas, the liver and the gall bladder. Chyme entering the small intestine contains partially digested carbohydrates, proteins and lipids; to complete the digestive process *pancreatic juice*, *bile* and *intestinal juice* are needed.

PANCREAS

The pancreas is sited in the epigastric and left hypochondriac areas of the abdominal cavity; it consists of a broad head, a body and a narrow tail. It is both an *exocrine* and an *endocrine* gland.

EXOCRINE FUNCTION

The pancreas consists of a large number of lobules which are made up of small alveoli, the walls of which consist of secretory cells. A small duct drains each lobule; these eventually unite to form the pancreatic duct, which extends the whole length of the gland and opens into the duodenum. Just before entering the duodenum, the pancreatic duct joins the common bile duct to form the *hepatopancreatic ampulla*. The opening into the duodenum is controlled by the hepatopancreatic sphincter (*sphincter of Oddi*).

The exocrine function of the pancreas is to produce pancreatic juice.

ENDOCRINE FUNCTION

Within the pancreas are groups of specialized cells known as the pancreatic islets, or *islets of Langerhans*, containing alpha cells, which secrete glucagon, and beta cells, which secrete insulin. These islets have no ducts, so the hormones diffuse directly into the blood.

The endocrine function of the pancreas is to secrete the hormones insulin and glucagon; these are mainly concerned with the control of blood glucose levels.

PANCREATIC JUICE

Pancreatic juice enters the duodenum at the hepatopancreatic ampulla and consists of:

- water
- mineral salts

- enzymes—amylase and lipase
- inactive enzyme precursors—trypsinogen, chymotrypsinogen and procarboxypeptidase
- sodium bicarbonate.

The presence of acid material from the stomach stimulates the secretion of the hormones secretin and cholecystokinin (CCK), which are produced by the endocrine cells in the wall of the duodenum; this stimulates the production of pancreatic juice.

Foods entering the small intestine are flooded with enzyme-rich pancreatic juice from the pancreas. The sodium bicarbonate makes the pancreatic juice slightly alkaline (pH 7.1–8.2), which:

- buffers the acidic gastric juice in chyme
- stops the action of pepsin from the stomach
- creates the correct pH for the digestive enzymes in the small intestine.

Protein digestion Trypsinogen and chymotrypsinogen are inactive enzyme precursors that are activated by enterokinase, an enzyme in the microvilli; this then converts them into the active enzymes *trypsin* and *chymotrypsin.* These enzymes convert polypeptides to tripeptides, dipeptides and amino acids.

If trypsinogen and chymotrypsinogen were not produced as inactive enzymes, they would digest the pancreas and the pancreatic duct.

Carbohydrate digestion Pancreatic amylase converts all digestible polysaccharides not acted upon by salivary amylase to disaccharides.

Fat digestion Lipase converts fats to fatty acids and glycerol. To aid the action of lipase, bile salts emulsify fats.

CLINICAL NOTES **DIGESTION AT BIRTH**

At 40 weeks' gestation the pancreatic secretions are sufficiently mature for a milk diet; lactose can be digested by a full-term baby. Amylase and enterokinase are also present at birth. During the first 3 months of life the pancreatic juice contains very little lipase; this limits the baby's capacity to convert fat into fatty acids and glycerol. Specific long-chain polyunsaturated fatty acids are present in breast milk to feed the large developing brain (MacGregor 2000).

LIVER

The liver is situated under the diaphragm to the right side of the body; it overlies and almost completely covers the stomach. Liver cells grow, divide, and become old only to be replaced by new cells, so that the size and weight of the liver shows little alteration throughout adult life. The average life of a liver cell has been estimated at 18 months (Sinclair & Dangerfield 1998).

FUNCTION OF THE LIVER

1. Carbohydrate metabolism—converts glucose to glycogen when insulin is present, and converts glycogen back to glucose when glucagon is present. These changes regulate the glucose level in the blood within relatively narrow limits.

2. Fat metabolism (desaturation of fat)—converts stored fat to a form in which it can be used to provide the tissues with energy.

3. Protein metabolism (deamination of amino acids):
   - Removes the nitrogens from the amino acids not required for the formation of new protein; urea is formed from this nitrogenous portion and is then excreted in the urine
   - Breaks down the genetic material from worn-out cells to form uric acid, which is excreted in the urine
   - Transamination—removal of the nitrogenous part of the amino acids and its attachment to other carbohydrate molecules to form new non-essential amino acids
   - Synthesis of plasma proteins and most of the blood-clotting factors from the available amino acids.

4. Breaks down erythrocytes and defends against microbes; this is carried out by the phagocytic Kupffer cells in the sinusoids as part of the macrophage system.

5. Detoxifies drugs and noxious substances; these include alcohol and toxins produced by microbes.

6. Inactivates hormones, including insulin, glucagon, cortisol, aldosterone, thyroid and sex hormones.

7. Synthesizes vitamin A from carotene.

8. Produces heat—the liver has a high metabolic rate and produces a great deal of heat. It is the main heat-producing organ in the body.

9. Stores—fat-soluble A, D, E and K, iron and copper, and some water-soluble vitamins (e.g. riboflavin, niacin, pyridoxine, folic acid and vitamin B12).

10. Secretes bile—the hepatocytes synthesize the constituents of bile from the mixed arterial and venous blood of the sinusoids; these include bile salts, bile pigments and cholesterol.

BILE

Bile is produced by the liver; it passes from the hepatic duct along the cystic duct to the gall bladder, where it is stored. Bile enters the duodenum through the hepatopancreatic sphincter in response to a meal being eaten. When food has been eaten, the duodenum secretes the hormone cholecystokinin; this stimulates the contraction of the gall bladder and relaxation of the hepatopancreatic sphincter, and allows bile and pancreatic juice to pass into the duodenum together.

Bile has a pH of 8; about 500–1000 mL of bile are secreted each day. It consists of:

- water
- mineral salts
- mucus
- bile salts
- bile pigments (mainly bilirubin)
- cholesterol.

Functions

- Bile salts, sodium taurocholate and sodium glycocholate emulsify fats in the small intestine.
- Bilirubin is a waste product of the breakdown of erythrocytes and is excreted in bile rather than urine because of its low solubility in water. Biliribin is changed in the large intestines, because of the microbes that are present. Some of this resultant urobilinogen, which is highly water soluble, is reabsorbed and excreted in the urine, but most is converted to stercobilin and excreted in the faeces.

- Fatty acids are insoluble in water; this makes them very difficult to absorb through the intestinal wall. Bile salts make fatty acids soluble, enabling both these and fat-soluble vitamins A, D, E and K to be readily absorbed.

- Stercobilin colours and deodorizes the faeces.

- The absence of bile causes increased amounts of fat to appear in the faeces (steatorrhoea) and deficiency of fat-soluble vitamins.

GALL BLADDER

The gall bladder is a pear-shaped sac; it is attached to the posterior surface of the liver by connective tissue.

FUNCTIONS OF THE GALL BLADDER

- Reservoir for bile
- Concentrates bile by up to 10–15-fold
- Releases stored bile.

INTESTINAL JUICE

About 1–2 litres of a clear yellow fluid is secreted each day. The mechanical stimulation of the intestinal glands by the presence of chyme is thought to be the main stimulus for the secretion of intestinal juice, although the hormone secretin may also be involved. Intestinal juice is slightly alkaline, with a pH of 7.6; it contains:

- water
- mucus
- mineral salts
- enterokinase

Both pancreatic and intestinal juices provide a vehicle for the absorption of substances in chyme as they come into contact with the microvilli. The numerous projections of the microvilli on the surface of the villi form the *brush border*. The absorptive epithelial cells that line the mucosa contain several digestive enzymes, called brush border enzymes. Among these are:

- four carbohydrate digestive enzymes: dextinase, maltase, sucrase and lactase
- protein digestive enzyme: peptide (aminopeptidase and dispeptidase).

These cells are constantly sloughed off from the apices of the villi into the lumen of the intestine. Some enzymatic digestion takes place at the surface of the epithelial cells rather than in the lumen as in other parts of the gastrointestinal tract. Enterokinase activates peptides such as trypsin, which converts polypeptides to amino acids and some smaller peptides. The final stage of breakdown of all peptides to amino acids occurs inside the enterocytes.

Table 7.2 provided a summary of the digestive activities discussed above.

ABSORPTION

Absorption of nutrients (Fig. 7.5) occurs by two processes:

1. Diffusion
2. Active transport.

About 90% of all absorption takes place in the small intestine, and 10% in the stomach and large intestine. The surface area through which absorption takes place in the small intestine is greatly increased

Table 7.2 Summary of digestive activities

Mouth	Stomach	Small intestine	Pancreas	Liver	Gall bladder	Large intestine
Food is mixed with *salivary amylase* and passed by peristalsis to the stomach via the cardiac sphincter	Mixing waves macerate the food, mix it with *gastric juice* and reduce it to *chyme*; it then passes via the pylorus into the duodenum	Chyme is mixed with *intestinal juice*; the food particles are brought into contact with the mucosa for absorption. Mild peristaltic contractions move chyme into the large intestine through the ileocaecal sphincter	Delivers *pancreatic juice* into the duodenum via the pancreatic duct	Produces *bile* for the emulsification and absorption of fats	Stores, concentrates and delivers bile into the duodenum via the common bile duct	Mass movement which sweeps along the transverse colon forcing the contents into the descending and sigmoid colons in preparation for defecation

Fig. 7.5
The absorption of nutrients.

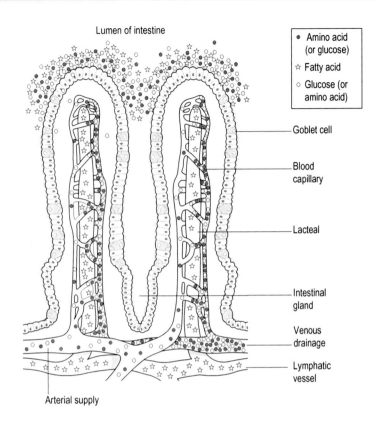

Lumen of intestine

- Amino acid (or glucose)
- Fatty acid
- Glucose (or amino acid)

Goblet cell

Blood capillary

Lacteal

Intestinal gland

Venous drainage

Lymphatic vessel

Arterial supply

by the circular folds of mucous membranes and the very large number of villi and microvilli. 'It has been calculated that the surface area of the small intestine is about five times that of the whole body' (Waugh & Grant 2001).

After digestion is completed, the simplified nutrients (end products) are ready for absorption:

- monosaccharides (glucose, fructose, galactose) from carbohydrates
- fatty acids and glycerides from fats
- small peptides and amino acids from protein
- vitamins and minerals are released as a result of digestion
- water and electrolytes contribute to the fluid food mass.

Monosaccharides, amino acids, fatty acids and glycerol *diffuse* slowly down their concentration gradients into the enterocytes from the intestinal lumen. Alternatively, they may be *actively transported* into the villi; this is a quicker process than diffusion. Disaccharides, dipeptides and tripeptides are actively transported into the enterocytes, where their digestion is completed prior to transfer into the capillaries of the villi.

- Monosaccharides and amino acids pass into the capillaries in the villi.

- Some proteins are absorbed unchanged, for example the antibodies in breast milk and oral vaccines.

- Fatty acids and glycerol pass into the lacteals.

- Following this, the end products of digestion enter the larger lymph vessels and then the portal blood flow at the thoracic duct, where further metabolism occurs.

- Exceptions are short- and medium-chain fatty acids, which can be absorbed directly into the blood circulation of the villi.

- Fat-soluble vitamins are absorbed into the lacteals with the fatty acids and glycerol.

- Vitamin B12 combines with the intrinsic factor in the stomach and is actively absorbed in the terminal ileum.

Large amounts of fluid enter the alimentary tract each day, approximately 9.3 litres in an adult. The majority of fluid is absorbed by the small intestine; this occurs by osmosis from the lumen of the intestine through the epithelial cells and into the blood capillaries. Water can move across the mucosa in both directions, depending on the absorption of electrolytes and nutrients, to maintain the osmotic balance in the blood.

CLINICAL NOTES	LACTOSE INTOLERANCE AND COELIAC DISEASE

Lactose intolerance

Following infectious diarrhoea, infants less than 6 months of age may have temporary lactose intolerance lasting from one to several weeks. Clinical features include:

- persistent fluid stools
- excessive flatulence
- excoriation of buttocks.

The infant is otherwise well. The formula milk should be replaced with a lactose-free formula for 3–4 weeks, after which time the normal milk formula can be reintroduced gradually (Royal Children's Hospital Melbourne 2000).

Coeliac disease

This results from a person's inability to tolerate gluten, a substance found in wheat and rye (Rudolf & Levene 1999). Clinical features include:

- usually presents before the age of 2 years
- failure to thrive

- irritability
- anorexia
- vomiting and diarrhoea
- abdominal distension and wasted buttocks
- steatorrhoea.

The condition is usually diagnosed by means of a jejunal biopsy, which will show subtotal villous atrophy. The prognosis is excellent provided the child adheres to a gluten-free diet for a minimum of 2 years to allow for full regeneration of villi.

LARGE INTESTINE

'The overall functions of the large intestine are the completion of absorption, the manufacture of certain vitamins, the formation of faeces and the expulsion of faeces from the body.'

(Tortora & Grabowski 1996)

The large intestine is approximately 1.5 m long; it extends from the ileum to the anus and is attached to the posterior abdominal wall by its *mesocolon*, a double layer of peritoneum. The large intestine is divided into four main regions:

- caecum
- colon
- rectum
- anus.

The *caecum* is the first part of the large intestine. It is a dilated area, which has a blind end inferiorly and is continuous with the ascending colon superiorly. Just below the junction of the two, the ileocaecal valve opens from the ileum. The vermiform appendix (*vermis* = worm; *appendix* = appendage), a tube-like structure about 8 cm long, is attached to the caecum at one end and has a blind end at the other.

The *colon* consists of four parts:

1. The *ascending colon* passes upwards from the caecum to the level of the liver where it curves to the left at the hepatic flexure to become the transverse colon.

2. The *transverse colon* is a loop that extends across the abdominal cavity where it forms the splenic flexure and becomes the descending colon.

3. The *descending colon* passes down the left side of the abdomen; it then curves towards the midline and after it enters the pelvis is known as the sigmoid colon.

4. The *sigmoid colon* is the **S**-shaped curve in the pelvis which then continues down to become the rectum.

The *rectum* is a slightly dilated piece of the colon that starts at the sigmoid colon and ends at the anus.

The *anal canal* is a short passage that leads from the anus to the exterior. Two sphincter muscles control the anus:

- the internal sphincter, which consists of smooth muscle fibres and is under the control of the autonomic nervous system
- the external sphincter, which is formed by skeletal muscle and is under voluntary control.

FUNCTIONS OF THE LARGE INTESTINE

Absorption

Water and sodium are absorbed until the familiar semi-solid consistency of the faeces is achieved.

Bacterial activity

The large intestine contains bacteria, which synthesize vitamin K, folic acid and some B complex vitamins. These bacteria include *Escherichia coli*, *Enterobacter aerogenes* and *Streptococcus faecalis*; they may become pathogenic if transferred to another part of the body. Bacteria also affect the colour of faeces, odour and gas formation. Large numbers of microbes are present in the faeces.

Mass movement

This occurs intermittently (about twice each hour). Waves of strong peristalsis sweep along the transverse colon forcing the contents into the descending and sigmoid colons. This mass movement is usually precipitated by the entry of food into the stomach; the sudden movement of the colonic contents into the rectum initiates the desire to defecate.

Defecation

The rectum is normally empty, but when a mass movement forces the contents of the sigmoid colon into the rectum, stretching stimulates the nerve endings within the rectum. The anus is usually closed by the internal and external anal sphincters. The external anal sphincter is under conscious control via the pudendal nerve. Defecation involves voluntary and involuntary contraction of the muscle of the rectum, and relaxation of the internal anal sphincter. When defecation is voluntarily postponed, the feeling of fullness and the need to defecate diminishes until the next mass movement occurs.

Faeces are a semi-solid brown mass; the colour is due to the presence of stercobilin. Faeces are made up of:

- 60–70% water
- fibre

Table 7.3   Summary of digestion and absorption (adapted from Waugh and Grant 2001)

	Mouth	Stomach	Small intestine		Large intestine
			Digestion	Absorption	
Carbohydrates	Salivary amylase converts cooked starches to disaccharides	Hydrochloric acid stops the action of salivary amylase	Pancreatic amylase converts cooked and uncooked starches to disaccharides	Into the blood capillaries of the villi	
Proteins		Hydrochloric acid converts pepsinogen to pepsin. Pepsin converts proteins to polypeptides	Enterokinase converts chymotrypsinogen and trypsinogen to chymotrypsin and trypsin. Chymotrypsin and trypsin convert polypeptides to dipeptides and tripeptides. Peptidases convert dipeptides and tripeptides to amino acids.	Into the blood capillaries of the villi	
Fats			Bile salts emulsify fats. Pancreatic lipase converts fats to fatty acids and glycerol. Lipase converts fats to fatty acids and glycerol.	Into the lacteals of the villi	
Water		Small amount absorbed		90% absorbed	Remainder absorbed here
Vitamins		Intrinsic factor secreted for the absorption of vitamin B12		Water-soluble vitamins absorbed into capillaries. Fat-soluble vitamins absorbed into lacteals of the villi	Bacteria synthesize vitamin K; some vitamin B complex and folic acid absorbed in colon

- dead and live microbes
- epithelial cells from the wall of the tract
- fatty acids
- mucus secreted by the epithelial lining of the large intestine.

Table 7.3 provides a summary of digestion and absorption.

CLINICAL NOTES	DEFECATION

Toilet training

Toilet training is often a difficult stage in the child's development; in the infant, defecation occurs as an involuntary action. Children are most ready to be toilet trained between the ages of 18 and 36 months, as during this period the nervous system matures and the child becomes aware of rectal pressure and anal sensitivity (Kinservik & Friedhoff 2000).

In practical terms this means that the brain can inhibit the reflex until it is convenient to defecate.

Constipation

Constipation is an alteration in the frequency, consistency and ease of passing faeces. Normal frequency in a child can be daily to every other day. Long intervals between bowel movements is known as *obstipation*; constipation with faecal soiling is called *encopresis*.

Constipation may arise secondary to a variety of organic disorders of the gastrointestinal tract; these include:

- strictures
- ectopic anus
- Hirschsprung's disease
- hypothyroidism
- hypercalcaemia due to hyperparathyroidism.

Constipation can also be a side-effect of drugs such as antacids, diuretics, antiepileptics, opioids and iron supplements.

The majority of children have idiopathic or functional constipation, as no underlying cause can be found. Chronic constipation can be initiated by environmental or psychological causes. During toilet training children may withhold a stool; repeated withholding can lead to stretching and dilatation of the rectum, which reduces the urge to defecate. Children with chronic constipation or encopresis may have abnormal defecation dynamics; the external sphincter contracts rather than relaxing during attempts to defecate.

Breast-fed babies

After the first few weeks of life, the fully breast-fed infant normally develops infrequent bowel movements. It is normal for them to have one bowel movement every 4–5 days, and one in 10 days is not unusual. The stools are soft and semi-liquid; the babies are not constipated (Rudolf & Levene 1999).

SELF ASSESSMENT

- Make a line drawing of the gastrointestinal tract and label each organ. Define digestion and describe the six processes involved.
- Describe the development of the foregut, midgut and hindgut. What are the origins of each part?
- Discuss the embryological and fetal development of the liver, and list the ten main functions of the liver after birth.
- Describe the digestion and absorption of proteins, fats and carbohydrates.
- Explain the structure and function of the villi.
- Why is it important that infants are given only milk for nutrition during the first 4 months of life?
- Explain the cause of and the difference between an omphalocele and gastroschisis.
- What are the causes of constipation in a newborn infant?

References

Hockenberry M, Wilson D, Winkelstein M, Kline N 2003 Wong's nursing care of infants and children, 7th edn. Mosby, St Louis

Huband S, Trigg E 2001 Practices in children's nursing. Churchill Livingstone, Edinburgh

Kinservik M, Friedhoff M 2000 Control issues in toilet training. Pediatric Nursing 26(3):267–272

MacGregor J 2000 Introduction to the anatomy and physiology of children. Routledge, London

Marieb E 1999 Essentials of human anatomy and physiology, 6th edn. Benjamin/Cummins Science Publishing, San Francisco

Moore K L, Persaud R V N 2003 Developing human clinically orientated embryology, 7th edn. W B Saunders, Philadelphia

Moules T, Ramsay J 1998 Children's nursing. Stanley Thornes, Cheltenham

Royal Children's Hospital Melbourne 2000 Paediatric handbook, 6th edn. Blackwell Science, Melbourne

Rudolf M, Levene M 1999 Paediatrics and child health. Blackwell Science, Oxford

Sinclair D, Dangerfield P 1998 Human growth after birth, 8th edn. Oxford University Press, Oxford

Tortora G, Grabowski S 1996 Principles of anatomy and physiology, 8th edn. Harper Collins, New York

Waugh A, Grant A 2001 Ross and Wilson anatomy in health and illness, 9th edn. Churchill Livingstone, London

Wong D 1999 Whaley and Wong's nursing care of infants and children. Mosby, St Louis

Bibliography

Carlson B 1999 Human embyology and developmental biology, 2nd edn. Mosby, St Louis

Coad J, Dunstall M 2001 Anatomy and physiology for midwives. Mosby, St Louis

Hubbard J, Mechan J 1987 Physiology for health care students. Churchill Livingstone, Edinburgh

Larsen W 1998 Essentials of human embryology. Churchill Livingstone, New York

Sukkar M, El-Hunshid H, Ardawi M 1998 Concise human physiology. Blackwell Science, Oxford

Chapter 8

Development of the renal system

Pauline Carson

CHAPTER OUTCOMES

This chapter will enable the reader to:

- Identify the various structures that comprise the renal system
- Discuss the formation of the renal system
- Identify the various stages of kidney development
- Discuss the formation of urine and the factors that affect it
- Identify abnormalities and conditions associated with the development of the renal system.

CHAPTER OVERVIEW

The aim of this chapter is to describe the normal embryonic and fetal development of the renal system. The chapter describes normal embryological anatomy and physiology, and outlines the development that takes place after birth. Clinical Notes address issues of clinical relevance and interest to the reader, and Self Assessment exercises assist in reflecting upon the chapter and guiding the relationship between theory and professional practice.

INTRODUCTION

The renal system is one of the excretory systems of the body; it plays an important role in maintaining the function of body systems by regulating water and electrolyte balance. It consists of two kidneys, two ureters, a bladder and urethra. The kidneys do the bulk of this work, producing urine that passes down through the ureters and is stored in the bladder until it is excreted from the body via the urethra.

Developmentally and anatomically the renal system is closely related to the reproductive system, especially in males and to a slightly lesser degree in females, and is therefore also referred to as the *urogenital system*. This chapter deals specifically with the formation and development of the renal system structures identified above. The formation and development of the reproductive system is addressed in Chapter 9.

THE EARLIEST DEVELOPMENT OF THE URINARY SYSTEM

The urogenital system develops within the first weeks of embryonic life from the intermediate mesoderm of the embryo that extends longitudinally along the dorsal body wall. When the embryo folds in the horizontal plane, this mesoderm is carried ventrally forming a longitudinal ridge on either side of the dorsal aorta called the *urogenital ridge*. This ridge, which has two main parts, forms the basis for the formation of the urinary system and the genital system. The gonadal or genital ridge will give rise to the genital system, while the second part, the nephrogenic cord or ridge, will give rise to the urinary system, which will begin development before the genital system.

DEVELOPMENT OF THE KIDNEYS

During embryonic development three sets of excretory organs or kidneys will develop in succession from the intermediate mesoderm:

- the pronephros
- the mesonephros
- the metanephros.

The first two sets, the *pronephroi* and the *mesonephroi*, are rudimentary and will largely disappear, while the third set, the *metanephroi*, will form the basis of the adult kidney. As the earlier forms of kidneys regress, some of their components are retained and will be reused by other components of the urogenital system (Carlson 1999).

THE PRONEPHROI

The pronephroi (singular, pronephros) develop early in the fourth week in the cervical region as clusters of cells and tortuous tubular structures that grow towards and open into the cloaca. These rudimentary and non-functional structures are transitory, degenerating and disappearing around day 24 or 25; however, their two ducts remain and will be used by the next set of kidneys, becoming the ducts of the mesonephros (Fig. 8.1).

THE MESONEPHROI

The second stage of kidney development is the formation of the mesonephroi (singular, mesonephros). These large elongated organs (Fig. 8.1), which appear late in the fourth week caudal to the pronephros, utilize the adjacent pronephric duct and are the second set of kidney structures to form in the intermediate mesoderm. The mesonephric kidneys are made up of mesonephric tubules and glomeruli, and thus, unlike the pronephroi before them, contain functional renal tissue that will act as interim kidneys until the third set of kidneys, the permanent kidneys, develop.

Fig. 8.1
Developing urinary system in 5-week-old embryo showing the pronephros disappearing and the developing mesonephros and metanephros. The allantois, division of cloaca and caudal ends of the mesonephric duct will all contribute to the development of the bladder.
(Adapted from Moore & Persaud 2003.)

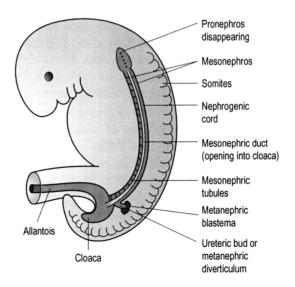

Fig. 8.2
Mesonephric excretory unit.
(Adapted from Moore & Persaud
2003.)

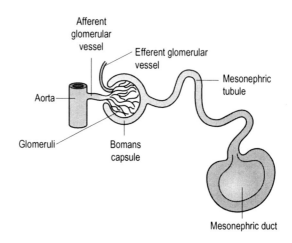

During weeks 5–11 nephrogenic cords canalize to form meso-nephric vesicles, these vesicles then form an S-shaped tubule, which in turn will join and fuse with the mesonephric duct (Matsumara & England 1992). This duct was formerly the pronephric duct, but during this second stage of kidney development is known as the mesonephric duct.

These tubules themselves also continue to develop, differentiating into excretory units that consist of a Bowman's capsule and glomeruli (Fig. 8.2) and resemble an abbreviated version of the adult nephron (Larsen 1998). The medial end of the tubule forms a cup-shaped structure called a *Bowman's capsule* or a *glomerular capsule* that sur-rounds a cluster of capillaries from the aorta called the *glomerulus*. The Bowman's capsule and glomerulus together form a renal corpuscle and this, along with the tubule, forms a mesonephric excre-tory unit. This new structure now forms a route from the excretory unit to the cloaca; it is functional and forms small amounts of urine between weeks 6 and 10 (Larsen 1998). Some of these tubules, especially the most cephalic of them, progressively degenerate; how-ever, new tubules forming at the caudal level ensure that a constant number is present between weeks 4 and 9, during the time when the third set of kidneys is forming and developing (Matsumara & England 1992).

After 10 weeks, when the third set of kidneys is established, the mesonephroi begin to degenerate and disappear, although some of the tubules and ducts persist. These remaining tubules and ducts form important parts of the male genital system. The tubules form the *efferent ductules* of the testes, while the ducts form the *epididymis*, the *ductus deferens* and the *ejaculatory duct*. In the female the ducts largely disappear, although the tubules may be retained near the uterus and in the broad ligament, forming the *paroöphoron* and *epoöphoron* respectively (Matsumura & England 1992). The further development of these structures is fully addressed in Chapter 9.

THE METANEPHROI: THE DEFINITIVE, PERMANENT KIDNEYS

The third set of kidneys to develop are the *metanephroi* (singular, metanephros). These kidneys, which begin to form in week 5, will give rise to the definitive, permanent adult kidney. These permanent kidneys develop from two primary sources:

- the *ureteric buds* or *metanephric diverticulum*
- the *metanephric blastema*, or metanephric mass of intermediate mesoderm (Moore & Persaud 2003).

The first of these sources, the ureteric buds or metanephric diverticula, sprout from the distal portion of the mesonephric ducts near the opening into the cloaca around 28 days, and begin to grow into the metanephric blastema, a portion of intermediate mesoderm adjacent to the buds (see Fig. 8.1). As they elongate and grow into the metanephric mesoderm, they begin to divide and branch, and at the same time induce the formation of a *metanephric mass* or cap over the end, producing a lobulated appearance. Thus, as the bud branches, each new growing tip, the *ampulla*, acquires a cap of metanephric blastema tissue, thereby giving a lobulated appearance (Larsen 1998). Both of these primordia give rise to the collecting system and the urine-forming units of the kidney, with the collecting system arising from the metanephric diverticulum and the urine-forming units, or nephrons, having their origin in the metanephric blastema.

The collecting duct system

The metanephric diverticulum gives rise to the *ureters* and the *collecting system—renal pelvis, calyces* and *collecting tubules*—with the stalk becoming the ureters and the cranial end forming the *renal pelvis* (Moore & Persaud 2003). Repeated branching of the ureteric bud produces the collecting duct system (Fig. 8.3). The first bifurcation of the ureteric bud forms the renal pelvis, while the subsequent repeated division of the straight collecting tubules forms successive groups, or generations, that converge to form the *major calyces* (the first four generations of tubules that enlarge and converge), the *minor calyces* (the second four generations that coalesce) and, finally, the *collecting tubules* or ducts.

The nephrons: the urine-forming units

The *nephrons* develop from the metanephric mass of mesoderm or metanephric blastema at the end of each arched collecting tubule (Fig. 8.4). This mass of mesoderm is induced to form small metanephric

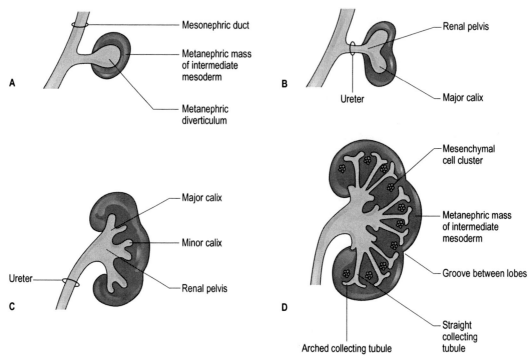

Fig. 8.3
Development of the permanent kidney showing the stages of development of the metanephric diverticulum weeks 5–8.
(From Moore & Persaud 2003, with permission.)

vesicles, which elongate to form metanephric tubules. As the vesicles develop into tubules, *capillary glomeruli* form and invaginate their proximal ends, forming a Bowman's capsule which surrounds the glomerulus. As was the case in the mesonephros, the Bowman's capsule and glomerulus form a renal corpuscle (Moore & Persaud 2003).

As the renal corpuscle is developing, the tubule continues to grow in length forming the proximal convoluted tubule, the loop of Henle, and the distal convoluted tubule, thereby forming a nephron. During the tenth week, the ends of the distal convoluted tubules connect and join to a collecting tubule or duct (Fig. 8.5), thereby making the metanephroi functional (Larsen 1998), with urine formation beginning around weeks 11–13.

FORMATION OF URINE BEFORE BIRTH

The fetal kidneys begin to function at around 10 weeks. The urine formed at this stage, however, unlike that formed after birth, is not used to get rid of waste products, because the placenta carries out this function (Larsen 1998). During fetal life the urine that is produced supplements the amniotic fluid volume, with production reaching up to 200 mL per day.

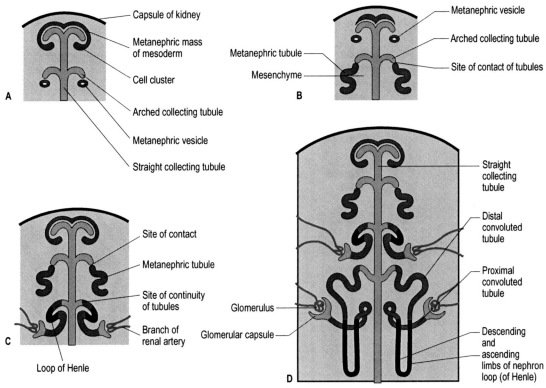

Fig. 8.4
Development of nephrons. **A–C** Nephrogenesis, starts around the beginning of the 8th week. **D** Between weeks 20–38 the number of nephrons more than doubles.
(From Moore & Persaud 2003, with permission.)

CLINICAL NOTES   **ANOMALIES OF THE RENAL SYSTEM**

Anomalies of the renal system are relatively common, affecting 3–4% of live births. Many of these, however, are asymptomatic or will manifest themselves only in later life (Carlson 1999).

Congenital anomalies that may occur during development of the kidneys include:

- renal agenesis—unilateral or bilateral absence of any kidney tissue
- renal hypoplasia—one or both kidneys are much smaller than normal.

DEVELOPMENT OF THE FETAL KIDNEYS

Initially the fetal kidneys are situated close to each other in the pelvis, but by week 10, as the pelvis and abdomen grow, they have migrated into the abdominal cavity to a position just below the suprarenal glands (Fig. 8.6). The main reason for this migratory ascent is growth in the caudal region of the embryo. As the embryo's body grows caudally, it grows away from the kidneys and thus the kidneys will progressively migrate and eventually occupy more cranial levels

Fig. 8.5
Diagram of a nephron including the arrangement of the blood vessels.

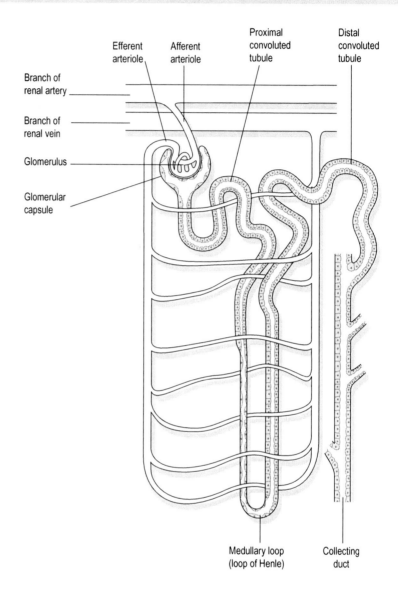

Efferent arteriole

Afferent arteriole

Proximal convoluted tubule

Distal convoluted tubule

Branch of renal artery

Branch of renal vein

Glomerulus

Glomerular capsule

Medullary loop (loop of Henle)

Collecting duct

(Moore & Persaud 2003). In the early stages of this migration the mesonephric kidneys are regressing, leaving behind the mesonephric ducts for further development in relation to the gonads (Carlson 1999).

At the same time as this migratory ascent is happening, three other processes relevant to the positioning of the kidneys are also taking place. During migration, the kidneys also rotate through approximately 90°, which eventually brings them to face the midline (Carlson 1999); at the same time the ureters increase in length, and the blood supply also undergoes change. Initially a branch of the common iliac artery supplies each kidney, but this alters as the kidneys ascend and receive their blood supply from the distal end of the aorta, receiving blood from new branches of the aorta as they migrate higher. Finally, when their migration stops, they receive their blood supply from

Fig. 8.6
Migration of the kidneys into the abdominal cavity to their position just below the suprarenal gland. The sites of the previous renal arteries are also indicated.
(Adapted from Moore & Persaud 2003.)

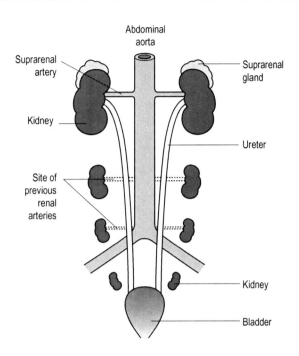

branches of the abdominal aorta. These branches will form the permanent renal arteries, and the inferior branches will eventually degenerate and disappear (Fig. 8.6) (Moore & Persaud 2003).

All of these changes take place behind the peritoneum. Thus, at the end of their migration, the kidneys are eventually situated in the abdominal cavity on the posterior abdominal wall behind peritoneum, thus making them *retroperitoneal* organs (Carlson 1999).

CLINICAL NOTES   **ANOMALIES ARISING DURING KIDNEY ASCENSION**

Several anomalies can arise as a result of the kidneys ascending, including 'pelvic kidneys', where the kidneys fail to ascend, 'horseshoe kidneys', where the two metanephroi fuse during ascent and form a U-shaped kidney, and malrotation of the kidneys, which is often associated with ectopic kidneys. Anomalies in the blood supply can also occur, including accessory renal arteries.

At this stage the kidneys also have a slightly lobular surface, as glomeruli and nephrons begin to form. The number of lobules increases as the kidneys develop and, although it diminishes near the end of the fetal period, the lobes are still visible in the newborn infant, gradually disappearing as the nephrons grow during infancy (Moore & Persaud 1998).

By the end of week 15 the kidney has also divided into two distinct regions, known as a medulla and a cortex. The inner medulla contains

Fig. 8.7
A longitudinal section of the right kidney.

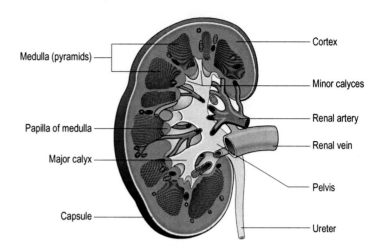

the collecting ducts and loops of Henle, and the outer cortex contains the nephrons. By the end of week 23 this division of the renal pelvis is complete, with the medulla and cortex almost fully developed (Fig. 8.7) by the end of the eighth month (Matsumara & England 1992).

The number of glomeruli increases gradually during weeks 10–18 of gestation, and then rapidly until week 32. Most of the glomeruli and convoluted tubules have formed by the time of birth, with each kidney containing 800 000 to 1 000 000 nephrons (Moore & Persaud 2003). After birth the increase in kidney size is due to enlargement of the existing renal tissue rather than the formation of new nephrons (Matsumara & England 1992). This largely involves the lengthening of the proximal convoluted tubules of the loop of Henle and, to a lesser degree, an increase in the amount of interstitial tissue (Moore & Persaud 2003).

DEVELOPMENT OF THE BLADDER

The bladder develops from two areas: the vesical part of the urogenital sinus, which forms the largest part of the bladder, and the caudal ends of the mesonephric ducts, which contribute to the development of the trigone region of the bladder (Fig. 8.8). The urogenital sinus, formed when the cloaca is divided by the urorectal septum, is divided into three parts, all of which are involved in the development of the bladder and urethra (Moore & Persaud 2003):

- a vesical or cranial part that is continuous with the allantois
- a pelvic or middle part that will eventually form the urethra in the bladder neck, the entire urethra in females, and the prostatic part of the urethra in males
- a phallic or caudal part that grows towards the genital tubercle.

Fig. 8.8
Development of the bladder
and ureters.
A Development of the bladder.
(Adapted from Moore & Persaud
2003.)
B Development of the ureters.
(Adapted from Moore & Persaud
2003.)
C The adult bladder.

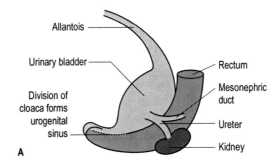

A

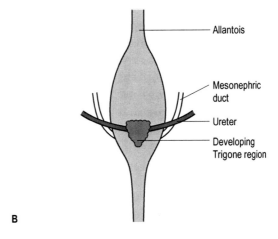

B

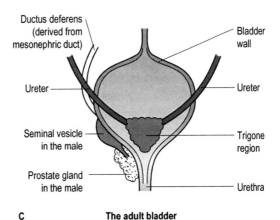

C   **The adult bladder**

It is the vesical part of the urogenital sinus that will form the main part of
the bladder and, as the vesical part is continuous with the allantois, this
means that, initially, so is the bladder. However, as the bladder grows,
the allantois, which extends into the umbilical cord, constricts and forms
a fibrous cord called the *urachus*, which runs between the two umbilical
arteries. This fibrous cord remains attached to the apex of the bladder

and the umbilicus, and in the adult becomes the median umbilical ligament which lies between the fibrous remnants of the two umbilical arteries known as the medial umbilical ligaments (Moore & Persaud 2003).

The second area of bladder development (Fig. 8.8) involves the mesonephric ducts. Two pairs of vessels, the metanephric duct (the future ureter) and the mesonephric duct enter the dorsal bladder wall. As the bladder enlarges, the distal parts of these ducts become incorporated into the wall in an area called the *trigone of the bladder*, identifiable in the adult as a smooth triangular area on the dorsal wall (Matsumura & England 1992). In becoming incorporated, these ducts contribute to the connective tissue formation of the bladder mucosa; however, the lining does not change and remains as the endothelium which is derived from the endoderm that lines the entire bladder. Initially the two vessels on each side lie quite close together, but as the mesonephric ducts become more absorbed into the bladder wall, so the ureters move superolaterally to pass through the bladder wall obliquely and open separately into the bladder. As the kidneys ascend, they exert a pull on the orifices of the ureters; it is partly because of this traction that this superolateral movement occurs and the ureters enter the bladder obliquely (Moore & Persaud 2003). The openings of the mesonephric ducts move closer together and, in the male, enter the prostatic part of the urethra where their caudal ends form the *ejaculatory ducts*; in the female the caudal ends degenerate (Moore & Persaud 2003).

THE BLADDER WALL

The bladder wall is made up of an inner layer of transitional endothelium and outer muscular layers. The inner layer of transitional endothelium, which lines the whole of the bladder including the trigone region, is derived from the endoderm of the vesical part of the urogenital sinus, the muscular layers of the bladder are derived from the surrounding splanchnic mesoderm. One of these muscle layers, which consists of bundles of smooth muscle arranged in three layers called the *detrusor muscle*, promotes the emptying of urine from the bladder when it contracts.

CLINICAL NOTES — ANOMALIES OF THE BLADDER

Anomalies that may arise as a result of bladder formation include:

- Extrophy of the bladder—a severe anomaly involving the anterior wall of the abdomen and the anterior wall of the bladder. The anterior bladder wall ruptures as result of incomplete formation and closure of the anterior abdominal wall, causing wide communication between the bladder mucous membrane and the exterior (Moore & Persaud 2003).
- Formation of a urachus cyst, sinus or fistula.

DEVELOPMENT OF THE URETERS

As noted above, the ureters arise from the ureteric buds or metanephric diverticula, with the stalk of the diverticulum giving rise to the ureters where it is surrounded by the metanephric mass. As the ureters are initially buds of the mesonephric ducts, this means that as the mesonephric duct is gradually incorporated into the trigone region of the bladder so too are the developing ureters (Fig. 8.8). As the ureters enter the bladder, they do so at an oblique angle, which helps to prevent the reflux of urine (Matsumara and England 1992), and, as noted above, they are pulled into their adult position in the bladder as the kidneys ascend to their position on the posterior abdominal wall.

DEVELOPMENT OF THE URETHRA

The urogenital sinus is also involved in the development of the urethra (Fig. 8.9), with the endoderm of the urogenital sinus forming the endothelium of the entire female urethra and most of the male urethra. During weeks 4–7 when the cloaca divides, the urogenital sinus extends to the base of the phallus as the urethral groove and then, as the urogenital folds fuse in weeks 9–12, the urethral groove forms a tube that, in turn, becomes the whole of the female urethra and part of the male urethra (Matsumara & England 1992).

As noted above, the endodermal urogenital sinus is responsible for only part of the male urethra. The remaining distal part of urethral

Fig. 8.9
Development of the urethra.
A In the female.
B In the male.
(Adapted from Moore & Persaud 2003.)

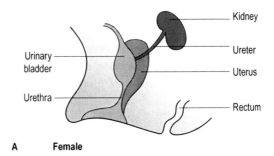

A   Female

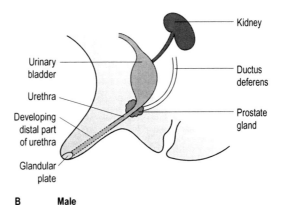

B   Male

formation in the male is derived from an ectodermal source, the *glandular plate*. This ectodermal plate grows from the tip of the glans penis into the developing glans penis, and eventually connects to the spongy urethra that has developed from the phallic part of the urogenital sinus. The glandular plate becomes canalized and therefore, when it joins with the spongy urethra, it allows the urethra to open out on to the glans (Matsumara & England 1992). As a result of these two different sources of male urethra development, the epithelium of the terminal part of the urethra is derived from surface ectoderm while the remainder is derived from urogenital endoderm. The other outer layers of connective tissue and smooth muscle in both the male and female urethra are, like the bladder, derived from the surrounding splanchnic mesenchyme (Moore & Persaud 2003).

DEVELOPMENT OF THE RENAL SYSTEM AFTER BIRTH

The kidneys and bladder continue to develop after birth, with kidney development not fully completed until the end of the first year after birth. Bladder development relates to control and also its location, with the latter not completed until puberty.

The kidneys

At birth, the structural components of the kidneys have formed and a full complement of nephrons has been established. Further development of the kidneys therefore involves the growth and enlargement of the renal tissue and the maturation of the nephrons, thus increasing their ability to filter and absorb. Prior to birth and in the neonatal period, the nephrons are small and immature with many of the tubular sections not yet fully formed. Consequently they are inefficient, with low glomerular filtration and an inability to reabsorb sodium and water. Adult values of glomerular filtration are not reached until 1–2 years of age, and so the newborn is unable to dispose of excess water and solutes rapidly or efficiently (Hockenberry 2003). Likewise, the short loop of Henle in the newborn also reduces the ability to reabsorb sodium and water, and is therefore responsible for the very dilute urine produced at this stage. As the tubules grow, however, their concentrating ability increases until by the third month they have reached adult levels (Hockenberry 2003). Other aspects of renal function in the newborn that differ from those in children and adults include reduced hydrogen ion excretion, lower acid secretion for the first year, low plasma bicarbonate levels and an inability to excrete water loads at rates similar to those in older persons. The reasons for this are as yet unknown; however, because of these inadequacies of kidney function, the newborn infant is more liable to develop severe metabolic acidosis (Hockenberry 2003).

In the first 24 hours after birth 95% of babies pass urine, with the newborn passing 20–35 mL four times a day while milk production is being established and intake is low. This quickly rises to 100–200 ml ten times daily by day 10, thus indicating that kidney maturity also relates to the load presented to it (MacGregor 2000).

CLINICAL NOTES   **SODIUM EXCRETION IN THE NEWBORN KIDNEY**

In the immediate newborn period, sodium excretion is reduced and the kidneys are less able to adapt to excesses and deficiencies. Consequently, because of this impaired ability to eliminate excess, an isotonic saline infusion may produce oedema. Alternatively, inadequate reabsorption of sodium from the tubules may increase sodium losses in conditions such as diarrhoea and vomiting (Hockenberry 2003).

CLINICAL NOTES   **COMPROMISED RENAL FUNCTION**

In the sick infant, renal function can quickly become compromised as dehydration, hypotension and hypoxia all result in a marked fall in glomerular filtration (Moules & Ramsey 1998).

The bladder

Before birth, in infants and in young children, the bladder is a cigar-shaped structure situated in the abdomen, even when it is empty. It does not take on its adult pyramid shape until about the age of 6 years, and it is also around this time that it begins to enter the pelvis minor. It is not until puberty that the bladder finally becomes located in the true pelvis (Moore & Persaud 2003). This change in position is a result of pelvic growth and the maturation of the pelvic bone, rather than a true migration of the bladder and urethra (Hockenberry 2003).

The ability to control bladder emptying is a learned process that also requires development of the nervous system. In infants and children less than 2–3 years old, neurones to the external urethral sphincter are not yet fully developed. Consequently, in this age group voiding is purely a spinal reflex action whereby the bladder voluntarily empties once it is sufficiently full to stimulate the *micturition reflex*. In the infant this stimulus occurs when the bladder is stretched by a volume of 15 mL; in the adult the stimulus occurs when the bladder exceeds 200–400 mL (Tortora & Grabowski 2003). As the bladder fills, stretch receptors on the trigone distend, and these in turn send signals to the sacral area of the spine via the autonomic nervous system. Nerve impulses from the spinal cord then stimulate contraction of the detrusor muscle and initiate relaxation of the internal urethral sphincter, leading to urine being expelled (Fig. 8.10).

In order for bladder control to be achieved, nervous system development is necessary. Impulses from the bladder need to be able to travel along the spinal cord to the micturition control centre in

Fig. 8.10
Diagram of simple reflex
control of micturition when
conscious effort cannot
override the reflex action.

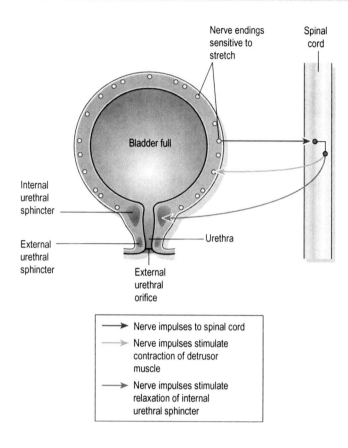

Nerve endings
sensitive to
stretch

Spinal
cord

Bladder full

Internal
urethral
sphincter

External
urethral
sphincter

Urethra

External
urethral
orifice

External
urethral
orifice

→	Nerve impulses to spinal cord
⇢	Nerve impulses stimulate contraction of detrusor muscle
⇾	Nerve impulses stimulate relaxation of internal urethral sphincter

the cerebral cortex of the brain, where they then create an awareness of the desire to micturate. Once this neurological maturation has occurred, the process becomes a controlled central nervous system activity, which then blocks the reflex arc (Fig. 8.11). Once children develop an awareness of the need to void, they can then learn to control bladder emptying. Through learning to control the external urethral sphincter and certain pelvic floor muscles, the cerebral cortex can initiate voiding or delay it for a limited period of time (Tortora & Grabowski 2003). In children, the ability to relax pelvic floor muscles voluntarily in order to void starts at about the age of 2 years.

URINE PRODUCTION AND EXCRETION

As explained in the section on kidney development, the nephrons are the functional units of the kidneys where urine is produced. Urine itself is formed in three phases:

- simple filtration
- selective reabsorption
- secretion.

Fig. 8.11
Diagram of the nervous control of micturition when conscious effort overrides the reflex action.

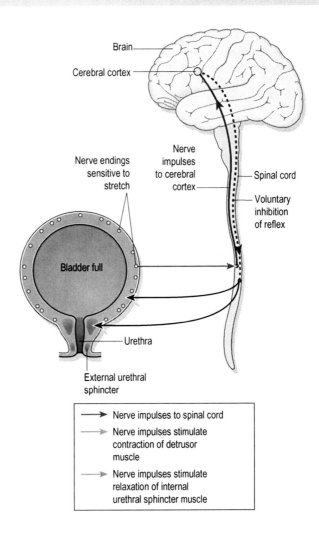

Brain

Cerebral cortex

Nerve endings sensitive to stretch

Nerve impulses to cerebral cortex

Spinal cord

Voluntary inhibition of reflex

Bladder full

Urethra

External urethral sphincter

→ Nerve impulses to spinal cord

⇢ Nerve impulses stimulate contraction of detrusor muscle

→ Nerve impulses stimulate relaxation of internal urethral sphincter muscle

Simple filtration

The first phase of urine formation is simple filtration. This process takes place through the semipermeable walls of the glomerulus and glomerular capsule (Fig. 8.12), with water and a large number of small molecules passing through into the glomerular capsule from the glomerulus. Large molecules, such as plasma and blood, that are unable to pass through remain in the capillaries (Box 8.1).

This process of filtration is governed by the same mechanism as filtration across other capillaries in the body, which includes the permeability of the capillaries and the hydrostatic and osmotic pressure gradients across the capillaries (Hockenberry 2003). The difference between blood pressure in the capillary and the pressure of the filtrate in the glomerular capsule assists the filtration process (Fig. 8.13). In this situation, blood enters the nephron at a much higher pressure than the pressure being exerted by the filtrate in the glomerular capsule. This high hydrostatic pressure in the capillary therefore forces water

Fig. 8.12
Diagram of the glomerulus and glomerular capsule.

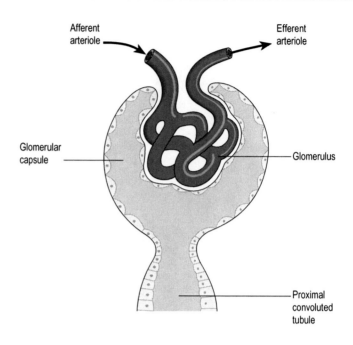

Box 8.1 Simple filtration	Blood constituents in glomerular filtrate	Blood constituents remaining in glomerulus
	Water	Leucocytes
	Mineral salts	Erythrocytes
	Amino acids	Platelets
	Ketoacids	Blood proteins
	Glucose	
	Hormones	
	Creatinine	
	Urea	
	Uric acid	
From Ross & Wilson	Toxins	
1996	Drugs	

and solutes through the capillary wall into the collecting unit. Once in the glomerular capsule, the filtrate travels through the renal tubules: the proximal convoluted tubule, the loop of Henle, and the distal convoluted tubule. As it travels along this route, selective reabsorption takes place.

Selective reabsorption

This is the second stage of urine formation and is the process whereby the volume and composition of the glomerular filtrate are altered by selectively reabsorbing constituents of the filtrate needed to maintain homeostatic equilibrium and fluid and electrolyte balance in the body

Fig. 8.13
Diagram of filtration in the
nephron.

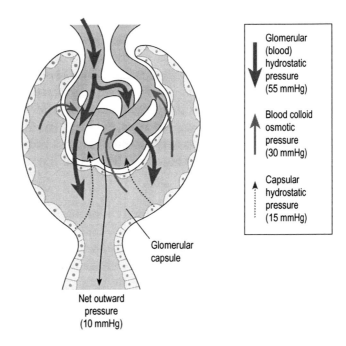

Glomerular
(blood)
hydrostatic
pressure
(55 mmHg)

Blood colloid
osmotic
pressure
(30 mmHg)

Capsular
hydrostatic
pressure
(15 mmHg)

Glomerular
capsule

Net outward
pressure
(10 mmHg)

Fig. 8.14
Diagram of selective
reabsorption and secretion in
the nephron.

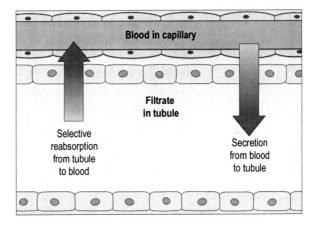

Blood in capillary

**Filtrate
in tubule**

Selective
reabsorption
from tubule
to blood

Secretion
from blood
to tubule

(Fig. 8.14). Some components of glomerular filtrate are never seen in urine because they are completely reabsorbed unless present in the blood in excessive quantities (Wilson & Waugh 1996). This process of reabsorption takes place either through osmosis (e.g. passive diffusion down a chemical or electrical gradient) or by active transport against these gradients. Amino acids, sodium, potassium, calcium, phosphate and chloride ions are all reabsorbed through active transport; some, such as sodium and chloride ions, can be absorbed by both active and passive mechanisms, depending on the site in the nephron (Wilson & Waugh 1996). Substances that are not normal constituents of blood and are not essential to body processes and homeostasis are not reabsorbed and are eliminated as waste.

Secretion

The third and final part of urine formation involves secretion. Substances that have not been filtered through the glomerulus, because of the speed with which the blood passes through the glomerulus and the short period of time that is spent in it, are secreted into the filtrate through the tubules (Fig. 8.14). Some substances, such as drugs, are secreted into the convoluted tubules and are then excreted from the body in urine, as the short period of time in the glomerulus often may not be long enough for them to be cleared from the blood by the normal filtration process.

EXCRETION OF URINE

Urine formed in the nephrons leaves the kidneys via the renal pelvis and the ureters. The main function of the ureters is to transport the urine to the bladder, and they do so via a process called *peristalsis*. Peristalsis is an intrinsic function whereby muscular movements that originate in the renal pelvis propel spurts of urine along the ureters to the urinary bladder for storage. Once in the bladder, the urine remains stored until the micturition reflex is stimulated or the cerebral cortex initiates micturition (see Development of the bladder). Once either of these processes has been initiated, the bladder empties as urine passes down the urethra and is excreted from the body.

A detailed discussion of renal physiology is beyond the remit of this chapter and the reader is advised to consult a physiology textbook for further reading in relation to urine formation and the hormonal role of the kidneys in relation to blood pressure control and red blood cell formation.

SELF ASSESSMENT

- Describe the earliest development of the renal system.
- Outline the development of the kidneys, clearly identifying each stage of development.
- Draw a diagram of a nephron and describe how urine is formed in it.
- Identify at least three congenital anomalies that may arise as a result of kidney or bladder formation.
- Describe the development of the bladder and ureters.
- Bladder control:
  a. Explain the 'micturition reflex' and why it is always present in children under the age of 2–3 years
  b. Explain how children develop bladder control
  c. Draw and label two diagrams that represent the nervous control in each of the above processes.

References

Carlson B M 1999 Human embryology and developmental biology. Mosby, St Louis

Hockenberry M J 2003 Wongs nursing care of infants and children, 7th edn. Mosby, St Louis

Larsen W J 1998 Essentials of human embryology. Churchill Livingstone, Edinburgh

MacGregor J 2000 Introduction to the anatomy and physiology of children. Routledge, London

Matsumara G, England M A 1992 Embryology colouring book. Mosby, St Louis

Moore K L, Persaud T V N 2003 The developing human clinically orientated embryology, 6th edn. W B Saunders, Philadelphia

Moules T, Ramsey J 1998 The textbook of children's nursing. Stanley Thornes, Cheltenham

Tortora G J, Grabowski S R 2003 Principles of anatomy and physiology, 10th edn. John Wiley, New York

Wilson K J W, Waugh A 1996 Ross and Wilson anatomy and physiology in health and illness, 8th edn. Churchill Livingstone, Edinburgh

Bibliography

Moore K L, Persaud T V N 2003 Before we are born essentials of embryology and birth defects, 6th edn. W B Saunders, Philadelphia.

Larsen W J 2001 Human embryology, 3rd edn. Churchill Livingstone, Philadelphia.

Silverthorn D U 2001 Human physiology: an integrated approach, 2nd edn. Benjamin Cummings/ Pearson Educational International, San Francisco

Vander A J, Sherman J H, Luciano D S 1990 Human physiology: international edition, 5th edn. McGraw-Hill, New York

Chapter 9

The reproductive tract

Mary Sandwell

CHAPTER OUTCOMES

This chapter will enable the reader to:

- Describe the embryology and fetal development of the reproductive tract
- Identify the organs that make up the reproductive tract
- Describe the functions of the organs of the female and male reproductive tract
- Explain the changes that take place in the female and male at puberty.

CHAPTER OVERVIEW

The aim of this chapter is to explore the development of the female and male reproductive tracts during the embryological stage of development (weeks 4 to 8 after conception), the fetal stage and at puberty. The Clinical Notes address issues of clinical relevance and interest to the reader. The Self Assessment exercises assist in reflecting upon the chapter and guiding the relationship between theory and practice.

INTRODUCTION

'Reproduction is the process by which new individuals are produced and the genetic material is passed from generation to generation'

(Tortora & Grabowski 1996)

Development of the genital system is one phase in the overall sexual differentiation of an individual; the subsequent phases of sexual development are controlled by the sex chromosome genes, hormones and other factors, most of which are found on the *autosomes*.

The female reproductive organs are divided into the external and internal organs (Fig. 9.1):

External:

- labia majora
- labia minora
- clitoris
- hymen
- vestibule glands
- perineum.

Internal:

- vagina
- uterus
- uterine (fallopian) tubes
- ovaries.

The male reproductive organs (Fig. 9.2) consist of:

- scrotum
- testes
- seminal vesicles
- ejaculatory ducts
- prostate gland

Fig. 9.1
The organs of the female reproductive tract.

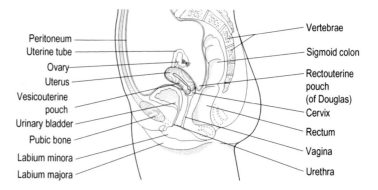

Peritoneum
Uterine tube
Ovary
Uterus
Vesicouterine pouch
Urinary bladder
Pubic bone
Labium minora
Labium majora

Vertebrae
Sigmoid colon
Rectouterine pouch (of Douglas)
Cervix
Rectum
Vagina
Urethra

Fig. 9.2
The organs of the male reproductive tract.

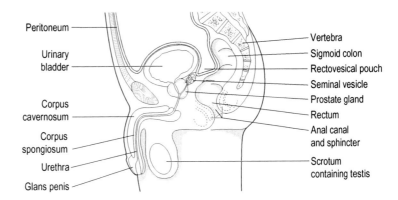

- urethra
- penis.

EMBRYOLOGY AND FETAL DEVELOPMENT

The genetic sex of an embryo is determined at fertilization when a Y chromosome or an additional X chromosome joins the X chromosome that is already in the ovum. For the first 7 weeks after conception, the gonads in both sexes appear identical. This period of early development is known as the *indifferent stage*. During this stage both male and female have two pairs of ducts: mesonephric and paramesonephric ducts.

Mesonephric ducts (also known as wolffian ducts) develop laterally to the mesonephric kidney. In the male they are retained to form the epididymis, the ducts deferens and the ejaculatory ducts. In the female these ducts mainly disappear, as testosterone is required for their development. A small part may be retained proximally as the appendix vesiculosa and distally as the duct of Gartner. This portion is equivalent to the part that forms the ductus deferens and ejaculatory duct in the male.

Paramesonephric ducts (also known as the müllerian ducts) develop laterally to the mesonephric ducts. In the male these ducts mainly disappear as the anti-müllerian hormone causes them to regress. A small cranial part of the duct may be retained, known as the appendix of the testes. In the female these ducts will form the uterine (fallopian) tubes, uterus and the superior part of the vagina.

Figure 9.3 shows the factors involved in sexual differentiation of the genital tact.

In week 4 of development, a *genital tubercle* develops at the cranial end of the cloacal membrane. Two pairs of swellings appear on either side of this membrane and surround it; there is an inner urogenital

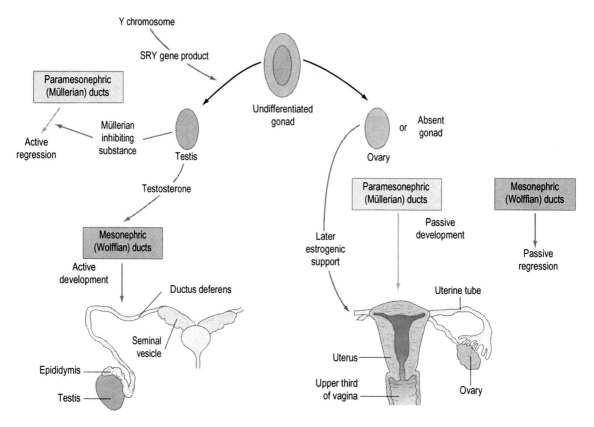

Fig. 9.3
Sexual differentiation of
the genital tract.
(From Carlson 1999.)

fold and outer urogenital swelling. The genital tubercle in both sexes elongates to form a phallus.

In week 6 the cloaca and cloacal membranes are divided by the urorectal septum into a urogenital sinus and a urogenital membrane, an anus and anal membrane.

Cells from the mesonephrons and coelomic epithelium invade the mesenchyme in the region of the presumptive gonads to form aggregates of supporting cells, the *primitive sex cords*, which completely ingest the *germ cells*. The primordial germ cells originate in the wall of the primitive yolk sac and migrate into the embryo and enter the sex cords; they eventually become the ova and sperm.

In weeks 7 to 8 the two membranes rupture and form the urogenital orifice, which contains the external surface of the phallus and anus.

DEVELOPMENT OF THE EXTERNAL FEMALE GENITALIA (Fig. 9.4)

- The phallus formed during the indifferent phase becomes the clitoris.

- The urogenital fold forms the labia minora and fuses posteriorly at the frenulum.

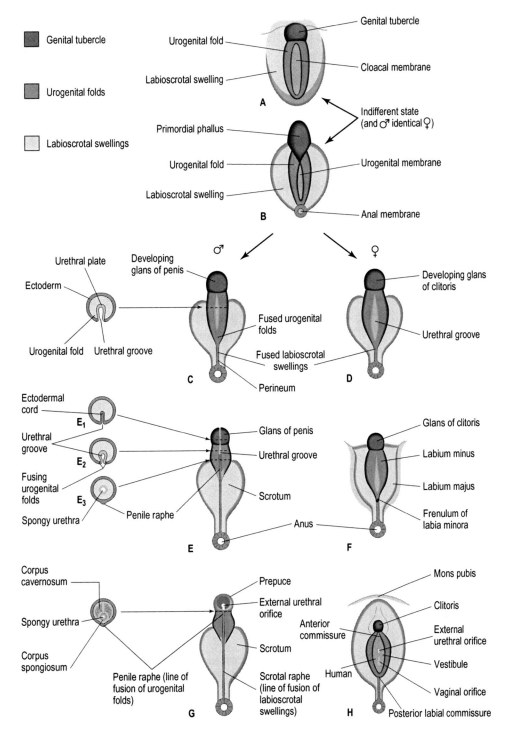

Fig. 9.4
Development of the external genitalia. (From Moore & Persaud 2003.) **A** and **B** illustrate the appearance of the genitalia during the indifferent stage (weeeks 4–7). **C, E, G** show the stages in the development of the male genitalia at weeks 9,11 and 12. To the left are transverse sections of the developing penis illustrating the formation of the spongy urethra. **D, F, H** show the stages in the development of the female genitalia at weeks 9,11 and 12.

- The labioscrotal swellings form the labia majora; they fuse anteriorly to form the mons pubis and posteriorly to form the postlabial commissure.

- The cephalic part of the urogenital sinus develops into the vestibule of the vagina.

- The hymen, which is sited across the vaginal lumen, usually ruptures in the perinatal period and so brings the lumen of the vagina into continuity with the vagina.

- The hymen is a thin membranous rim around the entrance to the vagina.

DEVELOPMENT OF THE INTERNAL FEMALE GENITALIA

The uterine tubes, uterus and superior part of the vagina develop from the paramesonephric duct.

The mesodermal epithelium invaginates, forming a tube where the edges of the invagination fuse. The open cranial ends of the tube are funnel-shaped and continuous with the peritoneal cavity; this area will form the uterine tubes. The caudal ends fuse in the median plane and form the interovaginal primoderm. The primoderm extends into the urogenital sinus; its position is located on the internal side of the urogenital sinus as the *sinus tubercle*. It connects with the urogenital sinus and activates two endodermal outgrowths called *sinovaginal buds*. These bulbs fuse and extend from the urogenital sinus up to the uterovaginal primoderm. This tube, which is called the interovaginal canal, becomes the superior portion of the vagina and the uterus.

The inferior part of the vagina forms from the urogenital sinus. The vaginal epithelium is developed from the endoderm of the urogenital sinus. The fibomuscular wall of the vagina develops from the surrounding mesenchyme. A solid cord of endodermal cells, known as the *vaginal plate*, forms; the central cells break down and form the lumen of the vagina. The peripheral cells remain as vaginal epithelium.

DEVELOPMENT OF THE OVARIES

In the female embryo gonadal development is slow; the ovary cannot be identified until week 10 of gestation. The primordial germ cells migrate from the yolk sac to the gonadal ridge. Primary sex cords grow into the medulla of the developing ovary. The cords are never obvious, but they form a *rete ovary*; this structure and the cords normally regress. The secondary sex cords (*cortical cords*) extend from the surface of the epithelium into the underlying mesenchyme where they incorporate primitive germ cells.

Each germ cell is surrounded by a layer of cells from its cortical cord. The cords break up into isolated cell clusters known as *primordial follicles*, which consist of *oögenia* drawn from the primordial germ cells surrounded by a layer of follicular cells. Active mitosis of oögenia occurs up to the fifth month of fetal life, producing thousands of these primitive germ cells. No further oögenia are formed after birth.

During the early stages of meiosis, all sex cells enter a dormant state and remain in meiotic suspension until sexual maturity (Tortora & Grabowski 1996). The flattened cells around the oögenia become cuboidal; the follicles are now known as primary follicles and will develop further at puberty. At birth there are between 200 000 and 2 000 000 oögenia and primary oöcytes in each ovary. During a woman's reproductive lifetime about 400 oögenia and primary follicles will mature; the rest will remain in the undeveloped state.

As the mesonephroi regress, each ovary is suspended by its own mesentery—the mesovarium. The surface epithelium is separated from the cortex and the primary follicle as a fibrous layer, known as the *tunica albuginea*, forms between the two layers. The cortex of the ovary is the dominant component as it contains the majority of the oöcytes.

DESCENT OF THE OVARIES

During embryological and fetal life the testes and ovaries both descend from their original positions at the tenth thoracic level. Although not as pronounced as the descent of the testes, the ovaries undergo a definite caudal shift.

The female fetus develops a *gubernaculum*, which has formed from the degenerating mesonephros. The gubernaculum extends from the inferior pole of the gonads to the subcutaneous fascia of the presumptive labioscrotal fold, and later penetrates into the abdominal cavity as the inguinal canal (Fig. 9.5A). In the more mature fetus, the gubernaculum is attached to the uterus near to the entrance of the uterine tubes.

The cranial section of the gubernaculum forms the ovarian ligament. The caudal part forms the uterine round ligament, which then passes through the inguinal canal and ends in the labium majus.

The ovaries descend from the posterior abdominal wall to a lower position to the pelvic brim and turn so that their caudal poles are directed medially. The descent of the ovaries is due to the movement of the cranial part of the abdomen as it grows away from the caudal part (Fig. 9.5B).

After birth, the ovaries are abdominal organs (Fig. 9.5C); they enter the ovarian fossae by about 6 years of age. There is little ovarian growth until puberty when they increase to 20 times the weight of the newborn organs.

Fig. 9.5
Descent of the ovary.
A Week 9.
B Weeks 12–13.
C Position of adult ovary.

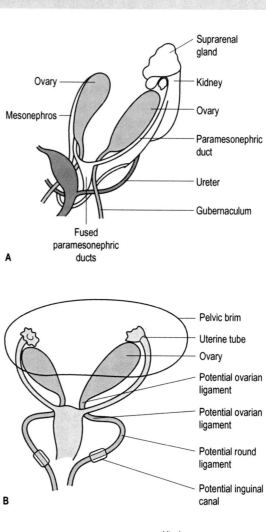

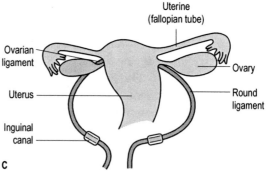

At birth the uterus lies in almost the same level as the vagina, as the bladder descends into the pelvis the uterus bends forward into the adult position of anteversion and anteflexion. The uterus is relatively large at birth, probably due to the influence of female hormones;

when these are removed the uterus shrinks and does not regain its birthweight until stimulated by hormonal activity at puberty. The cervix is considerably larger than the body of the uterus until adolescence; during this period the uterus outgrows the cervix and doubles its length. The uterine tubes grow at the same time as the uterus.

CLINICAL NOTES   **ABNORMALITIES OF THE FEMALE GENITAL TRACT**

A double uterus results from the abnormal fusion of the caudal portion of the paramesonephric ducts; a single or double vagina may be associated with a double uterus.

The vagina may be absent due to the vaginal plate failing to recanalize. This occurs in about 1 in 4000 females. The absence of a vagina and uterus are usually linked.

Imperforate hymen is a result of the hymen failing to rupture. It causes problems at puberty when the girl starts to menstruate, as the menstrual fluid cannot escape; surgical intervention is necessary.

DEVELOPMENT OF THE MALE GENITALIA (Fig. 9.4)

Masculinization of the indifferent genitalia is generated by testosterone, which is produced by the *Leydig cells* in the fetal testes.

As the phallus elongates to form a penis, the urogenital folds fuse along the ventral surface of the penis to form the (spongy) penile urethra. The external urethral orifice then moves to the glans penis. The labioscrotal swellings grow towards each other and fuse to become the scrotum. During week 12 the prepuce of the penis forms, when a circular ectodermal ingrowth of smaller diameter than the glans grows into the tip.

DEVELOPMENT OF THE PROSTATE GLAND

The prostate gland develops during the tenth week as a cluster of endodermal evaginates that bud from the pelvic urethra. The prostrate outgrowth initially forms at least five independent groups of solid prostatic cords. By week 11 the cords develop a lumen and glandular acini. During weeks 13 to 15, as testosterone secretion reaches a high level, the prostate begins its secretory activity. The mesenchyme surrounding the endoderm-derived portion of the prostate differentiates into the smooth muscle and connective tissue of the prostate. A glycogen-rich secretion appears in the ducts during the ninth month.

DEVELOPMENT OF THE TESTES

One of the first occurrences in the development of the male genitalia is the precise effect of the *SRY protein* (sex-determining region of the Y chromosome) within the sex cords. The influence of SRY cells in the medullary region of the primitive sex cords causes them to differentiate into *Sertoli cells*, which are derivatives of surface epithelium. During week 7 the Sertoli cells are arranged to form the *testes cords*.

As the primordial germ cells of male embryos reach the gonadal ridge on the posterior abdominal wall, prominent primary sex cords grow into the medulla. These cords anastomose and form the *rete testes*. The cords (now the seminiferous cords) are separated from the surface of the epithelium by a thick fibrous *tunica albuginea*. They give rise to:

- rete testes
- tubuli tecti
- seminiferous tubules.

The seminiferous tubules are made up of two types of cell:

- the spermatogonia, derived from primitive germ cells
- the Sertoli cells.

The mesenchyme lying between the seminiferous tubules gives rise to interstitial cells (Leydig cells), which produce testosterone. Fetal testes also produce the müllerian inhibiting hormone.

Between weeks 8 and 12 the initial secretion of testosterone stimulates the mesonephritic ducts to transform into the spermatic ducts called the *vas deferens*. The portion of the vas deferens distal to each seminal vesicle is called the *ejaculatory duct*.

DESCENT OF THE TESTES (Fig. 9.6)

Inguinal canals form in males and females, although in the female they play no part in genital development. In the male, the canal extends from the posterior abdominal wall into the scrotum and transmits the descending testicles.

Each testis is attached on its inferior ligament (*gubernaculum*). Both ligaments extend within the developing anterior abdominal wall to attach to the internal aspect of each labioscrotal swelling. To the front of each gubernaculum an evagination of peritoneum herniates along the path of the gubernaculum. Each herniation carries with it and in front of it extensions of certain layers of the abdominal wall that will form the walls of the inguinal canal. The deep inguinal ring forms where the herniation emerges through the abdominal wall. The superior inguinal ring forms in the aponeurosis of the external oblique muscle.

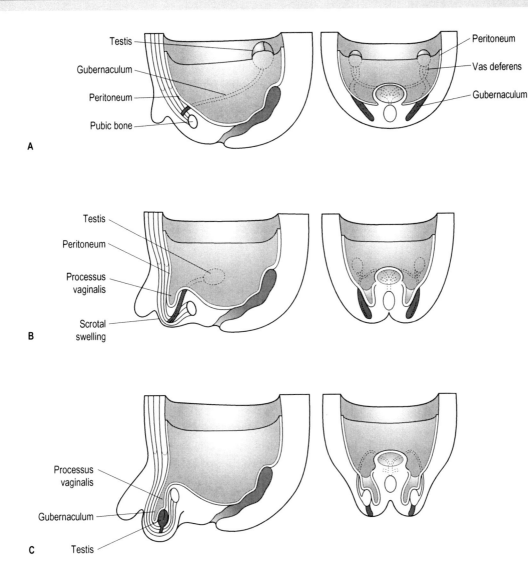

Fig. 9.6
A Testes before descent from the abdominal cavity (week 7).
B Testes in the inguinal canal (week 28–29).
C Testes secure in the scrotum (at term, week 40).

As the trunk grows the testes, the ductus deferens and vessels drop down from the posterior abdominal wall. As they descend, they are encased in fascial extensions of layers of the abdominal wall. The gubernaculum aids in securing the testes in the scrotum.

These processes begin at 28 weeks. The testes descend into the deep ring of the inguinal canal and complete their descent by the seventh to ninth month. It is believed that fetal androgens initiate and regulate the testicular descent.

CLINICAL NOTES   UNDESCENDED TESTES

Undescended testes (*cryptorchidism*) is the failure of one or both testes to descend. This occurs in about 3–4% of full-term baby boys, but falls to 1%

at 1 year of age. Retractable testes can be pushed into the scrotum, but true undescended testes rarely descend after the age of 1 year. Orchidopexy is usually performed before the child's second birthday.

After birth, the seminiferous tubules of the testicles are solid, until puberty when they become canalized. The testes remain small and grow slowly in childhood; the adult testis is about 40 times as heavy as that of a newborn baby. The prostate gland grows slowly until puberty and then doubles its size over a short period of time. The penis is relatively large at birth and the prepuce is imperfectly separated from the glans; the spongy tissue grows throughout childhood.

CLINICAL NOTES   **HYPOSPADIAS**

Hypospadias occurs in approximately 1 in 500 boys (Rudolf & Levene 1999); 10–15% of affected newborns have a father or brother with the same condition (Bukowski & Zemen, cited in Hockenberry et al 2003).

The condition occurs when the urethra is situated anywhere on the ventral side of the glans penis to the periscrotal junction or the perineum. The penis usually curves ventrally, a condition known as chordee.

Chordee results from the replacement of normal skin with a band of fibrous tissue, and most commonly affects the most severe forms of hypospadias. The foreskin is normally absent ventrally and, when combined with chordee, gives the penis a crooked and hooded appearance, which may leave the infant's sex in question at birth. The perineal position of the meatus may be mistaken for a urethra, and if the infant also has undescended testes the small penis may resemble an enlarged clitoris. If there is any doubt regarding the infant's sex, chromosome analysis is essential.

Management of the condition is surgical reconstruction before the age of 2 years. This will allow the boy to pass urine in a standing position, prevent future sexual malfunction and avoid any psychological consequences.

Epispadias occurs in about 1 in 25 000 males. In this condition, the urethra opens on the dorsal surface of the penis, caused by a failure of urethral canalization.

INTERSEXUALITY

An early embryo has the potential to develop as either male or female; errors in sexual development may result in various degrees

Table 9.1   Comparisons of normal and abnormal infant genitalia at birth

Normal findings	Abnormal findings
Male	
Penile shaft protrudes from the perineum and hangs freely	The penis is small, less than 2.5–3 cm in the newborn. It may be an enlarged clitoris
Urethral meatus is centred at the tip of the glans penis	The urethral meatus may be anywhere along the dorsal or ventral surface of the penis, especially on the perineum
Two scrotal sacs hang freely, covered with loose wrinkled skin	Small scrotum with smooth, tight skin and any degree of separation in the midline may be enlarged labia
Palpable testes in each scrotum	Absent testes may be undescended; if combined with small scrotum, may be evidence of enlarged labia
Female	
Small clitoris visible at anterior end of labia	Enlarged clitoris that protrudes from labia may be a small penis
Urethral meatus located between clitoris and vagina	Urethral meatus located in clitoris may suggest a small penis
Labia minora are prominent in newborn but atrophied and almost absent in the prepubertal female; they are completely separated from the clitoris to posterior vault of the vagina; on palpation there are no masses in the labia	Prominent labia, partially or completely fused with palpable masses on each side, may be a small scrotum with testes

From Wong 1999.

of intermediate sex, a condition known as *hermaphroditism* (Table 9.1). 'The infant's functional anatomy rather than genetic sex is the primary criterion on which the choice of gender should be based' (Wong 1999); therefore, a baby born with ambiguous genitalia creates a social emergency, as the parents need to know the baby's sex.

True hermaphrodite   True hermaphroditism is extremely rare. The person usually has 46XX chromosomes; both ovarian and testicular tissue are present at birth, either in the same or in opposite gonads.

Female pseudohermaphrodite   These individuals are genetically female and have 46XX chromosomes. The internal genitalia are female but the external genitalia are masculinized, either as a result of excessive androgenic hormones from the adrenal cortex (congenital adrenogenital hyperplasia) or because of inappropriate hormonal treatment of the mother.

Male pseudohermaphrodite

These individuals usually have 46XY chromosomes. This condition results from inadequate hormone production by the fetal testes, so the phenotype can vary. It is often associated with hypoplasia of the phallus.

Testicular feminization

These individuals are genetically male, having 46XY chromosomes. They posses internal testes but have normal external female genitalia. The testes produce testosterone but, due to a weakness in the receptors caused by a mutation on the X chromosome, the testosterone is unable to work on the appropriate tissues. Müllerian inhibitory substance is produced; therefore the uterus and upper part of the vagina are absent.

These individuals are usually raised as females; the condition is often not discovered until puberty when the individual seeks treatment for amenorrhoea.

PUBERTY

'Legally, puberty is the time at which the individual becomes functionally capable of producing a child; in England this state is recognised by the law courts to have been reached by the age of 12 for girls and 14 for boys'

(Sinclair & Dangerfield 1998)

The word puberty is used to explain a series of developments that are spread over several years, the order and timing of which vary in each individual. The process of sexual maturity begins during fetal development and continues until maturity is accomplished (Table 9.2).

Puberty begins before any physical signs are evident; it is instigated by the pulsed release of *gonadotrophic* hormones from the hypothalamus in the brain. These hormones can be detected in girls of about 7–8 years of age, and about a year later in boys.

- The rate of the pubertal changes varies in individuals by about 2 to 4.5 years.
- Approximately 50% of young people complete puberty in 3 years, virtually all in 5 years.
- A weight of 47 kg in girls has been suggested as a trigger for hormonal changes
- Changes usually begin with a growth spurt between the ages of 10 and 16 in boys, and about 2 years earlier in girls.

Table 9.2   Rough timetable of sexual maturation (Sinclair & Dangerfield 1998)

	Boys	Girls
Onset	• Testicular enlargement begins • Seminiferous tubules canalize • Primary spermatocytes appear • Fine, downy, straight pubic hair appears	• Ovarian enlargement begins • Breasts develop to 'bud' stage • Fine, downy, straight pubic hair appears
A year or more later	• Secondary spermatocytes present • Penile enlargement progressing • Pubic hair now coarser and curling	• Pigmentation of areolae • Pubic hair now coarser and curling
A year or more later	• Relative enlargement of the larynx beginning • First ejaculation	• Relative increase of pelvic diameter beginning • Menarche; first cycles may not produce ova
A year or more later	• Mature spermatozoa present • Axillary hair • Sweat and sebaceous glands very active	• Full reproductivity • Axillary hair • Sweat and sebaceous glands very active

FEMALE PUBERTY

Physical changes

- The uterus, uterine tubes and ovaries reach maturity.
- The menstrual cycle and ovulation begin (*menarche*).
- The breasts develop and enlarge.
- Pubic and axillary hair starts to grow.
- There is a growth spurt and the pelvis widens.
- Increased fat is deposited in the subcutaneous tissue, especially around the hips and breasts.

The menstrual cycle

During their reproductive years, from about the age of 14 to 50 years, non-pregnant females normally experience a cyclical series of events occurring about every 26–30 days, known as the menstrual cycle. The hypothalamus secretes luteinizing hormone releasing hormone (LHRH), which stimulates the pituitary gland to secrete:

1. Follicle stimulating hormone (FSH), which aids the maturation of ovarian follicles and the stimulation of oestrogen, leading to ovulation.

2. Luteinizing hormone (LH), which stimulates ovulation, the development of the corpus luteum and the secretion of progesterone.

The hypothalamus responds to changes in the blood level of oestrogen and progesterone. It is switched off by high levels and stimulated by low levels.

The menstrual cycle has three phases:

- menstrual phase
- proliferation phase
- secretory phase.

Menstrual phase: days 1–5

- If the ovum has not been fertilized, the corpus luteum begins to degenerate.

- Progesterone and oestrogen levels fall and the layers of endometrium are shed in menstruation.

- The menstrual flow consists of 50–150 mL blood from the broken-down capillaries and secretions from the endometrial glands. Menstruation usually lasts about 4–6 days.

- After degeneration of the corpus luteum, the falling levels of progesterone and oestrogen lead to anterior pituitary activity, rising FSH levels, and the initiation of the next cycle.

Proliferation phase: days 6–14

During this stage an ovarian follicle, stimulated by FSH, is growing towards maturity and producing oestrogen. Oestrogen stimulates the functional layer of the endometrium in preparation for the reception of a fertilized ovum. The endometrium becomes thicker due to rapid cell multiplication and because of the increased numbers of secretory glands and blood capillaries. This phase ends when ovulation occurs, usually around day 14, and oestrogen production declines.

Ovulation

Usually just one follicle within the ovary matures to become a vesicular ovarian (graafian) follicle. This follicle is quite large and forms a bulge on the surface of the ovary. A sudden burst of LH from the anterior pituitary gland triggered by a peak of oestrogen causes the follicle to rupture. It forces the ovum into the peritoneal cavity near the opening of the uterine tube. The ovum may survive for as little as 8 hours in a form that can be fertilized; if the ovum is not fertilized, it disintegrates within a couple of days.

CLINICAL NOTES   **SIGNS OF OVULATION**

The time of ovulation can be recognized by changes that take place in the woman's body:

- A rise in basal temperature.
- Near to the time of ovulation, increasing levels of oestrogen cause the secretory cells of the cervix to produce large amounts of cervical mucus.
- The mucus becomes very stretchy as ovulation approaches.
- The external os of the cervix dilates slightly; it rises and becomes softer.
- Pain in the area of one or both ovaries is felt by some women; this pain is called *mittelschmerz* (pain in the middle) and may last for several hours to a day or two.

During early menstrual cycles ovulation may not occur, but conversely cyclical release of ova may occur before the onset of menstruation.

Secretory phase: days 15–28

During this phase the levels of progesterone produced by the corpus luteum of the ovary rise and act on the oestrogen-primed endometrium to increase the blood supply. The endometrium becomes oedematous and the secretory glands produce increasing amounts of watery mucus, which is believed to assist the passage of spermatozoa through the uterus to the uterine tube, where the ovum is usually fertilized.

If fertilization does not occur, towards the end of this phase the corpus luteum begins to break down due to the decline in the level of LH. Lack of hormones in the blood causes the blood vessels supplying the endometrium to go into spasm. When deprived of oxygen and nutrients, the endometrial cells begin to die—this sets the stage for menstruation to begin on day 28 (Fig. 9.7).

MALE PUBERTY

Puberty in the male usually occurs between the ages of 9 and 15 years. The earliest sign is the growth of the testicle; this can be measured with an orchidometer, which is a string of ovoids of known volume. The average adult testicle has a volume of about 20 mL; a volume of 6 mL indicates that puberty has commenced. Luteinizing hormone from the anterior pituitary gland stimulates the interstitial cells of the testes to increase the production of testosterone. The rising level of testosterone in the blood of the young male stimulates the reproductive organs to develop to their adult size, and causes the secondary male sex characteristics to develop.

Changes that occur at puberty are:

- marked increase in height and weight and in the growth of muscle and bone
- larynx enlarges, and voice deepens and breaks
- hair grows on face, axillae, chest, abdomen and pubis
- penis, scrotum and prostate gland increase in size
- seminiferous tubules mature and spermatozoa are produced.

Hormonal control of spermatogenesis

At the onset of puberty, the anterior pituitary gland increases its secretion of the gonadotrophic leutinizing hormone (LH) and follicle stimulating hormone (FSH). Their release is controlled by the gonadotrophin-releasing hormone from the hypothalamus.

- LH stimulates the Leydig cells to secrete testosterone.
- FSH acts directly to stimulate spermatogenesis.

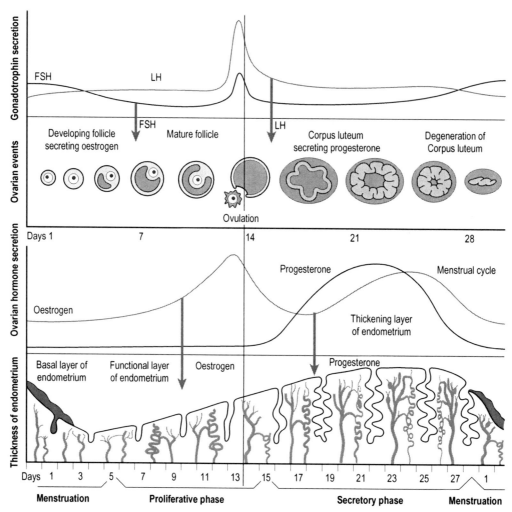

Fig. 9.7
The menstrual cycle. FSH,
follicle stimulating hormone;
LH, luteinizing hormone.

Spermarche is the onset of sperm emissions, indicating that spermato-genesis has been established. This an early pubertal event, with a median age of 13.4 years and a testicular volume of 11.5 mL. Sperm are formed in the semineferous tubule of the testes at the rate of about 300 million a day; sperm production begins during puberty and continues throughout life.

CLINICAL NOTES | **DELAYED PUBERTY**

A female is considered to have delayed puberty if there is a failure to menstruate beyond the age of 16 years.

A male is considered to have delayed puberty if more than 5 years have elapsed from initiation to completion of genital growth.

In about 90–95% of individuals with delayed puberty, the delay is constitutional; this diagnosis is made by excluding other causes, of which there are many including:

Gonadotrophin deficiency

- tumours
- trauma
- infections.

Congenital gonadal disorder

- Klinefelter's syndrome
- pure gonadal dysgenesis.

Chronic disease

- congenital heart defects
- asthma
- hypothyroidism.

Congenital syndromes

- Turner's syndrome (females)
- Noonan's syndrome (males and females)
- Prader–Labhart–Willi syndrome.

Malnutrition, either voluntary or not, will cause delayed menarche. This delay sometimes occurs in female dancers and athletes as they may be 10–15% below normal weight for their height.

Constitutional delay is often genetic. The young person and their parents need reassurance that growth and puberty will occur. If there are severe psychological problems, hormonal therapy may be given for 6 months. Most other causes of delayed puberty are irreversible (Neinstein 1996).

CLINICAL NOTES   **PRECOCIOUS PUBERTY**

A girl is considered to have precocious puberty if she has any breast development or pubic hair before the age of 8 years.

A boy is considered to have precocious puberty if he has pubic hair, penile and testicular enlargement, and textured scrotum before the age of 9.5 years.

Incomplete forms
These are generally self-limiting and will not progress as there is no early secretion of gonadotrophin.

True or complete forms

These result from the premature activity of the hypothalamic–pituitary–gonadal axis, which causes:

- early maturation and development of the gonads with the secretion of sex hormones
- development of secondary sex characteristics
- the production of mature sperm and ova.

Causes

- Organic brain lesions
- Postinflammatory disorders
- In most cases, no cause is found.

Treatment

If the specific cause is known it can be treated; otherwise precocious puberty is managed by monthly injections of luteinizing hormone releasing hormone. Treatment is discontinued at an appropriate age to allow puberty to resume.

SELF ASSESSMENT

- What is known as the indifferent stage of development?
- Which structures in the female reproductive system arise from the paramesonephric ducts? Which structures in the male reproductive tract arise from the mesonephric ducts?
- Describe the descent of the testes. When does spermatogenesis begin?
- What is the cause of hypospadias? Why is it important that the defect is corrected before the age of 2 years?
- What causes puberty to begin? List the physical changes that take place in the male and female during puberty.
- Explain the menstrual cycle.
- What signs and symptoms would cause you to think that a child's sexual development was premature? Why is it important to recognize and treat this?

References

Carlson B 1999 Human embryology and developmental biology, 2nd edn. Mosby, St Louis

Hockenberry M, Wilson D, Winkelstein M, Kline N 2003 Wong's nursing care of infants and children, 7th edn. Mosby, St Louis

Moore K, Persaud T Before we are born. W B Saunders, Philadelphia

Neinstein L 1996 Adolescent health—a practical guide, 3rd edn. Williams & Wilkins, Baltimore

Rudolf M, Levene M 1999 Paediatrics and child health. Blackwell Science, Oxford
Sinclair D, Dangerfield P 1998 Human growth after birth, 8th edn. Oxford University Press, Oxford

Tortora G, Grabowski S 1996 Principles of anatomy and physiology, 8th edn. HarperCollins, New York
Wong D 1999 Whaley and Wong's nursing care of infants and children. Mosby, St Louis

Bibliography

Larsen W 1998 Essentials of human embryology. Churchill Livingstone, New York
MacGregor J 2000 Introduction to the anatomy and physiology of children. Routledge, London
Marieb E 1999 Essentials of human anatomy and physiology, 6th edn. Benjamin/Cummins Scientific, San Francisco
Matsumura G, England M 1999 Embryology colouring book. Mosby, London

Money J, Ehchardt A 1996 Man and woman: boy and girl. Jason Aronson, Northvale
Rudolf M, Levene M 1999 Paediatrics and child health. Blackwell Science, Oxford
Van De Graff K 2002 Human anatomy, 6th edn. McGraw Hill, Boston

Chapter 10

Development of the immune system and immunity

Duncan Randall

CHAPTER OUTCOMES

This chapter will enable the reader to:

- Justify the importance of immunity in childhood
- Identify the elements of immune system in children
- Describe the development of various lymphoid structures and immune cells thoughout childhood
- Outline the differences between childhood and adult immunity
- Explore the functioning of lymphatic control of fluid balance in the fetus
- Justify why breast-feeding improves childhood immunity.

CHAPTER OVERVIEW

The aim of this chapter is to describe the development of immunity up to adult status, including normal embryonic, fetal and infant development. This chapter looks at the development of the cells that give rise to immune cells in the body (haematopoietic stem cells), the development of the main organs of the immune system, the thymus and bone marrow. It also addresses the development of secondary lymphoid organs such as the spleen and lymphatic system lymph nodes, as well as mucosa-associated lymphoid tissue (MALT). The development of immunity in childhood is considered, and the vaccination of children. Clinical Notes address complete DiGeorge syndrome and childhood vaccination. Self Assessment exercises are given to assist in reflection on the material in the chapter and its relevance to the reader's own area of professional practice.

The chapter does not cover the mechanisms of immunity in depth; these can be reviewed in Part One of Goldsby et al (2003). Other body systems that contribute to immunity, such as the natural barriers of the skin, mucosal membranes and the acidity of the gut, are covered in other parts of this book.

INTRODUCTION

The ability of the body to protect itself from invasion and colonization by other life forms and toxic substances (*antigens*) is essential to life. However, our understanding of the immune system appears to be reaching beyond simple defence. The fast developing field of immunology is now making links to the body's ability to regulate its own cells via the immune system, by describing immunological basis for cancers. The field of psychoneuroimmunology draws together neuroscience and behavioural psychology to relate them to the immune system. Proteins secreted by immune cells—*cytokines* such as interleukin 1 (IL-1)—induce inflammation when released by monocytes and macrophages in response to an antigen, but also act with other cytokines to induce fever, reduce food intake, sensitize nerve fibres to pain and increase slow-wave sleep. Cytokines, the message proteins of the immune system, are now being linked to memory and learning (Patterson & Nawa 1993). Thus immunity is not only important in maintaining the health of children but plays an important role in the development of children.

Allergic conditions in childhood are increasing—conditions such as asthma and specific allergic reactions such as peanut allergy (Burks 2003). Although these conditions result in few childhood deaths, the burden of morbidity to children, their families and the healthcare system is considerable (Austin et al 1999).

However, infectious diseases still kill many thousands of children worldwide. In developed countries global travel and controversial debates over immunization programmes, as well as poverty, have allowed some diseases that were once controlled to return. In the developing world neglect, conflict and poverty leave children unprotected from preventable disease (World Health Organization 1998).

EMBRYOLOGY

In utero the dangers to the embryo and fetus come, in the main, from the mother's own blood system, as the fetus is sealed in the amniotic fluid. The viability of the fetus depends on the immune system of both the mother and the developing child. A range of 'blocking' antibodies, including antibodies to specific fetal tissue (*leucocytotoxic, oncofetal* and *trophoblastic* antigens), have been identified in maternal blood. These may protect the fetus from immune reaction with the maternal body. The tissue of the maternal placenta (*syncytiotrophoblasts*—the major tissue type) is immunologicaly neutral as it does not exhibit *major histocompatibility complex* (MHC) proteins required for the recognition of the majority of T cells. A highly charged *sialomucin layer* covers the placenta, and reduces immune reactions. This, together with an immune active layer surrounding the cytotrophoblast and a lack of potential immune cells at the surface, helps to protect the embryo and the mother from immunological reactions.

Blood forms into islands as the embryo itself forms, and with them *haematopoietic stem cells* develop. During uterine life the production of immune system cells from haematopoietic stem cells occurs in the liver and spleen. Haematopoietic stem cells develop between the hepatic cells and the liver's encapsulating connective tissue between the third and sixth week of life. By the tenth week the liver accounts for 10% of the total bodyweight, in part due to the activity of the haematopoietic stem cells. The liver as a site of haematopoietic stem cell activity begins to diminish in the last 2 months of gestation, and by birth only small islands are left, the haematopoietic stem cells having migrated to the fetal bone marrow, which assumes the function of providing a *stromal* cell matrix for the haematopoietic stem cells to produce blood cells.

CELLS OF THE IMMUNE SYSTEM

Thoughout life new immune cells are generated from haematopoietic stem cells (Fig. 10.1), which differentiate into progenitor cells for myeloid immune cells (monocytes, macrophages, neutrophils, eosinophils, basophils and dendritic cells) as well as for lymphoid cells (natural killer cells, T cells, B cells and dendritic cells). Myeloid cells provide non-specific immune cells which destroy antigens by encapsulating them in their cell membrane (*phagocytosis*) and releasing chemicals that destroy the antigen (chemolysis). Lymphoid immune cells are specific in that they are able to recognize specific antigens and attack the antigen by using its own specific molecular structure. When the body detects a new antigen, lymphoid immune cells mature to attack the specific antigen; this process is mediated by cytokines.

Before the lymphoid immune cell can attack the antigen, the lymphoid cell must capture and bind to the antigen. Various mechanisms enable this process of binding to the antigen. Clusters of differentiated molecules (CD classification; e.g. CD4) on the surface of the immune cell attract and secure receptors on the antigen. Dendritic cells (both myeloid and lymphoid) are elongated cells with a structure similar to that of the nerve dendrite; they present antigens to immune-specific cells for binding and destruction.

Although haematopoietic stem cells are the source of the immune cells, some are modified and regulated either peripherally or in the organs of the immune system such as the thymus, which modifies T cells to respond to different immunological situations.

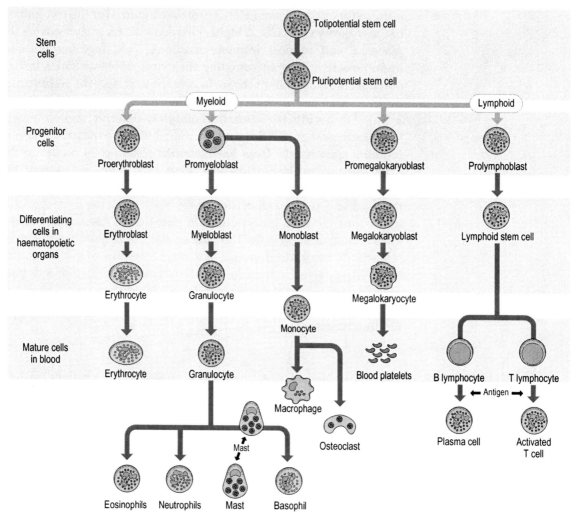

Fig. 10.1
Stem cells and their myeloid and lymphoid derivatives.

DEVELOPMENT OF THE THYMUS

In the fifth week of gestation, epithelial tissue in the pharyngeal pouces between pharyngeal arches 3 and 4 differentiates to form two lobes (Fig. 10.2), which migrate towards the thorax of the embryo. This migration causes the lobes to elongate and also draws tissue that develops into the parathyroid glands down to the thyroid gland. During week 8 the two lobes fuse and the bilobar structure is encapsulated by connective tissue from the neural crest. If this encapsulation fails, the thymus does not develop (as in complete DiGeorge syndrome; see Clinical Notes, page 268). Between 9 and 10 weeks of gestation, haematopoietic stem cells in the liver and spleen begin to differentiate into *prothymocytes*, which migrate and invade the thymus (Askin & Young 2001,

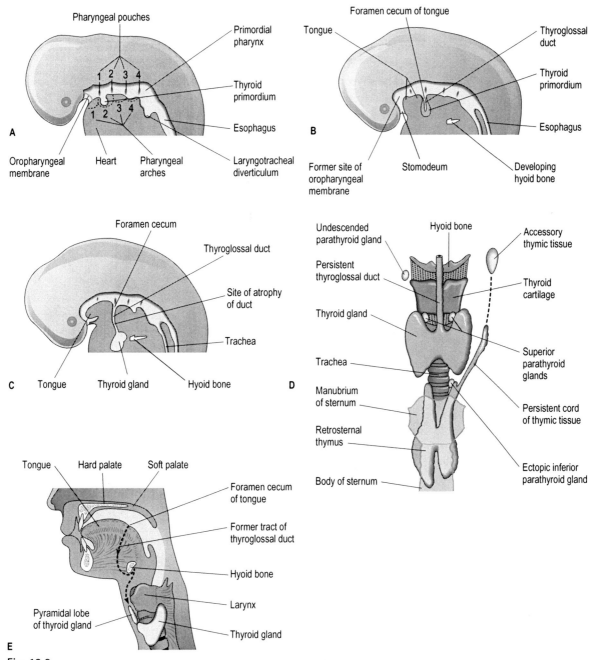

Fig. 10.2
Development of the thyroid gland and thymus.
A–C Development of the thyroid gland (4–6 weeks).
D Thyroid, thymus and parathyroid glands; an anterior view illustrating some congenital anomalies.
E Adult head and neck structures that relate to the thyroid gland, including path taken during embryonic development.
(From Moore & Persaud 2003, with permission.)

Holladay & Smialowicz 2000). The invasion of prothymocytes causes the thymus to restructure, with Hassall's corpuscles appearing between weeks 12 and 14. These concentric epithelial structures are thought to be involved in cytokine function (Nishio et al 2000).

The thymus begins to produce naive T cells between weeks 9 and 10 (Holladay & Smialowicz 2000). This production continues so that by birth a large pool of untriggered or naive T cells has accumulated, which De Vries et al (2000) suggest is required for the many primary immunological responses the neonate will need to mount. This activity prenatally goes some way to explaining why the thymus is so large at birth, occupying a large area in the thorax and clearly visible on radiography, where it can make the visualization of other structures difficult. The thymus continues to increase in size during childhood until adolescence, and then shrinks over the adult lifespan.

CLINICAL NOTES **DiGEORGE SYNDROME**

Children born with DiGeorge syndrome (chromosome 22q11.2 deletion syndrome) have anatomical abnormalities deriving from pharyngeal arch 3 and 4 development. These can include malformation or absence of the thymus gland. The syndrome is thought to affect 1 in 4000 live births. Cardiac abnormalities are also common, and are present in up to 75% of cases. T-cell populations in children with DiGeorge syndrome are seen to decline, associated with an increase in infections and autoimmune disease (Jawad et al 2001).

In complete DiGeorge syndrome no thymus forms (*congenital athymia*) and there is *hypocalcaemia* and cardiac defects. Bensoussan et al (2002) report such a child who suffered from repeated serious infections before successfully receiving a peripheral blood mononuclear cell transplantation from his sister, matched for human leucocyte antigen (HLA); T-cell responses were normal a few months after transplantion, allowing vaccination which produced vaccine-specific antibodies.

DEVELOPMENT OF THE SECONDARY LYMPHATIC ORGANS: SPLEEN AND LYMPH NODES

The primitive spleen forms from a proliferation in the mesoderm where the stomach attaches to the body wall (*dorsal mesogastrium*); as the stomach rotates into its mature position in the fifth week of gestation the spleen is pushed to the left above the kidney where it attaches to the inside of the peritoneum (Fig. 10.3). The mesenchymal cells from which the spleen originates are initially organized in islands, which form lobes in the developing spleen.

The lymphatic system of vessels that spread throughout the body and drain into the thoracic duct or the right lymphatic duct appear after the cardiac system, and are thought to develop from the

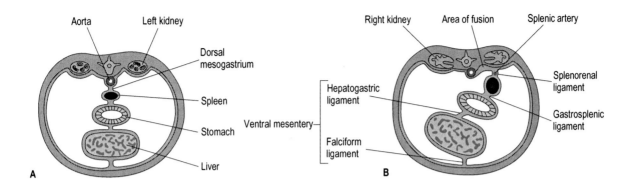

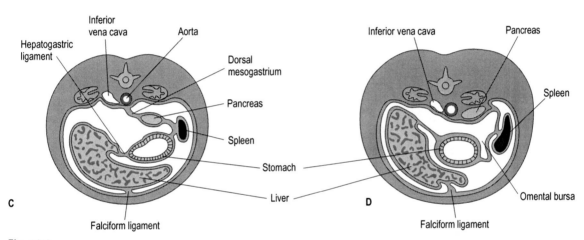

Fig. 10.3
A–D Transverse sections showing the development of the spleen from week 5 onwards.
(From Moore & Persaud 2003, with permission.)

endothelium of their associated veins in the cardiac system at about 5 weeks gestation (Fig. 10.4).

As well as its immunological functions, this system maintains the fetal hydrostatic fluid balance, preventing hydops fetalis or oedema in the fetus. As fetal interstitial compliance at 45 mL per mmHg per kg is ten times the adult level, oedema can be extensive. A greater degree of membrane permeability and higher plasma protein levels in the fetus are compensated for by higher capillary filtration rates and thus a larger volume of fluid delivered back into the circulation via the central veins (lymphatic outflow). The outflow pressure of the fetal lymphatic system is sensitive to positive changes in venous pressure at the subclavian and jugular veins. From studies in sheep it appears that small increases in venous pressure have dramatic effects on lymphatic outflow, with flow being stopped by a 15-mmHg increase. Sheep studies also suggest that hydration responses are mature in late gestation, as falling *haematocrit* (percentage of pack cells in plasma) induced proportional increases in lymphatic outflow rate. Thus fetal

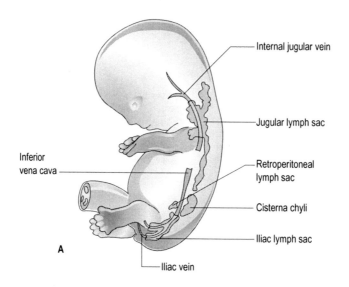

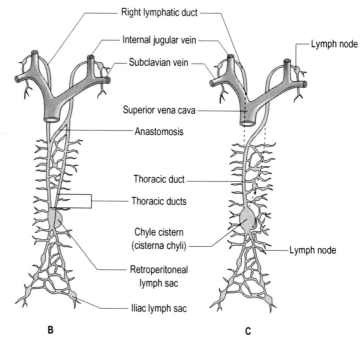

Fig. 10.4
Structure of the lymphatic system.
A Left side of an 8-week embryo illustrating primary lymph sacs
B Ventral view of lymphatic system at 9 weeks.
C Formation of thoracic duct and right lymphatic duct.
(From Moore & Persaud 2003, with permission.)

oedema may be related to small rises in blood pressure and/or significant changes in the permeability of capillaries. Although endocrine control of lymphatic outflow is similar to that in adults, with atrial natriuretic factor (ANF) suppressing flow and angiotensin II stimulating flow, it is not known when sympathetic nervous control matures.

FETAL DEVELOPMENT

DEVELOPMENT OF BONE MARROW AND MALT

The ontogenesis of bone marrow has been described elsewhere (see page 62–63). The bone marrow's immune functions begin at 20 weeks gestation when a network of reticular cells has been established that can support the proliferation of haematopoietic stem cells. From this time immune functions increase, replacing those of the liver so that at birth naive B cells are produced almost exclusively in the bone marrow. These B cells, like the T cells produced by the thymus in the fetal stage, are naive (i.e. not antigen specific).

At the 19-week stage, naive B cells are also being produced in the lining of the gut in Peyer's patches and other structures (Brandtzaeg 1998). These structures are part of the mucosa-associated lymphoid tissue (MALT), which consists of Waldeyer's pharyngeal ring (palatine tonsils, adenoids, etc.) derived from the epithelial lining of the second pharyngeal pouch and the nasopharynx, and gut-associated lymphoid tissue (GALT), areas of lymphoid tissue that differentiate from epithelial cells in the distal ileum, distal large bowel and appendix (Brandtzaeg 1998). These structures are invaded first by mesodermal tissue and then, during the second trimester, by lymphoid tissue. The separate tissues of the MALT system are joined by the lymphatic system and are thought to communicate through immune responses, so that antigens identified in one area initiate a response in associated MALT tissue, a process called homing (Brandtzaeg 1998). Thus B cells that encounter antigens in the tonsils produce cytokines, and enable cells in Peyer's patch to mature B cells specific to that antigen. However, the cells in the secondary follicles of Peyer's patch do not mature until after birth (Gebbers & Laissue 1990).

Immunity in the gut is functional before birth through maternal immunoglobulin (Ig) G, which crosses the placenta and is found in the fetal gut mucosa from 13 weeks. Some immunoglobulins (IgG and secretory IgA) and maternal antibodies enter the fetal gut from amniotic fluid and may provide a low-grade stimulus to enable GALT development. The fetus's own ability to produce immunoglobulins remains very low until birth, although salivary glands begin to produce IgA, IgM and IgG from 30 weeks (Brandtzaeg 1998).

IMMUNE RESPONSES IN THE NEONATE AND EARLY CHILDHOOD

At birth neonates are equipped with large populations of T and B cells; the production of immune cells in the primary and secondary lymphatic organs is established (i.e. thymus, spleen, MALT and bone marrow), and myeloid cells appear in similar numbers to adult levels. However, the competency of the neonate's immune system is poor in dealing with bacterial and fungal infection, especially in responding to viral antigens and producing protective antiviral memory (Holt 1995).

This pattern of response may be a delayed move away from the immune response needed during fetal life to ensure that fetal and maternal tissues do not interact immunologically.

Although there is a large pool of T and B cells at birth, these are naive cells, untriggered by antigens (De Vries et al 2000). Of the T cells in cord blood, 90% have the surface marker CD45RA (the naive form), compared with approximately 50% in adult samples. T cells with the surface marker of CD45RO T cells capable of triggering a memory response to antigens form only 5% or less of cord samples. This proportion steadily increases in childhood in response to environmental challenges (antigens entering the body), reaching adult levels (30–45%) between 15 and 20 years of age (Holt 1995). Holt suggests that the cellular immune system goes through an adaptive maturation after birth in which all immune cells develop the ability to respond to antigens more efficiently over time and with repeat exposure (Holt 1995).

Table 10.1 Immune cells: differences at birth and in adulthood

Cell type	At birth (cord blood)	In adulthood
Total lymphocytes[a]	4.7 (3.5–6.2)	2.1 (1.1–2.4)
T lymphocytes (CD3[+])[a]	2.6 (1.9–4.4)	1.5 (0.7–1.8)
B lymphocytes (CD19[+])[a]	0.8 (0.3–1)	0.2 (0.1–0.4)
Natural killer cells (CD16[+]/56[+]/CD3[−])[a]	1.0 (0.4–1.6)	0.2 (0.1–0.4)
Lymphoid dendritic cells	$3.3 \pm 0.7\%$[b]	$2.7 \pm 1.4\%$[d]
Myeloid differential counts		
Monocytes (mean)[c]	6%	7%
Neutrophils (mean)[c]	61%	55%
Eosinophils (mean)[c]	2%	3%
Myeloid dendritic cells	$4.6 \pm 1.4\%$[b]	$18.6 \pm 7.6\%$[d]

[a] Values are mean and range ($\times 10^9$/L) (De Vries et al 2000).
[b] Lymphoid BCDA-2[+], myeloid CD1c[+] (Schibler et al 2002).
[c] Data from Behrman & Kliegman 2002.
[d] Lymphoid BCDA-3[+], myeloid CD1b/c[+] (MacDonald et al 2002).

This is supported by the reduced ability of T cells to secrete cytokines, which activate B cells, and by the inability of B cells to respond to cytokine activation, as well as by the fall in natural killer cell numbers after birth and their poor reactivity, and by the poor presentation of antigens to T cells by monocytes and macrophages and their lack of response to inflammation. Neutrophil leucocytes are also deficient in their inflammation response and cell lysis, and eosinophils, although high in number at birth, show abnormal behaviour when invading areas of inflammation (Holt 1995).

During the first year of life naive T and B cells continue to be produced in large numbers, but T memory cells (CD45RO) increase to adult levels with peaks in the levels of T and B cells at 1 and 6 weeks after birth (De Vries et al 2000). The period in early childhood when the immune system is maturing has also been identified as the time at which primary sensitization to allergens takes place (Holt et al 1990).

CLINICAL NOTES	VACCINATION

Programmes of vaccination in childhood across the world have radically reduced mortality and morbidity. Some diseases have been eradicated (smallpox); others that were common features of childhood such as scarlet fever, measles and mumps, the symptoms of which were known to every mother and grandmother, are now limited to isolated outbreaks (World Health Organization 1998).

However, the success of vaccination is dependent on large numbers of children developing immunity to reach 'herd' immunity. When large numbers of a community are immune, pathogens, which rely on hosts to reproduce, cannot survive. Children's innate immunity may interfere with vaccine protection, making the timing of vaccination critical (Gans et al 1998).

Challenges to the safety of vaccination programmes have affected uptake levels in some communities. These challenges suggest a link between childhood vaccination and autoimmune disease. Large-scale population studies would seem to refute these claims (Madsen et al 2002). The real danger to children is that the scare factor will reduce uptake of vaccine. This not only places the individual child at risk of contracting the specific disease and its attendant risks of sequelae, but also risks an outbreak affecting children who are unprotected because medical conditions prevent vaccination (e.g. use of high-dose steroids) or those who have not responded to vaccination.

During infancy children also have the challenge of moving from placental nutrition to oral feeding. With food comes large numbers of pathogenic antigens. The newborn not only has to protect itself from these, but also has to develop oral tolerance, where nutritional proteins (or antigens) are allowed to cross the gut mucosa and enter lymph or blood vessels. Breast-feeding enhances both of these functions of the infant's gut. Secretory IgA and IgM migrate from the maternal GALT into maternal mammary glands and enter breast milk. These immunoglobulins enhance the infant's own secretory immune systems and boost vaccine response (Pabst & Spady 1990).

Oral tolerance is promoted by two mechanisms: the action of secretory IgA, which suppresses normal gut flora and thereby reduces the infant's gut immune response, and the action of the cytokine transforming growth factor (TGF) β, which also has an immunosuppressive effect on GALT (Brandtzaeg 1998). The enhancing effects of breast-feeding on the immune system can be seen in the reduced rate of infectious diseases in breast-fed children (Wold & Adlerberth 2000).

The infant's ability to produce its own immunoglobulins (IgA and IgM) within the gut appears to be dependent on challenges from antigens. This process begins, as already described, in utero. After birth production both in the lining of the gut and the salivary glands increases rapidly after 2–4 weeks. Salivary gland production peaks at 1–2 months, reaching adult levels within, on average, 15 months, whereas GALT production increases more rapidly, attaining the adult range at 12 months (Brandtzaeg 1998).

Large variation from individual to individual may be determined by genetic predisposition, as well as diet and antigen challenge. Some studies suggest that children with poor postnatal IgA development are at greater genetic risk of *atopy*, and that those with atopy have reduced gut IgA without increased IgM to compensate. A clinical picture of increased infection, atopic allergies and *gluten-dependent enteropathy* is seen in children with poor IgA production with secretory IgM compensation (Brandtzaeg 1998).

Immunity for children develops from early blood formation in utero, but at birth the immune system is not competent. Development during early childhood requires stimulation from the environment in the form of antigens entering the body.

The complexity of human immunity and its interaction with the environment throughout childhood is a highly active research area. It is also politically charged; a woman's choice to breast-feed is not based solely on the immunological science. These issues should become public health issues for children, as action is required to stem the increase in allergic and autoimmune disease (Austin et al 1999).

Understanding the development of children's immunity from the womb to the breast and in the school playground is just the first step.

SELF ASSESSMENT

- Why is development of the immune system important in childhood?
- Complete the table below, describing the development that occurs at each stage in the blank boxes.
- Identify a type of immune cell and describe its ontogenesis across the lifespan.
- Compare and contrast the immune systems of the newborn and adults.
- What factors affect the lymphatic outflow across the lifespan?
- How does breast-feeding affect the development of oral tolerance and immunity in children?

Developmental stage	Immune cells	Thymus	Spleen	Bone marrow	Lymphatic system	MALT	
						Waldeyer's pharyngeal ring (tonsils, etc.)	GALT
Embryological							
Fetal							
Neonatal							
Childhood							
Adulthood							

References

Askin D F, Young S 2001 The thymus gland. Neonatal Network 20(8):7–13

Austin J B, Kaur B, Anderson H R et al 1999 Hayfever, eczema and wheeze: a nationwide UK study (ISAAC, International Study of Asthma and Allergies in Childhood). Archives of Disease in Childhood 81:225–230

Behrman R E, Kliegman R M (eds) 2002 Nelson essentials of pediatrics, 4th edn. W B Saunders, Philadelphia

Bensoussan D, Le Deist F, Latger-Cannard V et al 2002 T-cell immune constitution after peripheral blood mononuclear cell transplantation in complete DiGeorge syndrome. British Journal of Haematology 117 (4) 899–906

Brandtzaeg P 1998 Development and basic mechanisms of human gut immunity. Nutrition Reviews 56(1):S5–S18

Burks W 2003 Peanut allergy: a growing phenomenon. Journal of Clinical Investigation 111(7):950–952

De Vries E, De Bruin-Versteeg S, Comans-Bitter W M et al 2000 Longitudinal survey of lymphocyte subpopulations in the first year of life. Pediatric Research 47(4):528–537

Gans H A, Arvin A M, Galinus J, Logan L, DeHovitz R, Maldonado Y 1998 Deficiency of humoral immune response to measles vaccine in infants immunized at age 6 months. Journal of the American Medical Association 280(6):527–532

Gebbers J O, Laissue J A 1990 Postnatal immunomorphology of the gut. In: Hadziselimovic F, Herzog B, Burgin-Wolf A (eds) Inflammatory bowel disease and celiac disease in children. Kluwer Academic Publishers, Dordrecht, p 3–44

Goldsby R A, Kindt T J, Osborne B A, Kuby J (eds) 2003 Immunology, 5th edn. W H Freeman, New York

Holladay S D, Smialowicz R J 2000 Development of the murine and human immune system: differential effects of immunotoxicants depend on time of exposure. Environmental Health Perspectives 108(suppl 3):463–473

Holt P G 1995 Postnatal maturation of immune competence during infancy and childhood. Pediatric Allergy and Immunology 6:59–70

Holt P G, McMenamin C, Nelson D 1990 Primary sensitisation to inhalant allergens during infancy. Pediatric Allergy and Immunology 1:3–13

Jawad A F, McDonald-Meginn D M, Zackai E, Sullivan K E 2001 Immunological features of chromosome 22q11.2 deletion syndrome (DiGeorge syndrome/ velocardiofacial syndrome). Journal of Pediatrics 139(5):715–723

MacDonald K P, Munster D J, Clark G J, Dzionek A, Schmitz J, Hart D N 2002 Characterization of human blood dendritic cell subsets. Blood 100(13):4512–4520

Madsen K M, Hviid A, Vestergaard M et al 2002 A population-based study of measles, mumps and rubella vaccination and autism. New England Journal of Medicine 347(19):1477–1482

Moore K L, Persaud R V N 2003 Developing human clinically orientated embryology, 7th edn. W B Saunders, Philadelphia

Nishio H, Matsui K, Tsuji H, Tamura A, Suzuki K 2000 Expression of the Janus kinases—signal transducers and activators of transcription pathway in Hassall's corpuscles of the human thymus. Histochemisty and Cell Biology 113(6):427–431

Pabst H F, Spady D W 1990 Effect of breast-feeding on antibody response to conjugate vaccine. Lancet 336:269–270

Patterson P H, Nawa H 1993 Neuronal differentiation factors/cytokines and synaptic plasticity. Cell 72:123–137

Schibler K R, Georgelas A, Rigaa A 2002 Developmental biology of the dendritic cell system. Acta Paediatrica. Supplementum 438:9–16

Wold A E, Adlerberth I 2000 Breastfeeding and the intestinal microflora of the infant—implications for protection against infectious disease. Advances in Experimental Medicine and Biology 478:77–93

World Health Organization 1998 Factsheet no. 200 Global infectious disease surveillance. WHO, Geneva

Bibliography

Ader R, Felton D L, Cohen N 2001 Psychoneuroimmunology: vol 1. 3rd edn. Academic Press, San Diego

Goldsby R A, Kindt T J, Osborne B A, Kuby J (eds) 2003 Immunology, 5th edn. W H Freeman, New York

Harding R, Bocking A D (eds) 2001 Fetal growth and development. Cambridge University Press, Cambridge

Sadler T W 1995 Langman's medical embryology, 7th edn. Williams & Wilkins, Balitmore

Walker S D 2002 DiGeorge syndrome in the neonate: helping parents understand its implications, Journal of Neonatal Nursing 8(6):191–194

Chapter 11

Development of the special senses

Carol A. Chamley

CHAPTER OUTCOMES

This chapter will enable the reader to:

- Define the term 'special senses'
- Outline the major structures that constitute the special senses
- Explain the primary functions of the special senses
- Explain the term 'chemosensation'
- Explain why the senses of gustation (taste) and olfaction (smell) are difficult to separate in utero
- Describe the sense of touch.

CHAPTER OVERVIEW

The aim of this chapter is to describe the normal embryonic and fetal development of the special senses, including the eye, ear, gustation (taste), olfaction (smell) and touch. This chapter discusses normal embryological anatomy and physiology, and outlines perspectives relevant to development and maturation of these senses. Clinical Notes address issues of clinical relevance and interest to the reader, and Self Assessment exercises assist in reflecting upon the chapter and guiding the relationship between theory and professional practice.

INTRODUCTION

The ability of the human organism to sense incoming stimuli and adjust to the physical (external) and homeostatic (internal) environments is essential to survival. The special senses, which include sight, hearing, taste, smell and touch, have receptor organs that are generally more complex in structure than receptors for more general sensations. The sense of smell in the human organism is the least specialized sense, in contrast to the sense of vision, which is highly specialized.

The fetal environment is busy and interactive. At birth, with the exception of vision, all the senses are functioning to a certain degree. Some refinement gradually occurs as the result of maturation of the nervous system and the ability of the child to interact and interpret the world in which they inhabit. As Slater & Lewis (2002, p 84) allude: '... the infant enters a new world, one that the child will experience for the rest of their life'.

DEVELOPMENT OF THE EYE

Eye development is evident during week 4 of gestation, when an optic sulcus appears on each unfused neural fold (Fig. 11.1A). The eye is derived from four tissue types:

- neuroectoderm of the forebrain
- surface ectoderm of the head
- mesoderm
- neural crest cells.

THE RETINA The posterior layers of the iris and retina are derived from the neuroectoderm of the ectoderm of the head, while the mesoderm between the neuroectoderm and the surface ectoderm form the vascular and fibrous coats of the eye. Furthermore, the mesenchymal cells are derived from mesoderm, whereas neural crest cells migrate into the mesenchyme and differentiate into the choroid, sclera and corneal epithelium.

During week 4 of embryonic development, the primordia of the neural components of the eye appear, when the *optic sulci* (optic grooves) develop in the neural folds at the cranial end of the embryo. As the neural folds fuse to form the diencephalon, the sulci form optic

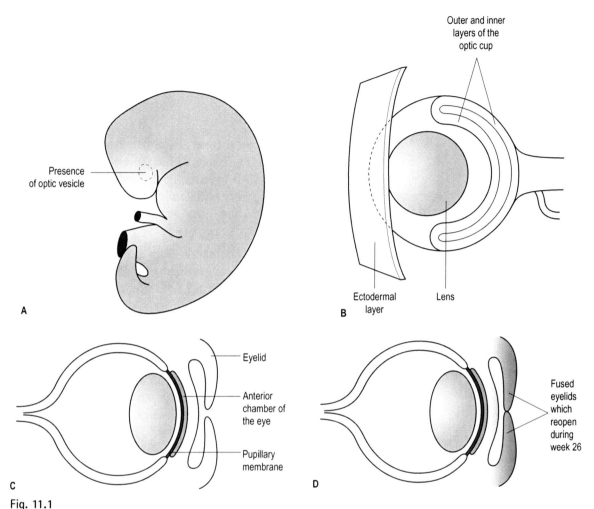

Outer and inner
layers of the
optic cup

Presence
of optic vesicle

Ectodermal
layer

Lens

A

B

Eyelid

Anterior
chamber of
the eye

Pupillary
membrane

Fused
eyelids
which
reopen
during
week 26

C

D

Fig. 11.1
A Development of the eye at
4 weeks' gestation.
B Layers of the optic cup.
C Pupillary membrane.
D Fused eyelids.

vessels, following closure of the rostral neuropore, and the optic sulci invaginate. As these optic vessels enlarge, their connection with the diencephalon narrows to form hollow optic stalks. Thickening occurs on the overlying surface ectoderm that is stimulated by the vesicles forming the lens placode—the primordia of the lens. The optic vessels and the lens placode invaginate, or indent, to form the double-walled *optic cups* (Fig. 11.1B). The inner layer of the optic cup forms the *neural retina* and the outer layer forms the *pigmented retinal epithelium*. The anterior portion of the cup forms the non-visual elements of the retina. The intraretinal space is reduced to a narrow split and each optic stalk develops a groove, or *optic fissure*. The original cavity of the optic cup is eventually obliterated as the inner and outer layers fuse, but this fusion is not secure and may detach (detached retina). The optic fissures contain vascular mesenchyme from which the hyaloid blood vessels develop. This artery is a branch of the ophthalmic artery and supplies:

- the inner layer of the optic cup
- the lens vesicle
- mesenchyme in the optic cup.

The hyaloid vein returns blood from these structures. The hyaloid artery and vein develop in the fissure of the mesenchyme; the distal elements of the hyaloid vessels eventually degenerate, but proximal parts remain as the central artery and vein of the retina.

THE OPTIC NERVE

The optic nerve forms when the axons from the cells in the neural retina grow into the optic stalks, migrating towards the diencephalon. They become myelinated later during fetal life, and this process is complete by 10 weeks into postnatal life.

THE LENS

The lens of the eye is derived from surface ectoderm. The epithelium of the anterior wall remains thin and develops into the anterior lens epithelium, while the posterior wall of the lens thickens and forms the anucleated primary lens fibre. As the layer thickens, the lumen of the lens vesicle is obliterated. Secondary lens fibres are formed from epithelial cells at the 'equatorial zone' of the lens.

CLINICAL NOTES **CATARACT**

Cataract is caused by opacity of the crystalline lens, which prevents light rays from entering the eye and refracting upon the retina. Cataracts may develop as a result of:

- antenatal infections
- trauma to the eye
- steroid therapy
- chromosomal defects
- hypothyroidism
- galactosaemia and galactokinase deficiency
- may be transient in preterm infants.

The treatment of cataracts may involve removal of the lens, correcting the vision with a lens implant, contact lens or spectacles.

THE CILIARY BODY AND THE IRIS

The ciliary body and the iris develop from the anterior portion (rim) of the optic cup that grows over most of the anterior portion of the lens. It forms the epithelium of the:

- iris
- ciliary body
- sphincter and dilatator pupillae muscles of the iris.

Furthermore, these structures are neurodermal in origin, whereas the mesenchyme around the rim of the optic cup forms the ciliary muscles and connective tissue. The iris is 'bluish' in most neonates, and the eye colour as pigment, which is genetically determined, is laid down in the months after birth.

THE CHOROID, SCLERA AND CORNEA

The optic cup and stalk are surrounded by mesenchymal cells that are continuous with the brain and condense to form two layers. The innermost layer forms the choroid layer of the eye, it is highly vascular and this layer is continuous with the pia and arachnoid layers of the meninges. The outermost layer forms both the sclera of the eye and the substantia propria of the cornea, and is continuous with the dura mater of the meninges.

CHAMBERS OF THE EYE

There are two separate aqueous chambers that develop in the eye; they are separated by the pupillary membrane (Fig. 11.1C). During week 20 of fetal development, the pupillary membrane degenerates as the pupil of the eye forms, and these two chambers communicate with one another.

The vitreous body is a gelatinous mass originating from mesenchyme. The vitreous humour is the fluid component of the vitreous body that is derived from the wall of the optic cup.

THE EYELIDS

The eyelids grow towards one another and fuse during week 8 of gestation (Fig. 11.1D). They are described as accessory eye structures, and develop as the surface ectoderm and underlying mesenchyme proliferate. The mesenchyme forms the connective tissue and tarsal plates. The eyelids remain closed during retinal differentiation, but open at week 26 of gestation. The glands of the eye and eyelashes form from surface ectoderm.

The cells of the visual area of the cerebral cortex have their peak burst of development during weeks 28 to 32 gestation. The visual analyser starts to myelinate shortly before birth and this process is completed by week 10 of postnatal life in order to cope with visual stimuli (MacGregor 2000, Tortora & Grabowski 2003).

CLINICAL NOTES — VISUAL HANDICAP AND CAUSE OF BLINDNESS

Most system and developmental disorders can be detected by examining the eyes of the infant or child for the following signs:

- purulent discharge
- abnormal shape of the eyelids or pupils
- presence of a squint—minor squints are common; a 'late' squint suggests a new origin of a cranial nerve disorder.

Visual handicap is quite common and most probably its prevalence is underestimated as it is very difficult to test vision accurately in babies, and visual assessment may be exacerbated if there is suspicion of developmental delay.

Causes of blindness in children may include (Candy et al 2001):

- retinopathy of prematurity
- cataract
- retinoblastoma
- optic atrophy
- congenital anomalies—optic nerve hypoplasia
- syndromic—septo-optic dysplasia
- malformations of the brain or acquired conditions, such as cerebral haemorrhage in neonates
- albinism
- retinal degeneration
- severe myopia
- untreated amblopia.

THE LACRIMAL GLANDS

The lacrimal glands (*lacrim* = tears) develop from solid buds that are invaginations of the surface ectoderm. The buds branch, becoming canalized to form the ducts and alveoli of the glands. The glands are small at birth and are not fully functional until approximately 6 weeks after birth.

The lacrimal apparatus is a group of anatomical structures that produce and drain *lacrimal fluid* (tears). Lacrimal fluid is a water-based solution containing salts, mucus and lysozyme, a protective bacterial enzyme (Tortora & Grabowski 2003). The primary functions of tears are to protect, clean, lubricate and keep the eyeball moist.

CLINICAL NOTES — GLAUCOMA

Most glaucomas are caused by the persistence of embryonic tissue in the outer rim of the iris, which results in increased intraocular pressure causing:

- photophobia
- excessive tear production (epiphora)

- spasm of the eyelids and spasmodic winking (blepharospasm)
- corneal haziness due to oedema
- enlarged eyeball (buphthalmos)
- halo effect around objects
- redness of the eye(s)
- mild pain or discomfort associated with increased pressure
- optic atrophy with reduced, or loss of, visual acuity.

Furthermore, glaucoma may complicate such conditions as retinopathy of prematurity and be associated with such conditions as Sturge–Weber syndrome, Lowe syndrome, neurofibromatosis, Marfan's syndrome and congenital rubella.

The treatment is surgery with the aim of improving drainage of the aqueous humour in order to prevent long-term damage to the optic nerve.

GROWTH AND DEVELOPMENT

At birth, the eye is approximately three-quarters of the adult size, the adult eyeball measuring 2.5 cm in diameter. During the first 12 months of life, growth of the eye is maximal, gradually decelerating in growth in the third year of life and continuing at a slower pace until puberty. Adult size is achieved at approximately 14 years; thereafter growth is negligible. Anatomically, different structures within the eye have different growth rates. Generally the structures within the posterior portion of the eye grow proportionally more than those in the anterior portion of the eye. A newborn infant has limited vision, and visual acuity is estimated to be in the order of 6/200.

In the infant the sclera is thin and translucent with a 'bluish tinge'. The cornea is approximately 10 mm, reaching adult size (12 mm) by the age of 2 years. The curvature of the eye gradually flattens with age, contributing to changes in refraction. The retina is well developed, but the fovea is immature (Lissauer & Clayden 2001).

In the newborn infant, the lens of the eye is spherical in shape, and continues to grow throughout life as new fibres are added to the periphery. The fundus of the eye in the newborn is less pigmented than in the adult eye, and the pattern of the pigmentation has a 'fine peppery' or 'mottled' appearance. The macular landmarks are less well defined and the peripheral retina may have a 'greyish' appearance, especially in premature infants where the nerve heads tend to be pale. By the age of 5–6 months, the fundus of the eye is more like that of an adult in appearance.

Newborn infants tend to keep their eyes closed for most of the time, but the normal infant can see and fix upon points of contrast, although the infant's vision is limited and the eyes move independently. One of the earliest positive signs of normal and intact vision, is the ability of the infant to engage visually with their mother's face.

By the age of 2 weeks the infant demonstrates greater and more sustained interest generally, and by the age of 8–10 weeks an infant has the ability to follow an object through 180°.

As the child continues to grow and develop there is gradual improvement in visual acuity. Following a period of uncoordinated eye movement, especially during the early days and weeks of life, by 6 weeks of age both eyes should move together and no squints should be present. Babies slowly develop their ability to focus, and visual acuity gradually improves from 6/60 at approximately 3 months to adult levels of acuity by 3 years of age.

CLINICAL NOTES	TESTING VISION AT DIFFERENT AGES (LISSAUER & CLAYDEN 2001)

Age	Test
Birth	Face fixation and following. 'Preferential looking'— a preference for patterned objects over and plain objects
6 weeks	Optokinetic nystagmus demonstrated when observing striped target
6 months	Reaches for toys
2 years	Can identify pictures of reduced size
3 years	Matches letters using a single-letter chart
5 years and over	Can identify a line of letters on a Snellen chart

DEVELOPMENT OF THE EAR

The ear is divided into three main anatomical regions:

- external ear
- middle ear
- inner (internal).

The ear is described as an 'engineering marvel' with sensory receptors capable of transducing sound vibrations with amplitudes as small as the diameter of an atom of gold (0.3 nm), and then transforming these vibrations into electrical signals 1000 times faster than photoreceptors can respond to light (Tortora & Grabowski 2003).

THE INTERNAL EAR

The inner ear (internal) is the first region of the ear to begin development at 22 days gestation, noticed as a thickening of surface ectoderm. This thickening forms the *otic placode*, found on either side of the myelencephalon (Fig. 11.2A). The otic placode invaginates deep into the surface ectoderm to form an *otic pit*, and the pits fuse to form an *otic vesicle* (otocyst) (Fig. 11.2B), which is the primordium of the membranous labyrinth. The otic vesicle develops a tubular diverticulum, which later forms the *endolymphatic duct* and *sac* (Fig. 11.2C).

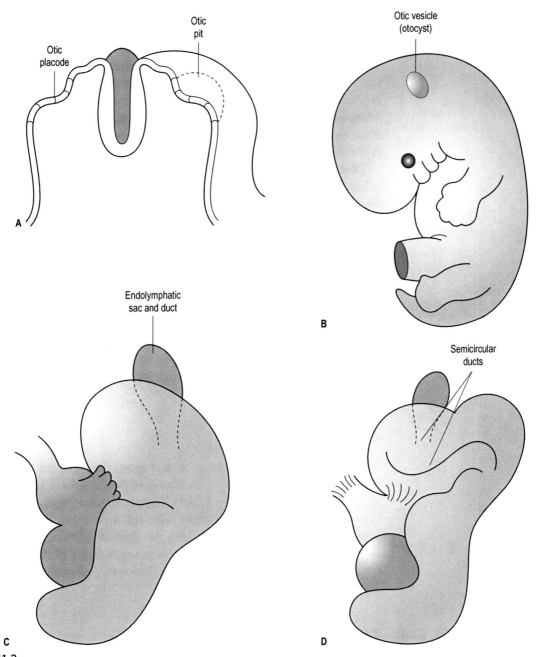

Fig. 11.2
A Otic pit and otic placode. B Otic vesicle (otocyst). C Endolymphatic sac and duct. D Developing semicircular ducts.

The otic vesicle becomes constricted near to its centre and two regions of the otic vessel are recognizable as:

- *Utricular portion*. Derivatives of the utricular part of the utricle are the endolymphatic duct and the three semicircular ducts
- *Saccular portion*. The saccular portion of the utricle gives rise to saccule and cochlear duct that spirals to form the organ of Corti.

The *semicircular ducts* (Fig. 11.2D) arise from the flattened outgrowths of the utricular portion of the otic vessel. The *cochlear duct* develops from the saccular portion of the otic vessel and forms the *cochlea* (KOK-le-a = snail shaped) and the spiral *organ of Corti*, which is a special neuroreceptor concerned with hearing. Ganglion cells from the eighth cranial nerve migrate along the membranous coils of the membranous cochlea, forming the spiral ganglion. Nerve processes extend from the ganglion to the spiral organ where they terminate on fine hair cells.

Derivatives of the otic vesicle form the membranous labyrinth containing *endolymph*—the fluid contained within the membranous labyrinth of the inner ear. The cartilagenous otic capsule ossifies to form the bony labyrinth that is located in the petrous portion of the temporal bone. The internal ear reaches adult size and shape by 20–22 weeks gestation.

THE MIDDLE EAR

The *tympanic cavity* is derived from an extension of the elongated first pharyngeal (branchial) pouch, an endoderm-lined outgrowth of the primitive pharynx. This forms the *tubotympanic recess* that approaches the floor of the first branchial groove. The tubotympanic recess gradually envelopes the auditory ossicles, which include:

- malleus
- incus
- stapes.

These are three very small bones that eventually extend across the middle ear; they develop by endochondral ossification of the first and second branchial arches (Fig. 11.3A). The proximal portion of the tubotympanic recess forms the *auditory tube,* and an extension of the tubotympanic recess later develops into the *mastoid antrum*. Most of the mastoid cells develop after birth, producing 'bulges' of the temporal bone (*mastoid processes*) that become fully developed at approximately 2 years of age (Fig. 11.3B).

THE EXTERNAL EAR

The external auditory (*audire* = hearing) ear (acoustic meatus or canal) develops from the dorsal end of the first pharyngeal groove.

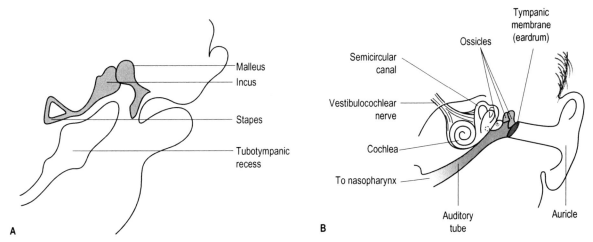

Fig. 11.3
A Ossicles in situ.
B The ear after birth.

Ectodermal cells proliferate to form a solid epithelial plate; the meatal plug degenerates late in the fetal period, forming the internal portion of the internal meatus.

The *tympanic (tympano* = drum) *membrane* develops from three sources:

- ectoderm of the pharyngeal groove
- endoderm of the tubotympanic recess, a derivative of the first pharyngeal pouch
- mesoderm of the first and second pharyngeal pouches.

The tympanic membrane, or eardrum, is located close to the surface of the meatus, as does the facial nerve. Therefore, birth trauma may cause damage to the drum and facial nerve (Sinclair & Dangerfield 1998). The colour of the tympanic membrane is translucent, light pearly pink or grey. Slight redness is normal in the newborn infant because of the increased vascularity of the membrane, and as a result of crying (Wong 1999).

CLINICAL NOTES   OTITIS MEDIA

Otitis media is one of the most commonest diseases of early childhood, with 20% of children under 4 years of age affected at least once a year. The incidence of otitis media is highest during the winter months, commonly affecting boys more than girls. The incidence is highest in children aged from 6 months to 2 years, gradually decreasing with age, except for a small increase between 5 and 6 years.

Otitis media is primarily the result of dysfunctioning eustachian tubes. The aetiology of the non-infectious type is unknown, although it is frequently the result of blocked eustachian tubes from oedema associated with upper respiratory tract infections, hypertrophic adenoids or allergic rhinitis.

The commonest infective organisms include:

- *Streptococcus pneumoniae*
- *Haemophilus influenzae*
- *Moraxella catarrhalis.*

The eustachian tubes have three important functions related to the middle ear, including:

1. Protection of the middle ear from nasopharyngeal secretions
2. Drainage of secretions produced in the middle ear into the nasopharynx
3. Ventilation of the middle ear to equalize air pressure within the middle ear with atmospheric pressure in the external ear canal and to replenish oxygen that has been absorbed.

Therefore, mechanical or functional obstruction of the middle ear causes accumulation of secretions in the middle ear. Any obstruction within the middle ear results in negative middle ear pressure and, if sustained, produces a transudative middle ear infusion. Drainage from the ear is impeded by sustained negative pressure plus impaired ciliary transport within the tube. When the passage is not totally obstructed, contamination of the middle ear can occur through reflux, aspiration or insufflation during crying, sneezing, nose blowing and swallowing when the nose is obstructed.

Clinical manifestations may include:

- hyperpyrexia
- holding and pulling the ears
- verbal children will complain of pain
- purulent fluid accumulates in the small space of the middle ear chamber and pain results from pressure on the surrounding structures
- treatment may include antibiotic therapy, antipyretics and analgesics.

The complications of otitis media may include:

- chronic suppurative otitis media
- adhesive otitis media (glue ear)
- tympanosclerosis (scarring of the eardrum)
- hearing loss
- tympanic membrane retraction
- mastoiditis
- labyrinthitis
- meningitis
- cholesteatoma.

The external auditory meatus is approximately 2.5 cm in length and is poorly developed at birth. The walls of the canal are pliable and 'floppy' due to underdevelopment of the cartilage and bone. The walls of the canal are pink, but may be more pigmented in darker-skinned children. Minute hairs are present in the outermost portion where the cerumen or wax is produced. The shape of the external canal changes with age. In children over 3 years of age, the canal curves downwards and forwards, and the tympanic membrane slopes inwards and upwards (Wong 1999).

CLINICAL NOTES	GERMAN MEASLES (RUBELLA)

Rubella, commonly referred to as German measles, is a markedly fetotoxic virus (Candy et al 2001), and the rubella virus may infect both the placenta and the fetus. Maternal infection during the first 3–4 months of pregnancy carries a high risk of embryopathy, with a typical pattern of congenital anomalies including deafness. Infection later on in the pregnancy does not cause embryopathy but may still result in assaults upon structures including the cochlea of the ear.

According to Haaheim et al (2002), approximately 30% of infants born who have acquired rubella during the first trimester of pregnancy will have congenital birth defects. Furthermore, this risk approaches 100% if the fetus is infected during the first 4 weeks of gestation, but reduces to 10–20% if the fetus is infected during the fourth month of fetal life. In approximately 15% of infected cases the fetus will be aborted spontaneously (Haaheim et al 2002).

SOUND WAVES

Sound waves are a series of alternating high- and low-pressure regions travelling in the same direction through air. Furthermore, the sounds heard by the human ear originate from sources that vibrate at frequencies between 500 and 5000 hertz (1 Hz = 1 cycle per second) (Tortora & Grabowski 2003).

The fetal environment is busy and noisy. The fetus normally responds to sound from 22 to 24 weeks gestation. Fetal response is influenced by the frequency, duration and intensity of the sound, and the fetus begins hearing at a lower frequency of 250–500 Hz (Slater & Lewis 2002).

The newborn infant has some primitive ability to locate the general direction from which a sound originates, and by 6 months most infants can generally locate and respond to sound. Children's hearing improves up until adolescence. It is generally recognized that infants' auditory acuity is superior to their visual acuity (Bee 1997, Bee & Boyd 2004).

CHEMOSENSATION

The senses of smell (*olfaction*) and taste (*gustation*) are chemical responses. These senses are difficult to separate in utero, because amniotic fluid bathes both receptors and simultaneously stimulates both senses. For this reason, fetal responses to smell and taste are considered together, under the heading of chemosensation (Slater & Lewis 2002).

During week 6 of fetal development, the *nasal pits* differentiate to form the epithelium of the *nasal passages*. The anatomical area of the tip of each cerebral hemisphere, where the axons of the primary neurosensory cells synapse, begins to form an outgrowth of tissue referred to as the *olfactory bulb*. As the developing face and brain change proportions and lengthen, the distance between the olfactory bulb and the point of origin in the cerebral hemispheres lengthens to form the stalk-like *olfactory tracts*.

The *olfactory nerve* develops when the epithelial lining of the nasal sac differentiates in the general area of the superior concha wall, into bipolar neurones. The unmyelinated axons form the 18 to 20 bundles of the olfactory nerve, and these bundles then pass superiorly and terminate in the olfactory bulb (Matusumara & England 1992). As the bundles pass superiorly to the olfactory bulb, the cribriform plate of the ethmoid bones grows and envelops the 18 to 20 bundles of axons of the olfactory cells (Fig. 11.4).

Fig. 11.4
Olfactory nerves and bulb.

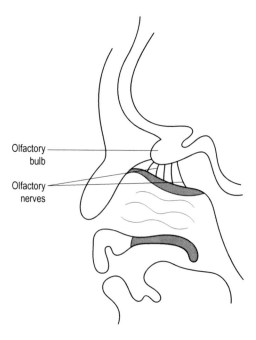

Olfactory bulb

Olfactory nerves

The fetus is able to discriminate between sweet and unpleasant noxious substances injected into the amniotic fluid. The fetal response is to increase the rate of swallowing, which is reduced when a less noxious substance is added to the amniotic fluid (Moore & Persaud 1998, Slater & Lewis 2002). The fetus swallows amniotic fluid from approximately 12 weeks gestation. At 26–28 weeks gestation, fetal chemosensation responses have been monitored through facial expressions when exposed to bitter-tasting substances, indicating further that reflex pathways between the taste buds and facial muscles are established. Thresholds for certain tastes increase with age; for example, the threshold for the taste of salt begins to increase at approximately 20 years of age (Sinclair & Dangerfield 1998).

TOUCH

This is the first 'special sense' to develop in the fetus, at about 8 weeks gestation. At 13 weeks the arm of the fetus will make contact with the face (Slater & Lewis 2002), and at 14 weeks gestation most of the fetus is responsive to touch. The sense of touch will be highly active between multiple womb partners such as twins or triplets.

SELF ASSESSMENT

Answer the following in relation to your area of professional practice:

- Define the term 'special senses'.
- List the major structures involved in the special senses.
- Outline the main developmental processes in relation to the eye and the ear.
- Define the term 'chemosensation'.
- Explain why the senses of taste and smell are difficult to discriminate in utero.
- Describe the sense of touch and its relevance during fetal development.
- Reflect upon this chapter and consider how you might relate your new knowledge to professional practice.

References

Bee H 1997 The developing child, 8th edn. HarperCollins, New York

Bee H, Boyd D 2004 The developing child, 10th edn. Allyn & Bacon, Boston

Candy D, Davies G, Ross E 2001 Clinical paediatrics and child health. W B Saunders, London

Haaheim L R, Pattinson J R, Whitley R S 2002 A practical guide to clinical virology, 2nd edn. Mosby, London

Lissaur T, Clayden G 2001 Illustrated textbook of paediatrics, 2nd edn. Mosby, London

MacGregor J 2000 Introduction to the developmental anatomy and physiology of children. Routledge, London

Matsumara G, England M A 1992 Embryology colouring book. Mosby, St Louis

Moore K L, Persaud T V N 1998 Before we are born: essentials of embryology and birth defects. W B Saunders, London

Sinclair D, Dangerfield P 1998 Human growth after birth, 6th edn. Oxford University Press, Oxford

Slater A, Lewis M 2002 Introduction to infant development. Oxford University Press, Oxford

Tortora G J, Grabowski S R 2003 Anatomy and physiology, 6th edn. HarperCollins, New York

Wong D L 1999 Whaley and Wong's nursing care of infants and children, 6th edn. Mosby, London

Bibliography

Candy D, Davies G, Ross E 2001 Clinical paediatrics and child health. W B Saunders, London

Haaheim L R, Pattinson J R, Whitley R S 2002 A practical guide to clinical virology, 2nd edn. John Wiley, Chichester

Lissaur T, Clayden G 2001 Illustrated textbook of paediatrics, 2nd edn. Mosby, London

Moore K L 1988 Essentials of human embryology. Blackwell Scientific, Oxford

Sinclair D, Dangerfield P 1998 Human growth after birth, 6th edn. Oxford University Press, Oxford

Slater A, Lewis M 2002 Introduction to infant development. Oxford University Press, Oxford

Tortora G J, Grabowski S R 2003 Principles of anatomy and physiology. John Wiley, New York

Waugh A, Grant A 2001 Ross and Wilson anatomy and physiology in health and illness, 9th edn. Churchill Livingstone, London

Chapter 12

Dentition

Carol A. Chamley

CHAPTER OUTCOMES

This chapter will enable the reader to:

- Explain the normal embryological development of mammalian teeth
- Discuss the process of eruption and the normal dental patterns during childhood
- Outline the normal functions of teeth
- Explore potential dental health-related issues and subsequent management.

CHAPTER OVERVIEW

The aim of this chapter is to outline normal dentition in childhood and discuss the normal embryological and fetal anatomy, and physiological processes involved in the development of human teeth. Furthermore, the teeth are accessory digestive organs (see Ch. 7) and also form part of the integumentary system (see Ch. 2). The chapter describes the four phases of dentition and addresses the development of the deciduous, or milk, teeth and the permanent teeth. Issues of teething and good dental health in childhood are explored. Clinical Notes are utilized to explain issues of clinical relevance and interest to the reader, and Self Assessment exercises assist in reflecting upon the chapter and guiding the relationship between theory and professional practice.

INTRODUCTION

There are many things that make teeth (*dentes*) special. Teeth contain the hardest biological substance known—enamel—and from an evolutionary–developmental perspective have four important features (McCollum & Sharpe 2001):

- cusp patterns
- tooth pattern intimately linked to feeding and hence to survival
- tooth development is a simple mechanism involving two embryonic cell types
- embryonic tooth *primordia* can be cultured in vitro to reproduce normal development.

Teeth are regarded as accessory digestive organs that are located in the sockets of the alveolar processes of the *mandible* and *maxillae* of the jaw. The alveolar processes are covered by the gingivae, or gums, which extend slightly into each socket to form the *gingival sulcus*. The sockets are lined by the periodontal ligament or membrane (*odont* = tooth), which consists of dense fibrous connective tissue that is attached to the socket walls and the cemental surface of the roots. This anchors the teeth into their normal anatomical position and acts as a shock absorber during mastication (Tortora & Grabowski 2003).

Furthermore, with regard to the development of the teeth and the jaws, there has been a significant increase in knowledge relating to embryonic development (*morphogenesis*) in terms of the development of different tooth types and control of dental patterns (Dean 2000). Tooth morphogenesis shares many genes with jaw skeletal morphogenesis. Disruptions that may affect dental patterning also produce abnormal skeletal development of the jaws (McCollum & Sharpe 2001). Therefore, changes in dentition may be genetically aligned to corresponding changes to the development of the face and skull. A series of complicated changes takes place in the jaws to allow room for the larger secondary teeth to occupy the limited amount of space left by shedding the primary teeth. It is at this time that many difficulties caused by crowding of teeth become apparent (Sinclair & Dangerfield 1998).

There is rapid growth of the face and jaws that coincides with eruption of the primary or deciduous (falling off) teeth. In addition, facial changes are more marked after eruption of the secondary or permanent teeth. The primordia of both the 20 deciduous teeth and most of the permanent teeth are present at birth, set in their alveoli (Matsumura & England 1992) (Fig. 12.1). The length of the developing face during childhood is affected by the development of the face and the paranasal sinuses. Dental age can supplement bone age in the estimation of maturity. Just as the condition of the skull sutures can

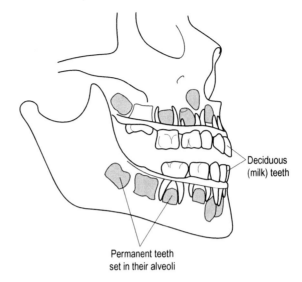

Deciduous
(milk) teeth

Permanent teeth
set in their alveoli

obtain a rough guestimate of the age of an adult, so can the condition
of tooth enamel.

Human beings have two sets of teeth that appear at different stages
of life. Dentition is divided into four phases:

1. Growth
2. Calcification
3. Eruption
4. Attrition.

The first set to emerge during childhood are the 20 temporary,
deciduous or milk teeth, all of which are present in each jaw:

- four incisors (two central)
- two canines
- four molars.

The second set are the 32 permanent teeth, all of which are present in
each jaw:

- four incisors (two central, two lateral)
- two canines
- two bicuspids
- six molars.

Each tooth consists of three portions:

- the *crown*—or body, projecting above the gum
- the *root* or fang—this is entirely concealed
- the *neck*—the constricted portion between the root and the crown.

The surfaces of the tooth are named:

- the labial surface—that which looks towards the lips
- the lingual surface—towards the tongue
- the proximal surface—towards the mesial line
- the distal surface—away from the mesial line
- the buccal surface—towards the cheek.

EMBRYOLOGICAL DEVELOPMENT

According to McCollum & Sharpe (2001), during development of the mammalian mandible, different hard tissues including teeth dentine (and cementum), bone and cartilage develop from neural crest-derived ectomesenchyme cells. The evidence now suggests that the ectomesenchymal cells of the developing mandible are capable of differentiating into other types of hard tissue-producing cells. This includes odontoblasts (dentine), osteoblasts (bone) and chondrocytes (cartilage).

The teeth are an evolution from the *dermoid system* and not the bony skeleton. The earliest evidence of tooth formation is at 6–7 weeks of gestation. Teeth develop from:

- oral ectoderm
- mesoderm
- neural crest cells.

The mucous membrane covering the embryonic jaw gives rise to a longitudinal ridge along the summit of each jaw. *Odontogenesis* (tooth development) is initiated by the influence of neural crest mesenchyme on the overlying ectoderm. Tooth development is a continuous process; however, not all teeth begin to develop at the same time, and odontogenesis continues for years after birth.

Enamel is derived from ectoderm of the oral cavity; all other tissues differentiate from the surrounding mesenchyme derived from mesoderm and neural crest cells.

BUD STAGE OF TOOTH DEVELOPMENT

The earliest indication of tooth development occurs in week 6 of gestation. The U-shaped bands—dental laminae—follow the curves of the primitive jaws. Each dental lamina develops ten centres of proliferation from which the *tooth buds* grow into the developing mesenchyme (Fig. 12.2A). These tooth buds develop into the first

Fig. 12.2
A Bud stage.
B Cap stage.
C Bell stage.

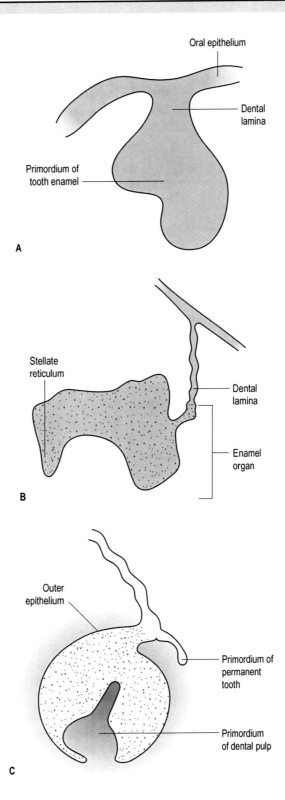

A

B

C

deciduous teeth, which are given this name because they are shed during childhood (Moore & Persaud 1998). During week 10 of gestation, the tooth buds of some of the permanent teeth appear lingual to the deciduous tooth buds. Maturation of the teeth is most advanced in the midline and progresses posteriorly in each jaw.

CAP STAGE OF TOOTH DEVELOPMENT

As the tooth bud grows it is invaginated by mesenchyme (the primordium of the *dental papilla*) and becomes cap shaped (Fig. 12.2B). The ectodermal portion of the developing tooth (enamel organ) eventually produces *enamel*, and the internal portion of the tooth, the dental papilla, is the primordium of the dental pulp. Together they form the *tooth germ*.

The cells of the inner enamel epithelium differentiate to form *ameloblasts*, whch deposit enamel over the dentin. The dental sac is the primordium of the *cementum* and *periodontal ligament*. The cementum is the bone-like portion of the root of the tooth, and the periodontal ligament is the fibrous connective tissue that surrounds the root of the tooth.

BELL STAGE OF TOOTH DEVELOPMENT

During this stage of tooth development, the tooth assumes a bell shape (Fig. 12.2C). The mesenchymal cells in the dental papilla differentiate into *odontoblasts* that produce *predentin*, which later calcifies to form *dentin*. As the dentin accumulates and thickens, the odontoblasts migrate towards the centre of the dental papilla leaving odontoblastic processes (Tomes' processes) embedded into the dentin. The hardest tissue in the body is enamel, which is protected by the second hardest tissue, dentin. Enamel contains calcium phosphate in the crystalline form and is the hardest biologically manufactured substance. Adequate amounts of calcium, phosphates and vitamin D during childhood are essential if the enamel coating is to be complete and resistant to decay.

Cells in the inner enamel epithelium differentiate into ameloblasts, which produce enamel in the form of prisms or rods over the dentin. Enamel and dentin formation begin at the tip (cusp) of the tooth and progress towards the future root. The root of the tooth forms when the epithelial root sheath forms the junction of the outer and the inner enamel. Epithelium grows into the adjacent mesenchyme and induces root formation. Odontoblasts adjacent to this sheath produce dentin, reducing the pulp cavity to a narrow *root canal* containing nerves and vessels.

Cementum is deposited over the dentin of the root, and meets the enamel of the neck of the tooth at the *cementoenamel junction*. The dental sac gives rise to the *periodontal ligament*, which is embedded in both the cementum and the alveolus (tooth socket), and anchors the tooth in its socket. As teeth develop, the jaws ossify and the outer cells of the dental sac become active in bone formation; each tooth becomes surrounded by bone, except over the crown.

ERUPTION

As the teeth develop, they begin a continuous slow movement towards the surface of the gum. By the time that the crown of the teeth have formed, each one is contained within a *loculus* of bone, which is open at the top towards the gum but sealed with fibrous tissue.

When calcification of the various dental tissues of the deciduous teeth is sufficiently advanced to enable it to bear the pressure to which it will be subjected, eruption takes place. This is a process whereby the tooth makes its way through the gum to the surface. The gum is gradually absorbed as the pressure of the crown of the tooth is pressed up by the increasing size of the fang.

The septa between the dental sacs ossify and form the loculi, or alveoli, and embrace the necks of the tooth, affording them a firm base and stability. The first teeth to erupt, at approximately 6 months of age, are normally the central mandibular incisors (Fig. 12.3).

Fig. 12.3
Tooth development at 6 months after birth: eruption of a central mandibular incisor.

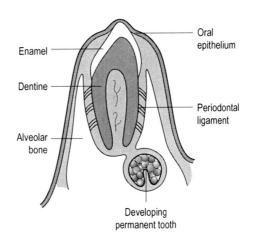

Enamel

Dentine

Alveolar bone

Oral epithelium

Periodontal ligament

Developing permanent tooth

BLOOD SUPPLY

Arterial blood is supplied via branches of the *maxillary arteries,* and venous drainage is via a system of veins that empty into the *internal jugular veins.*

NERVE SUPPLY

The nerve supply to the upper teeth is by branches of the *maxillary nerves,* and the lower teeth are supplied and branches of the *mandibular nerves.* These nerves are branches of the fifth cranial nerves—the trigeminal nerves.

FUNCTIONS OF THE TEETH

Teeth serve several important functions, including:

- accessory organs of digestion
- feeding
- mastication
- speech
- cosmetic effects
- contribute to the shape of the face
- a valuable and unique source of deoxyribonucleic acid (DNA).

CLINICAL NOTES | **TOOTH DECAY**

Dental caries are characterized by the destruction of the hard tissues of the teeth by organic acids. These acids are produced when bacteria in the mouth break down carbohydrates from food (Dairy Council 2001). Despite the fact that dental decay is preventable, 37% of 4–6-year-olds and 55% of 7–10-year-olds demonstrate evidence of dental caries in either primary or secondary teeth (Walker 2000).

Milk consumption is not shown to increase the incidence of tooth decay or erosion; however, dentists (including the British Dental Association) state that milk and plain water are the best drinks for teeth. Carbonated soft drinks, fruit squashes and fruit juice are all acid and therefore can be erosive to teeth (Dairy Council 2001). However, O'Sullivan & Curzon (2000) contend that the most critical factor in developing erosion from acidic drinks relates to consumption more than three times per day.

CLINICAL NOTES	HEALTH EDUCATION
	According to Ottley (2002), research demonstrates that simple health messages are the most effective. The following are recommended:

- Evidence-based research currently advises that teeth should be brushed twice a day with a fluoride toothpaste.
- Dental health education should be available to all families with young children. A healthy set of deciduous teeth is a strong indicator of future dental health and contributes to general health and well-being.
- Tooth decay in young children is becoming concentrated in deprived communities. Therefore, health visitors, midwives, community children nurses and child health nurses have an important role in health education and improving children's dental health.

TEETHING

The exact mechanisms responsible for the eruption of teeth are not fully understood, although action of the hormones pituitary growth hormone and thyroid hormone have been proposed as important.

Teething is a physiological process that occurs when the crown of the tooth breaks through the periodontal membrane. The age of tooth eruption may vary considerably, and there is a range of symptoms related to the teething process. Some infants appear to demonstrate minimal discomfort, whereas other infants appear irritable and unwell.

Table 12.1 shows the average age at which the various deciduous and permanent teeth erupt.

SIGNS AND SYMPTOMS OF TEETHING

- Pain
- Drooling
- Inflammation of the membrane overlying the tooth
- Facial flushing
- Gum rubbing
- Loss of appetite
- Ear rubbing
- Sleep disturbances.

MANAGEMENT OF TEETHING

Teething pain is the result of inflammation, and the symptoms of teething can therefore be managed in a variety of ways. This may include the use of teething rings, rusks, breadsticks, or cold or frozen objects, such as a metal spoon, frozen teething ring or ice cubes. The pain and discomfort of teething can be managed therapeutically with analgesics or topical anaesthetic agents.

Table 12.1 Patterns of dentition

Type of tooth	Age
Deciduous teeth	
Upper dental arch	
Central incisors	7.5 months
Lateral incisors	9 months
Cuspid	18 months
Primary first molar	14 months
Primary second molar	24 months
Lower dental arch	
Primary second molar	20 months
Primary first molar	12 months
Cuspid	16 months
Lateral incisor	7 months
Central incisor	6 months
Permanent teeth	
Upper dental arch	
Central incisors	7–8 years
Lateral incisors	8–9 years
Cuspid	11–12 years
First premolar	10–12 years
Second premolar	10–12 years
First molar	6–7 years
Second molar	12–13 years
Third molar	17–21 years
Lower dental arch	
Central incisors	6–7 years
Lateral incisors	7–8 years
Cuspid	9–10 years
First premolar	10–12 years
Second premolar	11–12 years
First molar	6–7 years
Second molar	11–13 years
Third molar	17–21 years

Systematic problems that may manifest, such as colds, coughs, pyrexia, vomiting and diarrhoea, are not symptoms of teething but of illness. The timing of tooth eruption (between 6 and 12 months) coincides with a reduction in the circulating maternal immunity that was conferred through the placenta (Ottley 2002).

Baby tooth care should be initiated as soon as the child's first tooth appears. According to Ottley (2002), babies' teeth are particularly vulnerable to decay as they erupt, and this is the time when decay-promoting bacteria begin to establish.

SELF ASSESSMENT

Answer the following in relation to your area of professional practice:

- Outline the developmental anatomy and physiology of normal dentition.
- Discuss the maturation and development of human teeth.
- Consider why tooth decay is concentrated in deprived communities and suggest how healthcare professionals may seek to address this.
- How would you encourage young children to clean their teeth regularly, twice a day?
- Reflect on your new knowledge and consider how this may benefit your patients/clients and their families.

References

Dairy Council 2001 Topical update: drinks and dental issues. Dairy Council, London

Dean C 2000 Progress in understanding hominoid dental development. Journal of Anatomy 197:77–101

Matsumura G, England M 1992 Embryology colouring book. Wolfe, London

McCollum M, Sharpe P 2001 Evolution and development of teeth. Journal of Anatomy 199:153–159

Moore K L, Persaud T V N 1998 Before we are born: essentials of embryology and birth defects, 5th edn. W B Saunders, London

O'Sullivan E A, Curzon M E 2000 A comparison of acidic dietary factors in children with and without dental erosion. Journal of Dentistry for Children 67:186–192

Ottley C 2002 Improving children's dental health. Journal of Family Health 12(5):122–125

Sinclair D, Dangerfield P 1998 Human growth after birth. Oxford University Press, Oxford

Tortora G J, Grabowski S R 2003 Principles of anatomy and physiology, 10th edn. John Wiley, New York

Walker A 2000 National diet and nutrition survey: young people aged 4–18 years. Vol 2: Report of the Oral Health Survey. The Stationery Office, London

Bibliography

Campbell S, Glasper A (eds) (1995) Whaley and Wong's children's nursing. Mosby, London

Candy D, Davies G, Ross E 2001 Clinical paediatrics and child health. W B Saunders, London

Dairy Council 2002 Topical update: drinks and dental issues. Dairy Council, London

Lissaur Y, Clayden G 2001 Illustrated textbook of paediatrics, 2nd edn. Mosby, London

MacGregor J 2000 Introduction to the anatomy and physiology of children. Routledge, London

Slater A, Lewis M 2002 Introduction to infant development. Oxford University Press, Oxford

Tanner J M 1990 Foetus into man: physical growth from conception to maturity, 2nd edn. Harvard University Press, Cambridge, MA

Waugh A, Grant A 2001 Ross and Wilson anatomy and physiology in health and illness, 9th edn. Churchill Livingstone, London

Index

Note: page numbers in *italics* refer to figures and tables